THE EDUCATIONAL PROCESS IN
CRITICAL CARE NURSING

THE EDUCATIONAL PROCESS IN
CRITICAL CARE NURSING

JoAnn "Grif" Alspach, RN, MSN, CCRN

Clinical Nurse Educator, Critical Care Nursing Service,
Clinical Center, National Institutes of Health, Bethesda, Maryland;
Adjunct Assistant Professor of Nursing, The Catholic University
of America, Washington, D.C.

With a foreword by

Vernice Ferguson, RN, MA, FAAN

Deputy Assistant Chief Medical Director for Nursing Programs,
Veterans Administration, Department of Medicine and Surgery, Washington, D.C.

With 33 illustrations

The C. V. Mosby Company

ST. LOUIS • TORONTO • LONDON   1982

MOSBY

A TRADITION OF PUBLISHING EXCELLENCE

Editor: Michael R. Riley
Assistant editor: Michelle Turenne
Manuscript editor: Dale Woolery
Book design: Susan Trail
Cover design: Suzanne Oberholtzer
Production: Kathleen Teal

The C.V. Mosby Company
11830 Westline Industrial Drive, St. Louis, Missouri 63141

Library of Congress Cataloging in Publication Data

Alspach, JoAnn.
   The educational process in critical care nursing.

  Bibliography: p.
  Includes index.
  1. Intensive care nursing—Study and teaching.
I. Title. [DNLM: 1. Critical care. 2. Education,
Nursing, Continuing. WY 18.5 A462e]
RT120.I5A42   610.73'61   82-2090
ISBN 0-8016-0141-X   AACR2

TS/VH/VH 9 8 7 6 5 4 3 2 1   02/A/231

To my parents
Joseph and Dora Griffin

Foreword

The phenomenal growth in critical care units and their sophistication over the past decade commands the attention of hospital administrators, physicians, nurses, planners, and particularly payers. Through the postanesthesia and nursing care units developed in the late 1950s as a response to more demanding surgery and an increased array of anesthetic agents and techniques, patients are provided with better care. Today, as an outgrowth of subspecialization, a variety of critical care units exist. Now more nurses than ever before give care in an environment that is continually changing with advances in technology and the application of new knowledge.

Nurses are integral members of the critical care team and are the "constants" in care. They therefore require continuous education to provide the care needed. The nursing service educator is responsible for developing programs to educate nurses for competency in critical care nursing.

The author of this book recognizes that a considerable amount of learning takes place where care is provided and that a planned approach to the educational process is required. She has provided a thoughtful view for teachers and learners in both service and academic settings. Such a didactic framework for teaching in the clinical setting is long overdue.

Pragmatic considerations for the service-based educator in collaborating with nurse administrators, nurse clinicians, and others in the hospital environment provide guidance to those responsible for staff development. This dimension, so often overlooked, becomes a significant contribution as this book joins others in addressing the education of nurses for critical care.

Vernice Ferguson

Preface

The majority of nurses responsible for teaching critical care nursing have limited or no formal preparation for their role as nurse educators. Even those with advanced degrees in nursing are more likely to be skilled as practitioners rather than as educators. Ever since graduate nursing education shifted from a functional to a clinical emphasis, this dissonance in role preparation has become more glaring. Nursing education has seemingly conceived a generation of nurse teachers who are not adequately prepared to teach and who often find themselves in need of such skills.

In the service setting, this dilemma is compounded in three ways. First, nurses who are unfamiliar with the traditional foundations of curriculum and instruction are even less likely to be well versed in the necessary areas of adult and continuing education. Second, nurses are generally not well prepared for either negotiating or actively collaborating with administrators and other groups within the hospital with whom they need to be able to work to achieve their common ends. Third, demands of patient care coupled with the staggering attrition rates associated with critical care nursing leave hospital employers unable to afford time for practitioners to develop the skills they should have possessed on entering into an educator role.

Although no one text can address the entire constellation of these issues, *The Educational Process in Critical Care Nursing* was written to address a number of them.

The primary purpose of the book is to provide critical care nurse educators with a single reference that describes both the essential elements of the educational process and their immediate application to critical care nursing. It is intended to provide for the information needs of experienced critical care practitioners who—by way of advancement, transfer, happenstance, or necessity—find themselves responsible for an educator role they are wont to fulfill.

The text is neither a compendium of educational methods nor a reference on critical care nursing practice. Rather, it aims at merging the salient elements of each into a functional unity so that hospital-based critical care nurse educators can get on with their work.

Readers will find that the text uses a collaborative approach to the nurse educator role. The need for this secondary focus emerged following an article I wrote in 1978 that described how collaborative efforts between hospital administrative, medical, and allied medical groups could effect educational programming that met administrative, educational, and practice goals. Nurse educators who wrote me after the article was published inquired as much about educational administration and hospital-based coordination of planning as they did about purely educational areas. *The Educational Process in Critical Care Nursing* attempts to incorporate some of the more problematic administrative issues nurse educators need to be knowledgeable about to perform their roles competently.

Nurses responsible for providing continuing education in critical care nursing will find the sequential consideration of each major element of the educational process helpful in acquiring a gradual understanding of how the educational process is put into operation in a service setting. Neophyte educators should find that the familiar four-step nursing process format facilitates understanding how each phase in the educational process relates to the others. The illustrations and the program syllabus (Appendix A) will be especially useful in seeing how the outcomes of each phase are developed. The detail and comprehensiveness of the program syllabus also offer busy critical care educators starting points to modify, abridge, or adapt for their own institution's needs and to readily transfer learned elements into their work.

Nurses who lack formal preparation in educational design may use the book to derive a clearer grasp of the fundamentals of curriculum and instruction. Nurses with some background in education can be selective in their focus on areas needing fuller development, whereas newcomers to the education field may find that smaller, more frequent doses of given segments are more manageable at first. Readers should be aware that the material within each section will need to be scaled and tailored to their institution's unique needs, although the principles and process presented generally hold as true for a short series of classes as they do for a year-long educational experience such as an internship.

Critical care practitioners who only intermittently assume an educator role may use the text as a reference to investigate areas of immediate concern. Nurses preparing to assume an educator role may use the book more as a textbook to learn the continuing education process.

Critical care educators who are preparing their colleagues to take the CCRN certification examination will find the correlation of the text and the syllabus with the American Association of Critical-Care Nurses' *Core Curriculum for Critical Care Nursing* helpful in its coverage of all major segments of critical care nursing.

Educational administrators and critical care nurse administrators will find the sections on administrative issues particularly meaningful in addressing how organizational concerns can be blended with those of staff education and nursing practice in a service setting.

Critical care educators who must prepare staff nurses or neophyte instructors to function as clinical preceptors or classroom teachers will appreciate the segments that address the preceptor role and the development of faculty.

Nursing school faculty who prepare nurses to teach in a service setting or nurse educators whose educational experiences are limited to academic settings are likely to find the text helpful in identifying how hospital-based settings for continuing education differ from academia in their strategy, approach, problems, implementation, resources, and evaluation.

The text is divided into five units, the first four of which represent sequential phases of the educational process. Unit I introduces the collaborative aspects of the nurse educator's role and considers the assessment of educational needs in a hospital setting. Chapters 1 and 2 describe the various groups who should be involved in assessing learning needs and the alternative methods and sources for compiling and organizing the needs assessment. Chapter 3 describes how to set priorities and scrutinize learning needs to determine program objectives.

Unit II covers the planning phase of the educational process and underscores the need for collaboration and cooperation with practitioners and administrators. It includes chapters on selecting a program format and preparing instructional objectives. The program syllabus again provides full illustration and application of these areas to critical care nursing. Chapter 6 considers the many and varied administrative aspects of the educator's role, including such topics as determining the learner group, the role of the program director, program funding, marketing, and proposal negotiation. A special section covers various means to enhance the cost-effectiveness of hospital-based programs and emphasizes the educator's responsibility in this regard to the employing agency. Chapter 7 completes the unit by describing how to sequence and allot instructional time, select and use media, coordinate and germinate fledgling faculty, and prepare useful class schedules.

Unit III progresses to the implementation of the educational process. Chapter 8 sets the stage by reviewing principles of the teaching-learning process and principles of adult education together with their implications for the critical care educator. Chapter 9 briefly highlights factors that influence selecting a teaching method, whereas Chapters 10 through 12 describe alternative teaching methods appropriate for classroom, laboratory, and clinical settings.

Evaluating continuing education programs is the subject of Unit IV. Because evaluating learning is notoriously a more problematic phase than its preceding phases, a moderate degree of attention is paid to it in the text. Chapter 13 reflects on the functions of educational evaluation and considers how evaluating continuing education in a hospital setting differs from its academic counterpart. Chapter 14 discusses the what, who, when, where, and how of evaluation and differentiates between evaluating achievement and evaluating mastery or competency.

Test construction and preparation of various test items are the subjects of Chapter 15. Chapter 16 introduces the application of fairly basic statistical analysis to educational evaluation, describes various grading systems, and offers suggestions on evaluating affective and psychomotor learning.

Other dimensions of a hospital-based nurse educator's role are considered in Unit V. Here responsibilities such as monitoring the status of continuing education within the profession, securing CEU approval, and weighing the merit of outside educational offerings are provided for the educator's expanded role.

The final segment of the book returns to the relationship between continuing education and nursing practice. Considering the dearth of data to support the impact of continuing education on practice, I vacillated between whether to locate this section at the very beginning or at the very end of the book. Having selected the latter to keep the preceding units in cohesion, I would suggest reading the last section first only if you are reality based enough to confront issues head on without becoming disillusioned or cynical. If you tend to be a more myopic pragmatist eager to get under way, start with Chapter 1. Do at least scan the final section, however, lest you leave this area yet naive.

A small group of highly dedicated people assisted in preparing this book. I am especially grateful to my husband, Rodger, whose enduring patience, encouragement, and logistical support awakened me to the previously unknown dimensions of computer text editing and word processing. A note of praise must also be struck for Pam Carroll, whose ability to decipher my dictation and script is deserving of no less than a meritorious service award. A very special thanks is also due to Dee Angleton, whose insight, mentorship, and ideas provided me with an opportunity to get into all of this in the first place.

JoAnn "Grif" Alspach

Contents

Unit V

EXTENSION

Unit I

ASSESSMENT

Chapter 1

The education of critical care nurses
assessing who cares

The individual charged with the continuing education of critical care nurses may occupy any number of organizational positions. The critical care educator may be a staff nurse, a head nurse or coordinator of a critical care unit, a clinical nursing specialist, a nurse clinician, or an in-service or staff development instructor. The possible job titles and their locations on the hospital's organizational chart are extremely variable from one health care institution to another. Regardless of the specific title worn by the critical care educator, however, this nurse's mandate is clear: to provide an effective process of educating critical care nurses so they possess the knowledge, skills, and attitudes requisite for safe, competent, and effective nursing practice in the critical care units. To fulfill this mandate the critical care educator must be cognizant of both the educational process and the administrative process as they exist in a service setting.

Reading the job description and knowing how to proceed in accomplishing its requirements are all too often events that occur asynchronously. One reason for this lag period is that the critical care educator usually envisions herself out on some limb of the organizational tree as the sole purveyor of the process of critical care education—the only person who really cares or directs its course. In reality, service-based nurse educators cannot afford to function in isolation from the administrative organizational structure that supports them. The second major reason for this early stumbling is that the nurse educator may not be adequately prepared in educational methods to know how to proceed with the educational process. Lacking such expertise, even a clinically adept nurse may be setting herself up for failure as an educator.

The following section will introduce the critical care educator to other individuals and groups within the hospital setting who share her concern for the education of critical care nurses. Knowing who these people are and how they participate in the education of critical care nurses is important throughout the educational process. The remainder of the book will explain each step of the educational process as it applies to critical care nursing.

Who cares about the education of critical care nurses? Read the following scenario and see if you can gain any insight.

Reflections of a critical care nurse educator

I sure wish somebody else cared—even just a little bit—about the in-service programs for the critical care units. But no, it happened again: after I spent hours getting these classes arranged, writing the objectives, confirming the details of where, when, and by whom, the end result is always the same—zip! It's no better whether I'm presenting the lecture or not; the response is always consistently lousy.

When the magic hour approaches, I invariably end up appalled, frustrated, and angry to see so few nurses in attendance. Why is it always the sharper nurses who attend rather than the ones who could really use it? If we ever have more than five nurses attend a single session, it will qualify as a miracle! I just can't see what I'm doing wrong! I just don't know any other way to do it!

One thing that could stand improvement is the cooperation level in this place. The lecturers, seemingly oblivious to the lack of an audience, invariably start late, and then rather begrudgingly do their thing. At times they are really miffed at me because they really wanted the nurses to hear this stuff.

The few day-shift people in the audience never ask any questions, but sit rather motionless and mute until it's time for their return to the unit.

As if all of this weren't bad enough, I've overheard the nursing staff complain about what a "waste" the in-service classes are—how they are boring and meaningless or "over their heads." They won't make plans to attend them because they don't get anything out of them and have other more important things to do. How can anything be more important than learning to do your job better? Some appreciation that is!

The head nurses are no different! They think I should be doing something more important—like giving bedbaths or just doing "something" to help out. I'm sure staffing is not the reason they don't see to it nurses are sent to the classes; they could spare the staff if they wanted to. They even have the gall to tell me I'm interfering with patient care when I hold classes on the units; they say I create too much confusion, noise, and crowds in the patient areas for them to be able to give good patient care.

The docs are voicing their complaints to the director of nursing that some of our staff aren't as adept at understanding and performing some of their functions on the units. I'm supposed to take care of all these little incidents! When I try to share some of this work load with the nursing in-service department, I'm told the units are my area of responsibility. Even the ancillary and paramedical services have joined the bandwagon; the lab, x-ray, and respiratory therapy departments would like to use some of our in-service time to clarify a few things with the nursing staff.

Today was really a bummer! I got called into the director of nurses' office to explain to her and the head nurses why they were looking at three resignations from the evening staff and two from the night staff. Each of the resignations claimed that, among other things, they were never provided with opportunities to attend in-service classes on their shifts. Before this little confrontation was over, the director of nursing also wanted to know how, in view of the aforementioned, I ever expected her to be able to justify an increase in the critical care in-service budget. Because the hospital administrator is about to face the Joint Commission on Accreditation of Hospitals, the State Cost Review Committee, and the hospital's board of trustees—all within the next 3 weeks—she'd like me to defend my continued existence around the place.

And just as I was leaving the unit today, the coordinator informed me that we've got two groups of orientees scheduled to arrive next month. Personnel promises them the world to recruit them and I'm stuck with having to deliver it within 3 weeks. I don't know why we bother. They only stay here an average of 6 months! I think I'll go home before anything else can happen. . . .

HOSPITAL ADMINISTRATORS
Hospital administration

Hospitals are extremely complex social systems designed to provide health care services to a given population of patients. This primary objective is achieved through the coordinated efforts of numerous departments and, ultimately, through the multitude of individuals who work within each of these departments. The hospital administrator, who has overall responsibility for management of the hospital, is responsible for this coordination. In community hospitals, the hospital administrator is ultimately accountable to a board of trustees.

The board of trustees is composed of businessmen and businesswomen, professionals, and local consumers of the community the hospital serves. This group is responsible for the long-range planning and financial solvency of the hospital. Do not overestimate your distance from this group nor underestimate the importance of your relationship to its members. Whenever hospital educational projects involve a substantial investment of time, money, or personnel resources, the board of trustees will probably be instrumental in determining the approval or disapproval of the proposal. The hospital administrator may sell your ideas to the board, or you may need to intercede directly with members of the board. In either case, it may be imperative for you to recognize this group and its influence on the hospital's day-to-day affairs for your plans to be realized. Personally communicating with key or all board members can be very effective in clarifying your intentions and enlisting their support.

Although you may presently perceive your relationship with the hospital administrator as antagonistic at worst and nonexistent at best, remember that the hospital administrator has a vested interest in the quality and nature of the work you provide. What you do and how well you do it will largely determine the degree of financial and administrative support you can anticipate receiving from the administrator. Although removed from the immediate patient care area, the hospital administrator receives feedback from patients, families, the community, physicians, and other hospital departments that may relate to the educational needs of the critical care staff. Cognizant of both the needs and the resources of the agency, the administrator is the pivotal figure for determining all major initiatives within the hospital. As will be discussed later, effectively selling your programs to the administrator, thereby gaining much needed support, usually makes the difference between envisioning what could be done and having the opportunity and resources to do it.

Broaden your perspectives to acknowledge more fully the possibility of establishing a working relationship with the administrator and the board of trustees. When you do, though, you must also confront certain realities: overrating the importance of your work to the hospital is no less disastrous than not recognizing the potential value of your services to the organization. Success and maturity result from striking a balance between naivete and presumptuousness. Because both are facts of life in the hospital setting, be mindful of the following:

1. You are only a single person among a multitude that exists within the hospital organization.
2. The hospital administration and the board of trustees may perceive of your position and work as more of an employee fringe benefit they are required to have for Joint Commission on Accreditation of Hospitals (JCAH) accreditation than as an integral component in the provision of health care services. As such, your position and programs may have a very low priority. Conversely, your role may be essential for the hospital to recruit and retain nurses in the critical care units.

At some hospitals, you may interact directly with the hospital administrator; more often, the administrators you work closely with are those within your department.

Nursing administration

The hospital administrator shares the responsibility for, and interest and influence in, critical care education with the director of nursing. Although you may more readily relate your individual and departmental role to the director of nursing, remember that the lines of responsibility extend above the director to the hospital administrator and the board. Because the usual chain of command requires that you communicate upward through your immediate supervisor, you must recognize that your relationship to this individual may be the crucial (i.e., only) means available to make the hospital administrator and the board of trustees aware of your proposals. Especially if you hold an independent staff position, your relationship with the director of nursing is vitally important because of the following:

1. The interest, support, and cooperation of the director of nursing is an essential component in the survival or success of any

educational endeavor within the department.

2. The director of nursing is usually the key person for communicating your proposal to higher levels of administration for their approval and support.

3. The director of nursing, who determines the goals of the nursing department, is responsible for determining the framework within which your educational goals are determined and realized; negotiating goals with her is important for your mutual satisfaction.

4. The director of nursing's demonstrated value system, expectations, attitudes, and style of leadership exert a profound effect on creating or deterring a climate conducive to facilitating your educational endeavors.

5. The director of nursing can supply the guidance, experience, and administrative know-how necessary to realize your plans.

6. The director of nursing is instrumental in directly determining the nature and amount of financial, clerical, audiovisual, and environmental support afforded to educational programs. This tangible support is an essential element in determining the feasibility of your proposals.

7. The director of nursing may be especially helpful in analyzing and validating critical care educational needs. The director's access to audit results and other forms of feedback can provide a reliable data base for substantiating educational needs.

This giving cannot, however, be a lopsided affair. In return for gaining these provisions, you are responsible for providing programs that

1. Are consistent with the goals, policies, and priorities of the nursing department

2. Are feasible given the resources they require

3. Recognize the financial and administrative impact of high turnover and burnout rates

among critical care staff members

4. Meet the requirements of regulating agencies such as the JCAH

5. Meet the educational needs of the staff nurses in your units

6. Meet expectations the director of nursing may have of you or your department

Ideally, an atmosphere of mutual trust, open and clear communications, and collaboration and cooperation exists in your relationship with the director of nursing. Assuming your situation exists somewhere along a continuum between full cooperation and antagonism, the aims of either or both parties are best met through the dual arts of communication and negotiation. If you expect to find unlimited support from the director of nursing, you will most probably be disappointed and thwarted. Do not expect the director of nursing to function as either your surrogate mother or as your scapegoat. Communicating mutual expectations and negotiating terms are typically the only plausible approaches to use.

Critical care head nurses. The head nurse's interest in critical care educational programs stems from her administrative responsibility for the patients, staff, and quality of nursing care provided on the unit. Well-conceived and well-executed educational programs should provide the head nurse with more competent staff nurses who will provide better patient care.

The head nurse is well attuned to the full spectrum of needs on her unit and can offer many valuable insights into the learning needs of the staff nurses. As they monitor the quality of care provided on the unit, head nurses are apprised of areas needing educational supplementation. Guided observations of staff nurses' performance, problematic or unusual patient care situations, crisis events, change of shift reports, patient care conferences, and even incident reports indicate where training experiences might be necessary.

Because the head nurse is instrumental in determining annual unit goals, she can anticipate needs for designing new educational programs necessary to achieve these goals. Being responsible for staffing, the head nurse knows which nursing personnel need additional training and which staff members need remedial or supplementary instruction. As new procedures, policies, and equipment are planned for, the head nurse can anticipate when in-service sessions on each would be most timely.

Head nurses also have access to determining each staff member's unique learning needs. Through counseling sessions and performance appraisals, she has the opportunity to elicit each individual's strengths and weaknesses in clinical proficiencies, educational needs, and career aspirations.

Since head nurses have a vested interest in educational programming for their staff nurses, the critical care educator should expect the head nurses' fullest cooperation. If the educator shares a common responsibility for improving the quality of care provided on the unit, the reverse should also hold true. In many instances, however, the head nurse–educator relationship is more accurately characterized as indifferent or adversary rather than collaborative. The reasons for this unfortunate situation are many and complex. Because a good working relationship can be mutually beneficial for the head nurse and the educator, some factors that precipitate problems and how each might be resolved are here briefly considered.

A critical care unit head nurse and educator can expect to find themselves at cross-purposes in a variety of situations. Foremost among these is when the educator fails to appreciate that meeting patient care needs will and should always take precedence over meeting the staff nurses' educational needs. This dictum applies not only to legitimate needs for adequate staffing to care for patients, but also at times applies with equal fervor to meeting far less life-threatening needs such as morning bedbaths. Rather than perceiving staffing needs as competing with educational needs, it is often less problematic

simply to accept this as historical precedent. Invest your energies into demonstrating the interrelation of education and patient care. Remember that practice will always take precedence over education.

A few other points are worth mentioning here. First, chronic staffing shortages in critical care areas create an agonizing problem for today's head nurses. Scheduling educational programs at times when the few staff nurses on duty cannot possibly leave the clinical unit is certain to cause a just measure of frustration. Ignoring or discounting true staffing deficits will not help you attain your ends. Investigating alternative and more flexible approaches to providing for staff nursing education may be more constructive.

Second, the perceived work load of the unit is a dynamic commodity; that is, at various times of the day, the anticipated volume of work could be judged quite differently. At 8 AM, the day's schedule always feels more heavy than it does at 11 AM, although patient care needs may remain comparable throughout. You may be able to negotiate even an onerous load by pitching in for awhile, assisting in redistributing assignments or working with the less experienced staff nurses.

Third, some unit personnel seem to take pride in always being (or appearing) overloaded with work. Some nurses, by well-established tradition, never have time to attend in-service sessions. Somehow, this busyness serves as a badge of honor that distinguishes critical care nurses. Saving lives and stomping out disease are rarely a continuous mode of unit operations, but overcoming this busyness attitude can be a thorny undertaking. The notion that continuing education is necessary for optimal practice can take some time to convey.

Situations such as these underscore the tendency for both the head nurse and the educator to become rather myopic within their own spheres of responsibility. Educators may neglect to realize that education is only one means to effect better patient care, whereas head nurses may neglect to realize that many educational endeavors could result in more efficient and effective use of staff. If unit educators can provide both *meaningful* and *feasible* learning experiences for the staff nurses, head nurses would likely be more open to appreciating the relationship between meeting staff education needs and meeting patient care needs.

As the educator, you should highlight the words "meaningful" and "feasible." You and the head nurse need at least an implicit consensus on what constitutes "a meaningful learning experience." From the head nurse's perspective, "meaningful" is directly related to its usefulness in improving the staff's ability to take care of patients. As a general rule, orientation of new and inexperienced personnel has top priority. This is especially true when units have staffing deficits and fully trained personnel are at a premium. In-service training in the use of new equipment or initiation of new procedures typically gets second billing, and last place is usually reserved for augmenting the nurses' general knowledge base through staff development. If your unit has more problems with retaining rather than recruiting staff, however, the list of priorities could be reversed. Whichever situation you confront, "meaningful" is directly related to having an adequate supply of trained nurses to care for the patients on that unit.

The other major element for the head nurse and the educator to agree on is how "feasible" the planned learning experiences are for the whole unit. Feasibility is the culprit when meaningful learning experiences that staff nurses and head nurses support continue to encounter obstacles to their successful culmination. The source of the problem is usually a failure to anticipate how the learning experience affects one or more areas of the unit's functioning. The critical care educator should recognize the potential impact instructional activities may have on unit operations. Some are discussed here.

Unit staffing. If classes are held during on-duty hours, the attending staff nurses will not be available for patient care; as the program involves more hours of instruction, the participants are less available for patient care assignments. In most critical care units, staff nurses who are not participants in the program will need to assume the responsibility for patient care during class hours.

Weight of patient assignments. Because educational programs influence staffing on the unit, they also influence the weight of patient care assignments assumed by staff nurses during periods of class instruction. The head nurse of the unit may reasonably balk at the need to realign patient assignments to accommodate individuals leaving for classes during the course of a workday. She may also fear that the ability of the unit staff to respond to an emergency, admission, or any unit crisis would be severely limited under these staffing situations. The remaining staff nurses who assume a heavier burden of patient care to accommodate other nurses' absence during classes may resent this burden. If the staff nurses responsible for carrying the weight of patient care assignments are not given an equal opportunity to attend educational programs, their support of the educational endeavor may be short-lived.

Unit budget. If staff nurses are paid for their attendance at educational programs during off-duty hours, or if additional staff nurses must be scheduled to accommodate the patient care requirements during educational programs, the actual cost of the programs escalates. The full impact of these additional costs must be calculated in addition to the outlay of funds from the unit or the department of nursing for external educational programs and tuition assistance or reimbursement paid as employee fringe benefits to staff nurses.

Work environment and work space. If the program places a number of students in the clinical area at one time, the present staff nurses may not wish to assume the extra burden of orienting large numbers of new personnel and may not relish the invasion of their work space. Staff nurses may rightfully object that they cannot "get to their patients" because of these additional personnel on the unit. Having to walk around extra people greatly increases the amount of time required to provide patient care and reduces the efficiency of work organization. The typical critical care unit has an extremely limited amount of work space; shrinking this work space by the addition of numerous other personnel only aggravates the problem.

Staff responsibilities. Many educational programs within critical care units directly involve staff members in some way. They may be called on to teach individual classes, to function as role models or as preceptors, or to assist in the orientation of new staff personnel. Whereas many critical care practitioners perceive of these responsibilities as part of their professional role, not all staff members will share in this opinion. Some staff nurses are exceptionally good practitioners; their enthusiasm and expertise for taking on an educator role, however, may not be equivalent. You are likely to encounter staff nurses who simply do not enjoy teaching or who are not very good at it. Even for staff nurses who enjoy the teacher role, adding these responsibilities to their role as practitioners may not always be feasible.

Staff morale. Staff morale can be expected to deteriorate if opportunities for attending educational programs are not provided equitably. If staff members must carry heavy assignments and work short-staffed during classes, if they feel crowded and thwarted in providing care, or if they are forced into assuming teaching functions they do not desire, the net effect becomes demoralizing.

• • •

In summary, critical care head nurses *care* about programs of staff education, but only when educational offerings effect a recognizable improvement in patient care, staff competence,

or unit operations. Otherwise, they *do* have more important things to care about.

Nursing in-service and staff development departments

The critical care educator may function within the nursing education department, be a peer associate with the department, or be completely independent of it. Regardless of your proximity to the nursing education department, you will likely coordinate your efforts with it because of the common responsibility you share for staff education. Ongoing interaction with other providers of nursing education assists in reducing unnecessary duplications of effort, expense, and resources such as the following:

1. Personnel: lecturers, preceptors, and clerical support
2. Work space: classrooms, clinical teaching areas, office space
3. Audiovisual materials: hardware, software, purchasing, or selection

As an individual educator, the scope and breadth of your responsibility is usually more limited than that of the nursing in-service department. Although you may provide educational services solely to nurses within your own subspecialty area, remember that your goals and plans may frequently overlap or complement those of the nursing in-service department. Just as in working with the administration, communicating your goals, needs, and expectations of the in-service department is necessary for a satisfying working relationship.

OTHER HOSPITAL DEPARTMENTS
Medical department

Until rather recently, nearly all of the instruction given to critical care nurses was provided by physicians. This was understandable because the content of these classes had previously fallen within the province of medical practice.

By the early 1960s, however, the responsibility for many of these sophisticated forms and measures of patient care were being assumed by critical care nurses. As nurses became increasingly more expert in the theory and practice of critical care nursing, there has been a comparable transfer of both the provision and the responsibility for teaching critical care nursing.

Some hospitals may have enough well-qualified nurses in each subspecialty area to assume these teaching responsibilities. Many, however, will continue to use staff physicians to share the teaching of unit staff nurses.

Physicians can be integral components in the education of critical care nurses for many reasons, including the following:

1. They may have the best preparation for teaching a given area. You may need to use their knowledge, expertise, and experience for a thorough coverage of selected topics.
2. They can more readily update current thinking on topics within their specialty area than can a critical care instructor who must keep abreast of changes made within many subspecialty areas of critical care nursing.
3. They may be excellent teachers.
4. They may particularly enjoy teaching nurses.
5. They are provided with a forum to discuss their personal and professional views on a range of topics about which they wish nurses to be informed.
6. Their participation provides a mechanism for informal communication between the two major professional groups responsible for patient care in the critical care unit. This fosters improved physician-nurse working relationships and provides opportunities for sharing viewpoints and approaches, understanding and clarifying issues, and resolving problems.
7. Physicians have a vested interest in the quality of care administered to the patients they admit to and manage in the units. The

more knowledgeable and skilled the nurse, the better the combined efforts of the team responsible for patient care.
8. Physicians will usually avoid admitting patients to hospitals when they are dissatisfied with the quality of nursing care. When competent critical care nurses care for their patients, physicians are more likely to support and participate in educational programs at that hospital.

Ideally in your hospital, an "us" (nurses) vs "them" (physicians) conflict about who provides for the education of critical care nurses does not exist. Just as in patient care, the process functions most proficiently through collaboration.

Allied medical departments

Few patient units within a hospital interact with such a multitude of hospital departments as do critical care units. Personnel from laboratory, radiology, physical therapy, social services, dietary, electrocardiography/electroencephalography (ECG/EEG), respiratory therapy, and other such departments are virtually permanent residents of busy intensive and critical care units.

At times the degree of interaction between the nursing staff and these allied professionals and technicians is so extensive that it is difficult to discern where the nurse's role ends and those of others begin. Role confusion and misunderstandings can then result. It is often helpful for part of a critical care nurse's education to include gaining an understanding of what each department is responsible for in light of the others' role, and how each can complement the other's work to provide optimal patient care and to facilitate interdepartmental rapport.

If you anticipate using faculty from other hospital departments for your program, you should allot adequate time for explaining the program and instructional objectives, answering questions, clarifying expectations, and specifying the details needed for confirming their participation. Even if members of these groups will not be serving as instructors, it is often helpful to meet with them so they may understand and lend support to your efforts and offer their suggestions.

Besides discussing your plans with individuals or committees on the medical staff, you may also wish to meet with individuals in the respiratory therapy, ECG/EEG department, operating room service, laboratory, radiology, dietary, and patient services departments.

CRITICAL CARE NURSING STAFF

The need to maintain current clinical proficiency provides a strong stimulus for critical care nurses to seek meaningful and continuous learning experiences in their area of practice. Whereas many nurses are self-directed in obtaining continuing education, others will rely heavily on the service institution for assistance.

Staff nurses are the most direct recipients of critical care educational programs. They are also usually keenly sensitive to how well the critical care educator fulfills the responsibilities of her position.

Your role as an educator is not divorced from your role as a practitioner of critical care nursing. In these days of rapid, nearly instantaneous obsolescence, an educator's loss of clinical proficiency and ability to empathize with staff nurses makes her credibility that much more vulnerable. Nurse educators with advanced degrees who have never worked as staff nurses in a critical care unit, yet attempt to function as an educator there, frequently confront this problem. Unless the staff members can see that you "know what it is like," your chances for establishing rapport are severely limited. Your effectiveness as a role model for staff members will be determined by their ability to respond to you as primarily a practitioner and secondarily an educator in critical care nursing.

Unless you hold a line position that provides you with administrative authority to institute changes in nursing practice, you will function from a staff position where any authority you earn derives from your clinical proficiency, advanced knowledge, and experience in the staff role. You can hardly expect to be considered an expert if you have no first-hand experience or know less than the staff members do about critical care nursing practice. Staff members need to see that you are different enough from them to recognize you as a resource, yet enough like them to be approachable and sensitive to their perspective and their problems.

In the teaching-learning process, your responsibility lies less in teaching and more in providing the conditions that facilitate learning. Depending on nurses' current competency in critical care nursing and aptitude for self-directed learning, your provisions may range from being very active to being very passive. In general, the more motivated, clinically proficient, experienced, and knowledgeable nurses are, the less active a role the educator will need to assume.

The instructor who is genuinely empathetic, helpful, and nonjudgmental in her relationship with staff members will usually be the most effective in facilitating learning. Instructors who are insensitive, detached, and critical of staff members are usually either ignored or resented.

Your relationship with staff nurses is crucial to your role and to creating a mutually satisfying experience in the teaching-learning process; it is the primary scale on which the effectiveness of your position is balanced. More experienced educators readily recognize that not all learning occurs on the part of staff nurses. The educator also participates in learning from and with staff nurses.

The reasons why staff nurses care about critical care staff education are very similar to those of their respective head nurses. For staff nurses, too, education is a means to an end—patient care. It should not be surprising that the staff nurse perspective may occasionally not mesh well with the educator's perspective. To identify how educators and staff nurses could interact more effectively, I will examine here each perspective and consider possible modes of collaboration in each major phase of the educational process.

The staff nurse viewpoint

Knapper has described some reasons for a persisting chasm between service and education personnel. Staff nurses may not sympathize with the inexplicable whims of educators. Staff nurses are generally more pragmatic and more concerned with work load than are educators. Staff nurses often view educators as unrealistic and idealistic critics of their performance who fail to recognize the supremacy of reality over theory.

In some clinical education programs, learners find themselves unwilling service providers. Staffing shortages, high turnover rates, and a deluge of demands placed on their time at work can quickly extinguish their zest for learning and can generate a cynical bias against other nurses not subjected to such problems. Some staff nurses will inevitably be threatened by unit instructors' preparation or demeanor.

The educator viewpoint

The educator may attempt to mask a lack of clinical competence by emphasizing cognitive rather than clinical proficiency. Educators may be intolerant of the goals and problems of nursing service, highly critical of the quality of care provided, and not amenable to negotiating their goals with those of staff nurses.

Stone and Berger remind us that whereas nursing service and education share in their philosophy of providing service to the patient, their varying orientation to this service can frequently breed conflict. Whereas nursing education prides itself on being future oriented, nursing service is of necessity present oriented. In the end, unless the two groups can negotiate sharing their support for one another, problems will inevitably arise.

What is to be gained from cooperation?

The issue of cooperation is not that education and service cannot function insulated from each another; sadly and often, this is the case. In actuality, mutual cooperation and attending to goals are possible without undue effort on either part, and both may realize many gains.

Hicks and Westphal identify a number of potential gains from this cooperative effort, as follows:

1. More realistic and up-to-date goals for patient care rather than the grandiose goals of academia or the resticted ones of tired staff nurses
2. More appropriate standards of care rather than the dated and trite ones of staff or the meaningless and unreachable ones of eduation
3. More competent clinical instructors who share their knowledge of theory with staff and continue to learn the current practice of nursing with staff.
4. More relevant educational programs than the task-oriented on-the-job-training of fellow staff members or the teaching of theory that has no referent in practice
5. The development of a cadre of excellent role models for participants to emulate and learn from
6. Validation of the relevancy of proposed educational programming to the work situation
7. Greater reinforcement of classroom instruction and a transfer of learning to the clinical situation
8. Creation of a climate where learning and teaching are an integral part of daily staff activities
9. Identification of more meaningful learning experiences participants can acquire to develop as functional staff members more efficiently
10. Increased strength of support for goals of the unit when both groups are working for the mutual benefit of patient care
11. Improvement of work environment, staff morale, and a sense of self-satisfaction and achievement
12. Greater cohesion among individuals involved

that fosters the rapport and team effort required for good working relationships

13. Representing the unit and its goals to the nursing department and hospital administrators with a more unified voice

FACILITATING A COOPERATIVE EFFORT IN THE EDUCATIONAL PROCESS

With so much to gain from a collaborative relationship between clinical educators and staff nurses, how could you then proceed to ensure this process? Each group incurs some responsibility here.

Enlisting the staff nurses' cooperation. Some ways the staff nurses may participate in the instructional process include the following:

Program planning

1. Contributing to the identification of realistic program goals and to the identification of educational needs and content
2. Suggesting feasible alternatives for program provision and for meeting stated goals
3. Sharing unit goals and problems with instructors
4. Adjusting staffing patterns and patient assignments to encourage staff participation in educational programs
5. Assisting instructors in updating their clinical proficiency
6. Identifying their areas of expertise and interest
7. Negotiating how responsibilities for patient care may be divided equitably
8. Conveying their reactions, concerns, and anticipated problems with proposed programs before the program's initiation
9. Clarifying unit policies, procedures, and equipment location to instructors
10. Maintaining an atmosphere conducive to innovation and improvement in nursing practice
11. Identifying irrelevant proposals for their deletion from programs

Program implementation

1. Serving as expert role models or clinical preceptors for participants
2. Serving as faculty for classroom instruction
3. Assuming responsibility for patient care so others

may assist in program provision or participate in learning activities

4. Fostering a spirit of inquiry and openness to learning on the unit
5. Assisting in reinforcing and transferring learning to the clinical setting
6. Identifying meaningful learning experiences for participants and conveying these to instructors
7. Facilitating logistical support of learning activities (using hospital forms, processing paperwork)
8. Serving as resources to participants and instructors during the program

Program evaluation

1. Assisting in peer evaluation of clinical proficiency from their perspective as fellow staff members
2. Sharing and recording observations concerning participants' performance with instructors
3. Providing direct feedback on performance to participants
4. Identifying areas most needing evaluation
5. Validating learning attained and competencies reached by participants
6. Providing timely evaluations

Enlisting the educator's cooperation. The educator's responsibility to the unit staff might include the following:

Program planning

1. Identifying how the proposed program will affect other educational programs presently offered
2. Seeking ways to accommodate staff nurses' needs for recognition, growth, development, and work satisfaction with program goals
3. Attempting to blend educational needs with unit goals, problems, needs, and routines to minimize disruptions
4. Remaining open to negotiations for problem solving
5. Explaining the purpose, objectives, and tentative plans for providing the program to staff nurses
6. Ascertaining staff nurses' perceptions of how the program will positively or negatively affect them and incorporating staff nurses' suggestions for reconciling these areas
7. Clarifying the roles, responsibilities, and expec-

tations among staff nurses, instructors, and administrators of the program

8. Preparing staff nurses for serving as role models and faculty by providing resources, information, and instruction as necessary
9. Being realistic in attitudes toward requirements necessary in the learning process
10. Communicating information to staff nurses: number of participants, clinical and class schedules, units to be used, kinds of learning experiences desired
11. Communicating a desire for staff nurses' involvement in all phases of program planning and implementation

Program implementation

1. Maintaining lines of communication open equally to criticisms, suggestions, and positive feedback
2. Providing up-to-date information and instruction
3. Assisting staff nurses in planning and executing the instructional process
4. Sharing lists of specific learning objectives sought and explaining any areas of ambiguity
5. Providing a liaison between the program and staff nurses
6. Recognizing the skills and expertise of practitioners
7. Assisting staff nurses in the supervision of participants
8. Serving as a resource person to staff nurses for accomplishing learning objectives and the instructional process
9. Maintaining frequent contact with head nurses and staff nurses regarding the program's impact on the unit
10. Clarifying responsibilities for various aspects of performance; differentiating supervision of patient care from meeting learning objectives
11. Attempting to merge meeting learning objectives with unit staffing needs

Program evaluation

1. Providing clearly understood mechanisms for obtaining and evaluating participants' performance
2. Specifying the nature and content of evaluation sought and criteria used in assessing satisfactory performance

3. Providing mechanisms for staff nurses to share with instructors problems related to the program
4. Demonstrating or explaining how staff nurses are to function in the evaluation process and how their evaluations will be processed and used
5. Providing a mechanism for ongoing and terminal feedback concerning how the program affects them and their work environment
6. Assisting staff nurses to prepare written assessments of participants' performance
7. Providing evaluation tools for staff nurses to use in making evaluations

Staff nurses of a critical care unit can provide relevance, timeliness, challenge, and spontaneity to an otherwise dull and unimaginative academic affair. Critical care educators who fail to recognize and use this resource waste an abundance of valuable contributions and usually soon find themselves isolated from the practice they purport to teach others.

CRITICAL CARE PATIENTS AND THEIR FAMILIES

Of all of the groups having an interest and influence in the education of critical care nurses, the population of critical care patients is probably the most salient and least often recognized. From a realistic standpoint, patients are both the ultimate recipients of the effectiveness of this education and the external criteria of the teaching-learning process. As such they deserve a prominent place within the framework of all educational programs in critical care nursing. From a pragmatic standpoint, the essence of what the staff nurses need to know is derived from the kind of patients they will be required to care for.

As a critical care nursing educator, you represent only one of many individuals and groups who share in a common concern for staff nursing education in critical care units. Recognizing and using this fact throughout all phases of the educational process will increase the assurance of your collective success.

REFERENCES

Alspach, J: A critical care nursing internship program, Superv Nurs **9**:31, 1978.

Banaszak, SM, and Willner RF: Clinical affiliations needed to augment educational experience, Hospitals **52**:169, 1978.

Continuing education—who cares? Nurs Admin Q **2**: entire issue, Winter 1978.

Coye, D: Organizational structures: considerations which facilitate effectiveness, J Contin Educ Nurs **8**:42, 1977.

Dexter, PA, and Laidig, J: Breaking the education/service barrier, Nurs Outlook **28**:179, 1980.

Ferguson, VD: The learning climate. In Popiel, ES, editor: Nursing and the process of continuing education, St. Louis, 1977, The C. V. Mosby Co.

Grubb, AW: Hospital takes systematic approach to educational programs, Hospitals **52**:78, 1978.

Hicks, BC, and Westfall, M: Integration of clinical and academic nursing at the hospital clinical unit level, J Nurs Educ **16**:4, 1977.

King, PJ: The hospital wide education department, J Nurs Admin **8**:13, 1978.

Knapper, EJ: The practitioner's responsibility in education. In Williamson, JA, editor: Current perspectives in nursing education, vol 1, St. Louis, 1976, The C. V. Mosby Co.

Kroh, LM: Standards for entering critical care? Life Support Nurs. **2**:24, 1979.

Medearis, ND: Planning for the training and development of the critical care nursing staff. In Hudak, CM, Lohr, T, and Gallo, BJ, editors: Critical care nursing, ed 2, New York, 1977, J. B. Lippincott, Co.

Pierce, SF: Clinical experience in the intensive care unit, Nurs Outlook **25**:650, 1977.

Pinkerton, SE: Administrative support for the clinical specialist organizationally placed in the CE department, Nurs Admin Q **2**:53, 1978.

Reuther, MA: Student experience in intensive care units: a faculty-staff collaborative venture, Heart Lung **8**:944, 1979.

Schweer, JE, and Gebbie, KM: Creative teaching in clinical nursing, ed 3, St. Louis, 1976, The C. V. Mosby Co.

Stone, S, and Berger, M: Nursing service and Education: an analysis of interorganizational relationships. In Williamson, JA, editor: Current perspectives in nursing education, vol 2, St. Louis, 1978, The C. V. Mosby Co.

Wagner, DL: Nursing administrators' assessment of nursing education, Nurs Outlook **28**:557, 1980.

Chapter 2

Establishing the need for educational programs

Now that you have assessed critical care nursing education from its broad, organizational perspective, you are ready to initiate the educational process. Leave the chalk and slides aside for now, though, because it is not time to teach just yet.

Teaching is, in reality, a secondary outcome of the educational process, not the entirety of the process. Learning constitutes the culmination of this process.

In contemporary definitions of the teaching-learning process, learning is recognized as a self-directed activity of the learner, evidenced by a change in what the learner knows, does, or feels. Learning occurs not as a necessary outcome of teaching, but as a purposeful, goal-directed activity of the individual learner. The role of the teacher is to assist the learner, that is, to initiate, stimulate, facilitate, guide, and sustain the learning process. If you wish your teaching endeavors to be successful, then long before you provide any form of instruction you the educator have some homework of your own to do.

Your homework consists of accomplishing a series of successively planned steps that ensure purpose, direction, and focus to your activities. If the purpose of your position is to meet the educational needs of the critical care nursing staff, your earliest responsibilities include knowing how to do the following:

1. Recognize an educational need

2. Differentiate among various types of educational needs
3. Identify sources for obtaining opinions on the educational needs of critical care nurses
4. Gather and summarize assessment data on educational needs
5. Validate an assessment of educational needs

If you are ready, it is time to start the assignment by discussing how you go about determining the need for educational programs in critical care nursing. Defining what is meant by an "educational need" is an appropriate beginning.

DEFINITION OF AN EDUCATIONAL NEED

An educational need may be defined as the difference between what people presently know and what they need to know. It is an interruption along a continuum between an individual's present level of competence or performance and the desired or necessary level of competence or performance. Moreover, an educational need is one that may be satisfied by an educational or learning experience.

CATEGORIES OF EDUCATIONAL NEED

Educational needs fall into one of three major categories: needs for in-service education, needs for staff development, or needs for continuing education.

Needs for in-service education. In-service educational needs are those that arise from an individual's need to fulfill the job description. They are recognized by an individual's awareness of an inability to perform all of the role expectations of the position without being supplied with a basic amount of information and training. An example might be a newly graduated nurse entering into critical care nursing practice who needs an extensive amount of orientation and training to be able to fulfill even the minimum requirements of her job description.

Needs for in-service education and orientation exist not only at entry levels, but also at more advanced levels. Examples of the latter would include the orientation an experienced critical care nurse from another hospital would need to a new unit's policies and procedures or the training a medical-surgical nurse would need to become a critical care nurse. Both entry and advanced needs for in-service education have the same basic requirement: provision of learning experiences that enable a nurse to fulfull her job description.

Needs for staff development. Besides needing to learn the essentials through in-service education, most staff nurses are also interested in learning to keep up with current developments and to enhance their scope of practice. Especially for more experienced staff nurses, meeting educational needs related to continuing professional development becomes increasingly important for job satisfaction and for preventing professional stagnation. An example of a need for staff development would be a coronary care unit nurse's desire to learn the skill of cardiac auscultation to increase her repertoire of clinical assessment skills.

Needs for continuing education. Nurses who seek to move up a career ladder, to specialize in one clinical area, to obtain a promotion, or merely to expand their general knowledge base often find that new skills need to be learned to attain these ends. The notion of continuing education in nursing may be broadly defined as consisting of any planned learning experience provided beyond basic nursing education. Given this definition, continuing education encompasses all three categories of educational needs. Insofar as the learner pursues her unique educational objectives in some systematic way, these planned learning activities constitute continuing education.

In summary, for fulfillment of one's job description needs of in-service education are most essential, needs for continuing education are least essential, and needs for staff development lie somewhere between these two.

SOURCES FOR COMPILING AN ASSESSMENT OF EDUCATIONAL NEEDS

Once you can recognize and categorize an educational need, you will have a clearer understanding of the kind of information sought during the assessment phase of the educational process. Educational needs of various types constitute the outcome of educational assessment.

The next step of the assessment process is deciding who will participate in determining the critical care nurses' educational needs. As any good investigator knows, some sources of information are more reliable and valid than others.

Primary sources

The primary sources for identifying the educational needs of critical care nurses can be determined on the basis of Sutton's law. Willy Sutton was a notorious bank robber in years past. Someone once asked Mr. Sutton why he robbed banks. Willy, looking somewhat incredulous, replied: "Because that's where the money is!" Such insight proves invaluable for resolving the problem at hand.

The most relevant and direct sources for deriving the educational needs of critical care nurses *are* the critical care nurses themselves. One common means for identifying these learning needs is by asking staff nurses to relate them in some manner. The validity and reliability of these felt needs for learning are, however, partly a function of nurses' knowledge and experience in clinical practice.

Experienced critical care nurses are typically adept at identifying the precise nature of their learning needs. A thorough grounding in the core matter of critical care nursing provides the seasoned practitioner with a background appropriate for differentiating what is known and understood from what is not. It takes some professional practice to recognize gaps in comprehension. Recent graduates and other neophytes to critical care, on the other hand, are generally less able to specify clearly the true nature of their educational needs. Indeed, one concern always present during the orientation of a neophyte staff nurse is that she will fail to recognize when to seek information and resources necessary for sound clinical decision making. When inexperienced staff nurses respond that "I do not know enough yet to know what I do not know," they are not likely to provide valid assessments of their learning needs.

A more accurate appraisal of staff nurses' educational needs might be garnered from systematically observing the quality of nursing care they provide. When compared to the nurses' job descriptions and the standards for nursing practice of a particular facility, clinical performance can be more validly assessed.

Inquisitive and self-directed staff members who continuously strive to better their level of practice will usually seek out the educator to find answers to perplexing patient care problems. For other staff nurses, the educator will likely assume a more active and direct role in identifying educational needs.

Some staff nurses may initially need help in identifying the quality of their clinical performance and their learning needs. The critical care educator should not assume that all staff nurses are equally proficient at identifying their educational needs.

Remember that the head nurse has access to many forms of information about the educational needs of unit staff nurses. As detailed in Chapter 1, the head nurse's formal and informal monitoring of nursing practice on the unit elicits a wide array of both objective and subjective indicators of where instructional support is needed. Educational needs elicited from staff nurses may then be compared with those identified by the head nurse to assess their consistency and validity.

Critical care educator. As the critical care educator, you usually have primary responsibility for determining the educational needs of unit staff nurses. This responsibility assumes you have both the clinical expertise and the educational preparation required to fulfill this function.

For you to be capable of identifying educational needs related to nursing practice, you must consider four factors: (1) the standard of nursing practice applicable in that situation, (2) the scientific basis for that standard, (3) the staff nurses' present levels of performance in relation to that standard, and (4) where performance deficits exist because of educational needs. The only notable modification to this approach is in setting realistic levels of expected performance. While the standard of practice remains constant, the level of performance expected of a newly graduated orientee and that expected of an experienced practitioner may vary somewhat. Each should be able to demonstrate the behavior essential for the situation, but elements of care beyond these essentials may be many for the seasoned nurse and few for the neophyte.

The assessment of educational needs should not, however, be limited to your own observations. Staff and head nurses' perceptions of these needs should be incorporated into a consideration balanced with your own impressions. Soliciting information from physicians, allied professional groups, administrators, and other nurse educators within the agency provides a useful base with which you can fortify your assessment findings. Although you may not always agree with other groups' assessments of educational needs, considering multiple objective and subjective sources of information is necessary for planning programs congruent with the combined professional aims of all members of the health care team.

Remember that local critical care practice originates from the patient population your agency serves. Take an accounting of the most common kinds and ages of patients cared for; their diagnoses and the spectrum of their clinical problems, their most frequent causes of morbidity, complications, and mortality; the nature and scope of services they require; and the agency's capability to provide these. When you consider nursing practice in light of patient care requirements, educational needs become more readily visible.

Secondary sources

Two secondary sources of information may be worthwhile to consult in assessing staff educational needs: related professional literature and area schools of nursing.

Related professional literature. In 1981 the American Association of Critical-Care Nurses published the second edition of its *Core Curriculum For Critical Care Nursing*. The *Core* serves as an outline compendium of what critical care nurses need to know to deliver competent patient care.

Other specialty nursing organizations such as the American Association of Neurological and Neurosurgical Nurses and the Emergency Department Nurses Association have also published their respective *Core* texts. Depending on the clinical base of your critical care unit, one or more of these publications may be a useful reference for determining common staff nursing educational needs in that specialty area.

The professional journals of critical care specialty nursing associations, related nursing and medical periodicals and texts, and basic research and science literature are all useful references for identifying potential and developing kinds of educational needs. As changes and improvements in the sciences underlying critical care nursing practice occur, learning needs arise from the necessity to keep staff nurses abreast of these.

Area schools of nursing. When one or a few schools of nursing consistently provide a significant proportion of critical care staff nurses to your agency, it may be useful to consult with their instructors regarding the common educational needs of their recent graduates. These instructors may be able to provide you with information about an individual student's strengths and weaknesses and common training needs their graduates require on entering critical care units. Collaboration and consultation between the critical care educator and local nursing school faculty may effect curriculum revisions that more adequately prepare new graduates for this kind of clinical practice.

Finally, the kind and quality of nursing programs available in your area may suggest educational needs likely to arise for graduates of these programs. Because the scope, breadth, and philosophy of nursing practice vary somewhat from one academic institution to another, nurses recently graduated from these institutions can be expected to vary in their clinical competencies as they enter into employment. Experience and exposure to graduates of each local program will eventually suggest common educational needs the employing agency must attend to.

An alternative source: the advisory committee

Rather than consulting with each of these separate sources every time an educational program for critical care nurses is considered, it may be more realistic and efficient to promote the notion of an ongoing advisory committee for critical care nursing education. A well-constituted advisory committee can serve as the primary vehicle of communication for all hospital groups sharing a common concern for the quality and provision of educational programs for critical care nurses.

Successfully using an advisory committee is contingent on securing an appropriate committee membership and a clear definition of the functions to be performed.

Advisory committee membership should be chosen primarily on the basis of providing proportional representation of all groups concerned with any aspect of critical care education. Chapter 1 outlined this membership to include hospital and nursing administration, unit administration, staff nurses, nursing in-service or staff development departments, medical and allied professionals, and, conceivably, consumers. The value of an advisory team is its ability to provide a broad base of information from a multitude of special interest groups. Committee meetings are an opportunity for discussion that can assist in reaching a consensus on what the educational needs of the critical care nurses are at a given time. The greater the variety and scope of perspectives, the more potential this committee has for providing useful assistance to the educator. Members should be able to represent responsibly and express clearly the viewpoints of their respective groups.

Although such a committee may be instrumental in offering perceptions related to educational needs, the advisory committee should not completely usurp the critical care educator's prerogative in these determinations. Neither should the educator attempt to shift the responsibility for educational needs assessment to the advisory group. The educator retains responsibility and accountability for the outcomes of these deliberations, whereas the advisory team provides the multiple perspectives necessary for sound decision making. Should you decide to use an advisory committee, hospital politics and group dynamics often require that the committee's role in decision making be clarified from the outset.

The purpose of an advisory committee may be limited to identifying critical care educational needs, but may also encompass conceptualizing, promoting, planning, provisioning, and evaluating programs. The range of functions this committee may assume includes the following:

1. Identifying and verifying educational needs and ideas for programs
2. Determining long-range goals for staff education
3. Defining program objectives and format
4. Delimiting program content
5. Securing necessary faculty and material resources
6. Problem-solving in the educational process
7. Communication of ideas to all who need to know
8. Supporting and publicizing the program to others within and without the hospital
9. Promoting a shared responsibility for education of critical care nurses
10. Evaluating the program

All phases of the educational process require participative decision making. Whichever approach you use to secure participation, be especially certain to provide for it in these very early stages. The complexity of the hospital system makes it a sound educational investment.

METHODS FOR ASSESSING EDUCATIONAL NEEDS

A variety of methods are available to the critical care educator for compiling staff nurses' educational needs. The methods available may be direct or indirect in their approach.

Direct methods provide this information by means of a straightforward solicitation of perceived learning needs. Examples of direct techniques include interviewing, discussion groups, and written questionnaires.

Indirect methods use analyses of the work situation and various hospital records to yield information related to staff nurses' educational needs. Examples of indirect techniques include guided observations, purposeful listening, and reviewing hospital and unit forms and statements.

Direct methods

Interviewing. Interviewing critical care staff nurses to elicit their perceived learning needs is a necessary step in the process of adult education. For experienced critical care nurses, this self-evaluation usually provides an enumeration of specific, concrete learning needs—some of which may be met through educational programs. With neophyte critical care nurses, interviewing may be a less useful technique, inasmuch as they may not know enough about critical care nursing practice to be able to identify readily their specific educational needs.

Appointments need not be formally scheduled for interviewing staff nurses. In fact, interviews may be most effective when they occur spontaneously during lunch, breaks, or during or after work. If you are not able to meet with an adequate or representative number of staff nurses informally, however, you may find that scheduling a meeting with them at a mutually convenient time may be more effective.

Personal contact enables you to clarify the nature, scope, and depth of perceived educational needs, as well as staff nurses' present levels of competence in relation to those needs. Interviews also provide an appropriate time for determining the immediacy of various learning needs and for conveying your accessibility and willingness to assist staff nurses in meeting these needs.

Discussion groups. Rather than interview staff nurses individually you may approach them as a group. Individual interviews usually yield more detailed information on the specific needs of individual learners. Group meetings often obscure the unique needs of individual learners in favor of eliciting more common needs of a major-

ity of the staff nurses. If your management of these group sessions is sensitive and skillful, you should be able to derive a mixture of individual and collective staff educational needs.

Written questionnaires. Another method for eliciting individual educational needs is the written questionnaire or survey. The questionnaire format may provide you with more descriptively detailed responses than group methods of data collection.

When using a questionnaire or survey, you can anticipate some inherent problems. Construction of a survey form that is neither too brief nor too cumbersome can be a challenging task. Staff nurses may be reluctant or too busy to complete the forms and retrieval may be difficult. If less than half of all forms are returned, the sampling of responses may be too small to be valid for the group. Some of these potential difficulties can be minimized by structuring the format so that it extracts information in its most usable form.

A questionnaire or survey may be developed in a number of different formats such as the following:

1. Open-ended, nondirective questions
2. Direct questions
3. Projective questions
4. Checklist

Open-ended, nondirective questions. Open-ended, nondirective questions are most useful for nurses who are highly motivated to learn, well-attuned to their own learning needs, and able to express themselves clearly and effectively. For these nurses, an open-ended question such as "The areas of respiratory care nursing I most need to learn about are . . . " may be all that is required effectively to determine their perceived educational needs.

Nondirective questions require minimal preparation time, and only a few of these cover all potential areas of need. The effectiveness of this format, however, is highly dependent on the learner's willingness and skill to invest the time, energy, and interest necessary to provide you with relevant information. The information it yields may be too broadly stated to be useful. Respondents may not be willing to allot time for "filling out another form." To avert these problems and to provide a mechanism for gathering information from the less than highly introspective nurse, more structured formats may be preferable.

Direct questions. Directly questioning staff nurses about their relative needs may be more efficient than using open-ended questions when you are attempting to solicit information about specific aspects of critical care nursing. For example, a question such as "Do you need to learn about nursing care of the MI patient in cardiogenic shock? (yes) (no)" is more direct than "Areas of coronary care nursing I need to learn more about are. . . ."

Direct questions may then go on to delineate which aspects of care the nurse is interested in learning about. The nurse may need to learn more about fluid management, clinical signs, and psychosocial aspects of care, whereas she may not need instruction in ECG interpretation or drug therapy. One advantage of using direct questions instead of open-ended questions, then, is that direct-questions elicit greater detail about specific needs and avoid unnecessary instruction. One disadvantage of this method is that it assumes you have a thorough knowledge of likely areas of learners' educational needs. If you do not know your learners as individuals, it is difficult to anticipate their learning needs. A second disadvantage of this method is that a comprehensive coverage of potential areas of educational need may generate an unwieldy volume of paper and require much time for compiling responses. If you have a small number of nurses to survey, have access to computer processing of responses, or intend to restrict your focus to a circumscribed content area, the direct question method may be a very pragmatic way to elicit the straight answers you seek.

Projective questions. Projective questions, which stimulate recalling past situations when educational gaps were perceived, is an alternative approach for determining learning needs. Especially for experienced critical care nurses, providing a context may assist them in more precisely identifying learning needs. Some examples are the following:

1. "When I am responsible for the care of a patient with an acute spinal cord injury at the cervical level, the aspects of care I feel least secure in are _____."
2. "When talking with families of patients who are dying, my main problem is usually in _____."
3. "Whenever the Code Blue (cardiac arrest) team is activated, my major problems in carrying out this procedure center on _____."

For nurses who lack the necessary experience to draw on, this device is accordingly less useful. For these nurses, a more structured and inclusive design will usually prove more efficient in assisting them to determine their learning needs.

Checklist. A checklist enumerating all of the potential learning needs you anticipate staff nurses could have can provide staff nurses with an easily and quickly completed form to indicate their educational needs. The format may be limited only to specific subject headings such as the following:

1. Arterial blood gas analysis
2. Assessment of breath sounds
3. Care of patient on mechanical ventilator
4. Intermittent positive pressure breathing (IPPB), positive end expiratory pressure (PEEP), continuous positive airway pressure (CPAP)
5. Methods of weaning from mechanical ventilation

The items can also be stated in terms of learning objectives such as the following:

1. To differentiate metabolic from respiratory disturbances of acid base balance
2. To identify vesicular breath sounds

3. To demonstrate aseptic bronchopulmonary suctioning technique
4. To recognize the effects of IPPB, PEEP, and CPAP on cardiac output
5. To compare and contrast the advantages of IMV over traditional weaning techniques

Although checklists are relatively easy to design and complete, their usefulness extends only to the areas included. Other equally pertinent areas may be inadvertently omitted. When working with a large number of staff members, using checklists may result in an inordinate amount of data to tabulate. One possibly feasible method of tabulation is computer processing of response forms or cards. Another tabulation device, a matrix, is described later in this chapter.

Indirect methods

Indirect methods of gathering information about educational needs may be more useful than direct methods, because direct methods all assume learners can more or less readily recognize their learning needs. Educational needs, however, are not always so visible to learners. At times, even specific introspective responses do not portray the full picture of what learners need to know. In such circumstances, gathering other types of information from less subjective sources is often helpful. Some of the methods available for this purpose include guided observations, purposeful listening, and review of forms and documentation.

Guided observations. Guided observations are useful if you have determined the competencies that represent satisfactory job performance in various work situations, because you may then compare what you actually see performed by staff nurses with this standard of performance. As a clinically expert observer, the educator may use guided observations to evaluate more objectively the quality and consistency of staff nursing performance in relation to the expected outcomes of care. This form of systematic observation can indicate areas needing instructional attention.

Observations may be obtained informally while you work with various members of the staff or during specific times such as nursing rounds. By comparing your observations with the standards of nursing practice, you can deduce many areas of educational need that might otherwise go undetected.

Purposeful listening. Purposeful listening can be rewarding because during change-of-shift reports, nursing rounds, and patient care conferences, many educational needs will surface if you are listening for them. Thinking through situations, problems, mistakes, and daily occurrences for their educational implications requires a sensitivity to subtle clues, insight, and deductive reasoning. Using purposeful listening, the critical care educator tunes her ear to detect situations reflecting educational needs. Unless you listen with an educator's ear, you may miss hearing many clues about learning needs that occur in daily unit functioning.

Reviewing hospital forms and documentation. Review of hospital forms and documentation is another method for collecting data on the educational needs of critical care nurses. Periodic appraisal of the critical care unit's goals, policies, procedures manuals, and written standards of care will reveal many potential areas of educational need. Comparing the job descriptions of each level of nursing personnel will assist you in differentiating among the learning needs for each level. Auditing nursing care plans, Kardexes, and nursing notes may illuminate areas of educational need regarding the quality, inclusiveness, and consistency of planned and provided care. Even if you are not a member of the peer review or nursing audit committees, you can readily incorporate any deficiencies noted in these reports into your needs assessment.

SUMMARIZING NEEDS: A MATRIX ASSESSMENT

After this discussion of the numerous methods with which you can gather data on educational needs among critical care nurses, it is now time to discuss how to organize the data into some manageable form. One way to accomplish this is by constructing a matrix assessment.

A matrix assessment consists of an orderly arrangement of learners and their perceived learning needs, constructed in such a way that as each nurse indicates her specific learning needs, those needs common to the group simultaneously emerge. This is accomplished by listing each of the learners vertically down the left margin of a form and the potential areas of educational need in blocks horizontally across the top of the page. Additional room may be left across the horizontal areas to leave room for educational needs not previously identified that may be supplied by the learners. As specific learning needs of each individual are identified, a mark is made for that individual within the box corresponding to that particular learning need.

As you can see in Table 1, the matrix assessment has the potential both for obtaining an overall needs assessment and for indicating the relative priority or commonality of needs among

Table 1. Matrix assessment of learning needs

NURSE	LEARNING NEEDS					
	ECG and axis interpretations	*Breath sounds*	*ABG interpretation*	*Hemodynamic monitoring*	*Patient with head trauma*	*DKA*
RNs						
1. *D. Griffin*	X	X		X	X	
2. *S. Supernurse*	X			X		
3. *T. Hoover*		X		X		X
4. *C. Mager*		X		X		
5. *A. Tessier*	X	X		X	X	
6. *J. Wheatley*				X		
7. *R. Gorr*	X		X	X		X
8. *E. Ciesinski*		X		X		X
9. *C. Boyle*				X		
10. *D. Finney*	X	X	X			
GNs						
1. *B. James*	X	X	X	X	X	X
2. *L. Ng*	X	X		X	X	X
3. *C. Bergamo*	X	X	X	X		
4. *J. Burks*	X	X	X	X	X	
5. *V. Dodds*	X	X	X	X	X	X
LPNs						
1. *J. Harris*	X			X	X	
2. *M. Maher*		X	X	X	X	
3. *C. Romano*		X	X			X
4. *P. Vazquez*				X	X	
5. *P. Griffith*	X		X	X	X	
TOTAL	12	13	9	18	10	7

the staff. Unless the array of selected educational needs can be limited to a manageable number, however, it could potentially expand to infinity.

VALIDATION OF EDUCATIONAL NEEDS

Up to this point, I have described the information gathered as perceptions of educational needs, that is, what the nursing staff, head nurses, and others perceived these needs to be—each from their unique perspective. Before you begin to use these perceptions for program planning, however, it is necessary that you do the three following things:

1. Differentiate needs that can be met through a learning experience from other types of needs
2. Verify that the derived needs are educational
3. Validate all educational needs

Differentiating educational needs from other types of needs

As you gather information from relevant individuals and groups, you often begin to recognize that not all of the needs expressed were truly educational needs. Remember that for a need to be an "educational need," it must be one that can be met through some kind of instructional program. For example, the director of nursing may note that two medication errors occurred with the same patient within a 4-week period. The director of nursing then transmits a memo to you relating that the staff nurses need a program on the action of cardiac drugs. If you fail to investigate this further, you might not find out that the first incident involved an extremely busy coronary care unit (CCU) nurse. In the midst of her hurried shift, this nurse observed a lethal ventricular dysrhythmia and reflexly administered lidocaine (Xylocaine) rather than the procainamide (Pronestyl) that was ordered. You might also find that the second incident involved a newly graduated R.N. who administered Lidocaine because she thought that Procainamide was just another name for Lidocaine. Assuming that both incidents can be remedied through instruction is obviously erroneous. The first incident may have been attributable to any number of reasons: not taking the time to first check the physician's order, the nurse's confusion and tension involved with another patient's deteriorated condition just before the incident, the inadequacy of staffing that day, or the nurse involved was working her tenth straight duty hour "to help out." This nurse's error did not reflect an educational need. As an experienced CCU nurse, she clearly knew the differences between the drugs; correcting the circumstances of the error and some appropriate counseling would likely be more beneficial in correcting the deficiency than having her attend a mandatory lecture on drugs used in the coronary care unit. The second nurse, on the other hand, whose error was directly attributable to her lack of knowledge, could be said to have had a true educational need.

One needs to make a recognizable differentiation between needs that arise because of lack of knowledge, attitudes, or skills, and those that arise because of attendant or associated problems in the execution of a known task. Unwarrantedly providing educational instruction to individuals not truly in need of instruction is a waste of time for both parties. So do not automatically assume that the need is educational. Differentiate between educational and noneducational needs.

Verifying educational needs

Once you are able to distinguish between educational needs and other types of needs, you must verify that all the needs you will address from this point on fit the criteria of an educational need.

Remember that as a nurse educator in a health agency, the needs you should be most intent on addressing are those consistent with what the staff nurses must know to fulfill their responsibilities to patients, families, and the agency. Providing for the "must knows" of inservice education takes priority over both staff development and continuing education.

Validating individual educational needs

The third step of validation consists of validating individual educational needs. To accomplish this, each need must be defined, mutually understood, and substantiated as a deficiency from the desired or necessary level of knowledge or competence. The educator and the learners must reach a consensus on what the desired state is, what the current state is, and what the intervening gap consists of. Perceived needs should be checked to assure they truly exist before time and energy are expended toward meeting these needs.

Once these educational needs are validated, the educator should review the final list once more, but this time with an evaluative eye. After consulting many sources to determine what these educational needs were, you may well find yourself looking at a very long list and wondering where to start. You can determine your starting point by now ranking each educational need based on its priority in the hospital.

REFERENCES

Assessing learning needs

American Association of Critical-Care Nurses: Core curriculum for critical care nursing, ed 2, Philadelphia, 1981, W. B. Saunders Co.

American Association of Critical-Care Nurses: Standards for nursing care of the critically ill, Reston, Va., 1981, Reston Publishing Co.

American Nurses' Association: Guidelines for staff development, Kansas City, 1976, American Nurses' Association.

Bell, DF: Assessing educational needs: advantages and disadvantages of eighteen techniques, Nurs Educ 3:15, 1978.

Bille, DA: Successful educational programming: increasing learner motivation through involvement, J Nurs Admin 9:36, 1979.

Binger, JL, and Huntsman, AJ: Keeping up: the staff development educator and the professional literature, Nurs Educ 4:19, 1979.

Chatham, MA: Discrepancies in learning needs assessments: whose needs are being assessed? J Contin Educ nurs 10:18, 1979.

Clark, CC: The nurse as continuing educator, New York, 1979, Springer-Verlag New York, Inc.

Cooper, SS: Continuing education: some definitions, J Contin Educ Nurs 10:36, 1979.

Crockett, J: Restructuring an orientation program for nurses utilizing management by objectives principles, J Contin Educ Nurs 9:19, 1978.

Curran, CL: What kind of continuing education? Superv Nurs 8:72, 1977.

Dixon, JM, et al: A computerized education and training record, J Contin Educ Nurs 6:20, 1978.

Dutton, D: Should the clientele be involved in program planning? In Popiel, ES, editor: Nursing and the process of continuing education, ed 2, St. Louis, 1977, The C. V. Mosby Co.

Hicks, BC, Blackman, SS, and Westphal, M: A need-oriented approach to staff development, J Nurs Admin 7:46, 1977.

Johanson, BC, et al, editors: Standards for critical care, St. Louis, 1981, The C. V. Mosby Co.

Koonz, FP: Identification of learning needs, J Contin Educ Nurs 9:6, 1978.

Lenburg, CB: Nontraditional approaches to learning, AORN J 26:48, 1977.

Lorig, K: An overview of needs assessment tools for continuing education, Nurs Educ 2:12, 1977.

Nelson, R: Needs assessment: essential to relevant programs, Focus 6:13, 1979.

O'Connor, AB: Diagnosing your needs for continuing education, Am J Nurs 78:405, 1978.

Pascasio, A: Interprofessional Continuing Education. In Popiel, ES, editor: Nursing and the process of continuing education, St. Louis, 1977, The C. V. Mosby Co.

Petersen, J, Jackle, M, and Ceronsky, C: Nursing students' experience in critical care, J Nurs Educ 16:3, 1977.

Pocklington, DB, Thomas, CR, and Srsic-Stoehr, KM: The development of a nursing education record keeping system, J Contin Educ Nurs 11:34, 1980.

Popiel, ES: Assessing and determining training needs. In Popiel, ES, editor: Nursing and the process of continuing education, ed 2, St. Louis, 1977, The C. V. Mosby Co.

Ranzou, ML: Identifying the consumer of continuing education. In National League for Nursing: The community college and continuing education for health personnel, New York, 1978, The League.

Rockwell, SM: What is inservice education? In Popiel, ES, editor: Nursing and the process of continuing education, ed. 2, St. Louis, 1977, The C. V. Mosby Co.

Rothweiler, TM: Needs assessment in nursing education, Nurs Educ 3:18, 1978.

Rufo, KL: Guidelines for inservice education for registered nurses, J Contin Educ Nurs 12:26, 1981.

Smith, JO, Ross, GR, and Smith, IK: Statewide continuing education needs assessment in nursing: the SNAP system, J Contin Educ Nurs 11:40, 1980.

Spitzer, D: "Remember these dos and don'ts of questionnaire design, Training HRD 16:34, 1979.

Staropoli, CJ, and Waltz, CF: Developing and evaluating educational programs for health care providers, Philadelphia, 1978, F.A. Davis Co.

Stross, JK, and Bellfy, LC: Continuing education for coronary care nurses, Heart Lung 8:318, 1979.

Tobin, HM: Staff development: a vital component of continuing education, J Contin Educ Nurs 7:33, 1976.

Yunek, M: Self-assessment of learning needs: a tool to assist nurses in self-directed learning, J Contin Educ Nurs 11:30, 1980.

Advisory committee

May, FE: Planning committees: an asset in continuing education, J Contin Educ Nurs 10:41, 1979.

Mayer, EA: Organizing and using advisory committees for adult education. In Popiel, ES, editor: Nursing and the process of continuing education, ed 2, St. Louis, 1977, The C. V. Mosby Co.

Spikes, F: Planning continuing nursing education programs: a guide for the practitioner, J Contin Educ Nurs 9:5, 1978.

Chapter 3

Generation of educational program objectives

For educational needs to be useful to the educator, they must be transformed into workable program objectives. Knowles suggests this may be accomplished by ordering educational needs into a priority system, screening them through discriminating filters, and transforming the residual needs into program objectives.

PRIORITIES OF EDUCATIONAL NEED IN A HOSPITAL SETTING

Ordering educational needs according to their relative importance is a pivotal step in the educational process. It is required for determining the starting point, focus, direction, and subsequent development of all organized educational programming.

To appreciate this notion more fully, you should understand why the priority-setting process is necessary, where educational priorities originate in a hospital setting, what factors influence the significance of an educational need, and how to set priorities at your institution.

Rationale for setting priorities of educational needs

Why is it necessary to set priorities of educational needs? Consider the following list of educational needs and see if you can decide:

1. To demonstrate how a nurse assists with a pericardiocentesis scheduled 1 hour from now

2. To set up a seminar on the managerial functions of critical care nurses who wish to become head nurses
3. To instruct staff nurses in the care of a patient who will require peritoneal dialysis this evening
4. To work collaboratively with other hospital departments in planning for a 6-month internship program in critical care nursing
5. To orient 10 graduate nurses who will supplement evening and night shift staffing

After reviewing this list, you can see how some educational needs immediately take priority over others.

In very practical terms, the necessity for setting priorities of educational needs derives from three major realities we face:

1. Educational needs are not of equivalent importance; some directly affect the quality of patient care and others do so to a much lesser extent.
2. Educational needs are more or less infinite; they are variable and will change with time.
3. The resources available to meet educational needs are more or less finite; the time, money, personnel, equipment, and facilities available to the educator rarely approximate the need for such resources.

As an educator, you must be able to set priorities of educational needs. Otherwise you may find yourself planning for management seminars when a nurse orientee needs to learn how to assist with a pericardial tap within the next hour.

Factors influencing the priority of an educational need

In weighing the significance of an educational need, some factors to consider are its potential benefits, impact, requirements, justification, plausibility, and contingency. Seeking answers to the following questions will be helpful for placing educational needs into a priority system:

1. What will be gained in patient care by meeting this educational need? What can you realistically hope to accomplish for patients, the unit, the hospital, and the staff by attempting to meet this need?
2. What are the nature and extent of potential consequences to patients, the hospital, and staff if this unmet need persists?
3. What resources would be required to meet this need? How much time, money, personnel, expertise, equipment, and facilities would be necessary? What would meeting this need require of the educator, the hospital, the learners, or others?
4. Are the necessary resources immediately available for meeting this need? Could they feasibly be secured? What would securing these resources necessitate?
5. What is the likelihood you will be successful in your attempts to meet this need? If you were unsuccessful in meeting this need, would your lack of success impede your ability to meet other educational needs?
6. Considering items 3 to 5, is the expenditure of resources to meet this one need justified by items 1 and 2?
7. Would meeting this educational need assist in meeting other important needs of the staff, hospital, or patients?

Derivation of educational priorities

The educational priorities within a hospital derive from the basic mission of a hospital. It was stated in Chapter 1 that the primary function of a hospital is to provide health care services to the community of patients it is intended to serve. Ultimately, patient needs dictate the hospital's organizational needs, which in turn determine what departments and the individual employees within these departments need to do to meet patient needs. To the extent that patient needs are met, the hospital accomplishes its mission. To the extent that employee needs are met, moreover, the more likely that patient care needs are met. Successful and effective educational programs attempt to incorporate simultaneously meeting patient, hospital, and employee needs.

Within this context, three major groups of needs emerge: those of the community at large (patient population), those of the institution and its subgroups (hospital and its departments), and those of the individual (staff members).

Regarding accountability, educational endeavors within the nursing department of a hospital are not ultimately directed to the staff nurses per se, but to the patients who receive their services. This perspective reminds us that any service provided by the health agency—including the education of its employees—has as its ultimate goal the improvement of patient care.

The needs of patients, therefore, should always take precedence over those of the hospital organization or its member departments and employees. The word *should* is used here because this assertion is often overlooked in day-to-day activities.

As emphasized in Chapter 1, the educational process is a highly collaborative one that acknowledges the organizational context within which it functions. When you set priorities of educational needs, consider whether meeting one educational need might simultaneously assist in meeting other important needs of the staff, hospital, or patient population.

At the staff nurse and unit level, the quality, accessibility, and frequency of educational programs can represent a major employee benefit that produces increased job satisfaction, professional growth, and morale. For professionals, increased experience coupled with greater knowledge and clinical competence may lead to clinical advancement and upward career mobility with correspondingly higher pay. Especially for critical care staff nurses, the availability of a sound continuing education program that enables staff nurses to keep abreast of changes in nursing practice is of the utmost importance in maintaining a positive self-image.

At the administrative level, high-quality educational programs may contribute to reduced staff turnover, may improve trained staff retention, and may serve as a recruitment incentive. When you are meeting the educational needs of staff nurses, the nurses' endorsement and participation contribute to the resolution of administrative problems that in turn often make your endeavors self-perpetuating. Educational programs that provide these complementary effects will usually engender greater administrative approval and support. If you can objectively verify the effects your programs have on variables such as the cost of orientation, recruitment, retention, and quality of trained staff, you are less likely to encounter administrative resistance to your proposals. Although not all recruitment and retention problems are attributable to deficient staff education, some may be. And it is well within your role to assist here.

Guidelines for setting educational priorities

After considering each educational need within this framework, it is time to summarize some guidelines on setting priorities of educational needs. Maslow's "hierarchy of human needs" may be used as a guide to differentiate between needs of various priority as they exist for staff nurses and for patients. We can rank educational needs similarly. Educational needs aimed at benefiting a patient's physiological condition are of the first order, whereas a patient's needs related to safety, belonging, self-esteem, and self-actualization follow respectively. Our primary educational energies, therefore, should be focused on in-service education, with commensurately lesser amounts focused on staff nursing development and general continuing education. Table 2 summarizes the derivation of priorities of educational needs for the hospital setting.

Table 2. Priorities of hospital-based educational needs

Needs:	Maslow's hierarchy	Derivation of needs	Category of education	Priority for provision
	Self-actualization	Staff nurse	Continuing education	Nice to know
	Self-esteem	Unit staff		Useful to know
	Belonging	Nursing department	Staff development	Desirable to know
	Safety	Hospital		Important to know
Priorities:	*Physiological*	*Patients*	*In-service*	*Essential to know*

SCREENING EDUCATIONAL NEEDS

Setting priorities of educational needs does not make them rigid; it merely gels them more clearly into areas deserving preferential attention. In a sense, ordering needs forces weighing what one ideally should do first.

When you consider the factors influencing an educational program objective, however, you will find that not just one, but two offsetting forces are balanced: not only the *ideal* of what should be done, but also the *reality* of what can be done in a particular setting.

Formulating realistic program objectives is rather like pouring the foundation of a large building. It requires a well-blended mixture of the right ingredients in the right proportions:

1. The ideal is like the water added to powdered cement. It affords a usefulness, purpose, and form the powder alone cannot provide.
2. Reality is the cement that affords the strength and support necessary in the mixture for the building's emerging existence and future endurance.

An excess of either ingredient or an inadequately mixed solution of the two produces two notable effects. First, the structure subsequently erected usually collapses under stresses, and, second, the cost of rebuilding after mistakes is usually higher than doing it right in the first place.

So let the priority of educational needs serve as the fluid of your foundation mixture, affording the program its focus and direction. Blend it thoroughly with the cement of reality so it may withstand the weight and burden that will be placed upon it.

Essential attributes

How do you know if meeting a particular educational need falls within the realm of what you reasonably could do in your setting? Knowles suggests that the educational need should possess the three following essential attributes:

1. Appropriateness: to the primary mission of the organization
2. Desirability: to potential participants
3. Feasibility: to the operational and educational resource limits of the organization

Filters

Filters are the last hurdle educational needs must overcome if they are destined to become realistic program objectives. These filters are

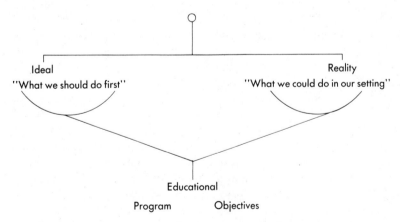

Fig. 1. Factors influencing program objectives.

not so much obstacles as issues to confront in the reality of your setting. Dealing with what is rather than merely with what should be lends a credibility to your intentions that becomes paramount for gaining administrative approval of your plans.

Organizational filter: checking on appropriateness. Hospitals participate in educating their employees for three reasons: first, on the assumption that the better prepared the employee is to do a job, the more likely that employee is to provide higher quality patient care services; second, on the mandate requiring in-service and staff development programs for accreditation of the hospital by the JCAH; and third, on the hope that a hospital's reputation for good educational programs may lead to better recruitment and retention of well-trained staff members.

The programs you propose for meeting the educational needs of critical care nurses need to be consistent with your hospital's philosophy and degree of commitment to staff education. If you work in a large university teaching hospital, where the support and commitment to educational endeavors are positive, pervasive, and persistent, you may aim high. If you work in a small community general hospital, where the support for staff education is blunted, thwarted, or largely ignored, your sights must realistically aim at a lower level. Although some educational needs may be a high priority for you, they must also be reasonable in light of what your hospital and its administration are likely to support. Learn from the past experience of others; talk plainly with your supervisor or the director of nursing. Do not make assumptions one way or the other.

In their attempts to plan educational programs, hospital-based nurse educators at times become disoriented. If you forget you are located in a hospital setting, you may find yourself planning programs that really should be provid-

ed through a school of nursing, university, college, or some outside community agency. It is unreasonable to expect hospitals to subsidize educational programs that have little or nothing to do with effective job performance by employees. Do not expect support for such endeavors. Be sure the needs you address are appropriate for a hospital to meet. Maintaining competency is basically the employee's responsibility; education beyond that required for job performance is a nice educational benefit, but it is neither a hospital's responsibility nor an employee's right.

In these days of cost containment, hospitals have the responsibility for avoiding duplication of services. If you are proposing a program already offered by neighboring hospitals, you are not likely to engender hearty support from the front office unless you can fully substantiate a sound rationale for it. If, however, the programs of neighboring institutions are successful, you may wish to adopt something similar if your needs, purposes, and resources are comparable. Likewise, if you are creative enough to have developed an educational program that is unique in your area, you may use this as a pacesetting endeavor to secure administrative support. A substantial amount of flexibility usually exists in determining a program's appropriateness, but be realistic in your assessments. Keeping up with the Joneses or with current vogues in nursing education is neither cost effective nor sound rationale.

Whether you agree with the educational philosophy of your institution or not, if you are to function effectively within its physical and philosophical walls, you must develop a sensitivity to its priority system and the prevailing attitudes toward your area of responsibility. Being reality based is not the same as being defeatist; reality can only be changed by those who first acknowledge its existence.

Participant filter: checking on desirability. The participant filter identifies the origin of educational needs to distinguish which of these needs originated from the critical care nurses. Because the critical care nurses comprise the learner participants, their perspectives and desires for specific educational programs should merit special attention.

Remember that these educational needs were solicited from a wide variety of sources inside and outside the hospital. The critical care staff nurses were only one source, albeit a very important one, for determining the final list of needs. By rearranging these needs into a priority system, the needs of the patients, the hospital, and the administration were placed well ahead of those of the staff nurses. In so doing, the resulting list of needs could become constructed in such a way that the bits contributed by the likely participants are now so interwoven with those of others that they are difficult to isolate and appreciate in their original form. The participant filter retrieves the information provided by the likely participants.

In planning for adult education, it is necessary for learners to seek out and actively participate in learning experiences. Adults are likely to do this only when they think a learning experience will be useful for resolving practical work problems they encounter. Educational programming that focuses exclusively on meeting organizational and administrative goals that are incongruent with or not shared by staff nurses often prove to be perfunctory exercises largely ignored by the staff nurses.

It is necessary to recognize educational needs that originate beyond staff nurses, but this is not to say that the needs identified by participants are or should be usurped by other hospital groups. The educator must recognize alternatives and additional viewpoints to gain a necessary organizational perspective. The precepts of adult education, however, strongly urge that the educational needs expressed by the participants be used as focal junctures within which and on which related organizational, administrative, and community needs hinge.

As mentioned previously, you will find it is often possible to incorporate meeting a number of needs simultaneously. This is possible when the educational needs identified by the groups of nonparticipants can and should be blended together with those of the participants into a workable educational endeavor that reflects the composite needs. Meeting educational needs within an organization as complex as a hospital is rarely an either-or process; arbitration and negotiation are not equivalent to acquiescence and concession.

Mark those needs attributable to critical care staff nurses. Insofar as it is appropriate and feasible, you will want to concentrate on meeting as many of these needs as possible.

Logistical filter: checking on feasibility. The logistical filter is the last one your educational needs must successfully penetrate. The logistical filter considers the here-and-now feasibility for meeting each need.

Logistical feasibility is addressed from two perspectives: operational and educational.

Operational feasibility. Operational feasibility considers the organizational resources necessary for meeting each educational need. Meeting a specific educational need is operationally feasible if the necessary resources are within the scope of the organization. Some specific resource areas you will want to survey to decide on this feasibility include the following:

TIME. Time is an exceedingly precious commodity that has pervasive effects on your educational plans:

1. Are there any necessary restrictions on the time available to meet any of these needs?
2. If some needs have time limits, what are these limits?
3. Should a time limit be imposed on any of these needs?
4. How urgent are your high-priority needs?

5. How much lead or preparation time is available for meeting these needs? Is it adequate?
6. How long should it take to provide for these needs individually and collectively?
7. How much time will realistically be available for staff nurses to attend educational programs without compromising patient care?
8. Will programs be held on hospital time, the staff nurses' own time, or some combination of the two?
9. Will intended instructors have time available to participate in your program? How much time can they give to teaching?
10. As the educator do you have time available simultaneously to teach, coordinate, precept, and administer the program?
11. Is there sufficient time available to develop modules for individualized instruction? Computer-assisted instruction? Programmed texts? Lectures? Clinical skill instruction?

FINANCIAL BASE

1. How much money is presently available for critical care staff nursing educational programs?
2. What is the projected budget for critical care staff nursing education?
3. Are further adjustments likely to be made in this budget?
4. How much money is available for paying instructors, providing support personnel, securing teaching materials and equipment, and advertising programs?
5. Is the hospital willing to share a full or partial burden of the financial responsibility for educational programs?
6. What are the current educational fringe benefits for the critical care staff nurses?
7. Can employee educational benefits overlap with projected program costs?
8. Are there estimates available of other noneducational costs (costs of recruitment, staff turnover, sick time, job dissatisfaction) that may be offset by the provision of sound educational programs for the critical care staff nurses?

PERSONNEL. The educator should be cognizant of three different categories of resource personnel: faculty, support personnel, and assistants.

Faculty

1. Who would be available and willing to teach the critical care staff nurses?
2. How many potential instructors are available from within the hospital, its staff, and its employees?
3. Would instructors be paid if they are not hospital employees?
4. Would it be necessary to secure outside faculty?
5. Are faculty appropriate for a nurse audience?
6. Are potential experts also effective teachers for nursing practice?
7. Are instructors available for all necessary content areas?
8. Do instructors know how to write or provide instruction based on written instructional objectives?

Support personnel

1. Will someone be available to relieve the nurse-educator of clerical and secretarial chores such as:
   a. Typing correspondence, records, and reports
   b. Keeping records
   c. Filing
   d. Xeroxing, collating
   e. Answering telephones
   f. Scheduling and notifying arrangements of meetings, rooms, and activities
   g. Logistical processing of applicants and participants

Assistants

1. Who will be responsible for supportive activities if no secretary is available?
2. Will anyone be available to assist in teaching, administering, and coordinating the program?
3. With what aspects of the program will this individual be able to provide assistance?

PHYSICAL FACILITIES

1. What types of classroom facilities (classroom, conference room, auditorium) are available with-

in the hospital? Are these available for nursing personnel? Who controls or regulates the use of these facilities?
2. What is the seating capacity in these rooms?
3. Do the rooms have individual movable desks or are tables and chairs provided?
4. Are rooms well lighted, heated, and ventilated?
5. Do the rooms have lecterns, microphones, or podiums if necessary?
6. What facilities are available for clinical instruction?
7. Are the clinical units (halls, patient rooms, cubicles) spacious enough to provide adequate room for small or large group beside teaching?
8. Is clinical laboratory space available for instruction on specific clinical skills? Are these facilities supplied with standard hospital equipment such as a bed, standard suction, oxygen, and power equipment?
9. Would office space be available to the educator? Are facilities adequate to provide room for filing records and teaching materials?

INSTRUCTIONAL MATERIALS

1. What types and numbers of audiovisual materials are currently available or budgeted for?
2. What is the range of available audiovisual materials: pamphlets and duplicated handouts, computerized teaching programs, closed circuit television?
3. Are audiovisual materials static or dynamic? Does the hospital have access to developing its own audiovisual materials or must these be purchased?
4. How many media forms are currently available for instructional use?

AUDIOVISUAL EQUIPMENT

1. What types and numbers of audiovisual equipment are currently available or budgeted for?
2. What is the range of audiovisual equipment currently available (chalkboard, projector, closed circuit television, computer capability)?
3. How many other groups need to use this equipment? How readily available will the equipment be for nurses?

4. Does the hospital have its own audiovisual department or must outside vendors be used?

SUPPLIES

1. Are basic office equipment and supplies available for program use (typewriter, filing cabinets, telephone, miscellaneous office supplies)?

After surveying the resources available to you for educational programs, you should have a more accurate gauge with which to estimate your potential for providing for the educational needs of your staff. It may be helpful for you to summarize this information in some way so that you may refer to it later. Table 3 is an example of how you might do this.

Educational feasibility. Educational feasibility relates to the educational requirements for designing and providing a program that meets the educational needs of staff nurses.

CONSIDERATIONS. A number of different considerations need to be weighed in determining educational feasibility: commonality among educational needs, range or span of learning needs, depth of learning needs or level of instruction, nature of learning needs, source of the educational need, preferred learning style, and the time frame available for instruction. Table 4 summarizes the kinds of information you will need to determine concerning each of these considerations and provides the options available to you for determining educational feasibility.

COMPETENCIES. In addition to considering program features for determining educational feasibility, the educator must also recognize her own capabilities and limitations. As a provider of educational programming, the critical care educator has three functional roles: as practitioner, as educator, and as educational administrator. In relation to educational feasibility, the educator must determine her relative competencies in each of these roles. Because each functional role

Table 3. Summary of operational feasibility

Resource	Current status	Projected needs	Options	Feasibility decision(s)

1. *Time*
  Preparation
  Instructional
  Administrative				

2. *Financial base*
  Allocations
  Educational benefits
  Offsetting factors				

3. *Personnel*
  Instructors
    Intramural
    Extramural
    Numbers-areas
    Quality
  Support
    Categories
    Numbers
  Assistants
    Categories
    Numbers				

4. *Physical facilities*
  Classroom
  Laboratory
  Clinical
  Office				

5. *Instructional materials*
  Types
  Numbers
  Availability				

6. *Audiovisual equipment*
  Types
  Numbers
  Availability				

7. *Supplies*				

Table 4. Considerations for educational feasibility

Consider	Ask	Weigh	Decision
1. *Commonality:* similarity among learning needs	How much variation exists among the needs? Are any needs similar, related to, or inclusive of larger areas of need? Is there an identifiable core of common needs sought? How many needs could be grouped within the same or more inclusive categories?	Group learning format vs. individualized learning format	
2. *Range:* span, extent or breadth of needs	How extensive is the area of educational need? In relation to the whole of critical care nursing, are identified needs limited to a few, many, or nearly all areas?	*Restricted range:* Limited number of topics Few classes Discrete learning experiences *Comprehensive range:* Many topics Units-courses-programs Integrated learning experiences	
3. *Depth:* level or scope of instruction	Are many nurses beginning critical care practitioners who need to learn the essentials? Need orientation? What proportion of staff nurses need development beyond essentials? What proportion of staff nurses need highly advanced programming? Is programming aimed at professional and career advancement warranted? Are discernable patterns present— Many needs with lesser scope and depth? or fewer needs with greater depth?	In-service education vs. staff development vs. continuing education *Combinations:* Beginning—intermediate Beginning—advanced Intermediate—advanced	

Continued.

Table 4. Considerations for educational feasibility—cont'd

4. *Nature*: characteristics of behavioral change sought	Do educational needs relate to cognitive, affective, or psychomotor learning? What proportion of educational needs relate to acquisition vs. application of knowledge? Can educational needs be differentiated according to location and type of learning experience required?	*Needs for:* Knowledge *vs.* attitudes *vs.* skills *vs.* integration of these three *Provided by:* Didactic instruction *vs.* laboratory/clinical instruction Combined forms of instruction
5. *Source*: origin of educational need	From what source were these educational needs derived—patients, staff, administrators?	*Priorities of each need in hospital setting (listed in order):* Patients Hospital Department Unit Staff
6. *Learning style*: method by which education is gained	What are the learners' preferred learning styles? How much variation exists in preferred learning style? What have been learners' reactions to nontraditional methods of instruction? How accustomed are learners to self-directed modes of learning?	Traditional, more passive instructional methods vs. contemporary, more active and interactive methods Supplementation by nontraditional methods of instruction
7. *Time frame*: when available for instruction	How much time is necessary to meet each group of educational needs? Do any significant restrictions exist for meeting any of these groups of needs? How much time is needed to complete classes, a series of classes, units, courses, or programs?	*Short-term episodes for learning:* Finite number of hours Narrow objectives *Long-term schedule of learning experiences:* Weeks to months Broad objectives *Ongoing schedule of learning experiences:* Weekly Monthly

possesses its own unique attributes, each should be considered separately.

THE EDUCATOR'S COMPETENCY AS A PRACTITIONER

1. In relation to identified educational needs, am I familiar with all facets and areas of current clinical practice? Where are my strengths? Where are my weaknesses?
2. Can I feasibly gain clinical expertise in areas I am unfamiliar with or lack clinical proficiency in? Will I be able to accomplish this within the time limits available to me?
3. Are others available for instruction in my areas of clinical weakness? Do I know how to function as an effective role model in all areas of critical care nursing practice?
4. Is my knowledge of clinical practice current?

Options

1. Employ sole vs. shared teaching responsibility.
2. Acquire further clinical competency vs. utilize available resources.
3. Use self as role model or utilize other staff as role models.
4. Acquire an updating of clinical knowledge or delegate teaching responsibility to other resources.

THE EDUCATOR'S COMPETENCY AS AN EDUCATOR

1. How well do I recognize my assets and limitations as an educator?
2. Do I enjoy functioning in an educator role?
3. Am I thoroughly prepared for the educator role?
4. Am I proficient in curriculum planning, design, implementation, and evaluation for a large-scale educational program? A small-scale program?
5. Am I capable of evaluating both teaching and learning?
6. Do I have a working knowledge of
   a. Principles of learning and teaching
   b. Principles of adult education
   c. Teaching methods
   d. Use of instructional media and aids
   e. Test construction and validation

7. Am I open to new ideas for the teaching-learning process?
8. Can I plan a curriculum cooperatively with others?
9. Can I be enthusiastic and supportive of learners?
10. Am I a student myself?
11. What is my teaching experience thus far?
    a. Content areas
    b. Didactic vs. clinical teaching
    c. Formal vs. informal classes
    d. Audience composition
12. Can I function as a facilitator of learning rather than as a provider of information? Can I communicate ideas effectively?
13. Is my knowledge of all relevant areas up to date and accurate?
14. Am I an effective teacher with individuals and with groups?

Options

1. Acquire further knowledge of the educator role or attempt to function as an educator with a limited background
2. Function as the only evaluator of learning or use pooled evaluation methods
3. Use principles of teaching that I was taught or acquire new approaches to teaching and learning

THE EDUCATOR'S COMPETENCY AS AN EDUCATIONAL ADMINISTRATOR

1. What experience do I have as an educational administrator?
2. Have I been successful in coordinating a program that lasts for hours? Days? Weeks? Months? Years?
3. Am I capable of coordinating a limited number of faculty? A large number of faculty?
4. Am I able to set priorities and manage time effectively?
5. Do I interact well with others as individuals and in groups?
6. Can I effectively delegate responsibilities, supervise, evaluate, and counsel others?
7. Am I an effective leader and manager?
8. Can I both listen and communicate effectively?

9. Am I goal oriented in my work?
10. Can I effectively manage conflict, handle stress, and accept criticism and blame?
11. Do I have a sense of humor?
12. Can I effectively function as a group leader?
13. Do I possess good judgment and decision-making skills?
14. Do I know how to manage a budget?

Options

1. Defer responsibility for educational administration or attempt to obtain gradually background as an educational administrator
2. Coordinate only my own activities as an educator or attempt to coordinate those of faculty members
3. Function in isolation as an educational administrator or use system resources available to me for this purpose

• • •

Now that you have scrutinized the priority of educational needs for appropriateness, desirability, and feasibility, summarize your findings and decisions in each area. Your summary sheet should contain the salient points your educational programs must reflect, that is, the areas of educational need at once appropriate for you to pursue, desired by participants, and feasible in your setting. Needs not appropriate for your organization or not operationally or educationally feasible in your setting must be discarded or deferred to some later time. Educational needs that have survived this discriminating scrutiny are destined to become program objectives.

FORMULATION OF PROGRAM OBJECTIVES
Nature of program objectives

Program objectives as terminal objectives. Once educational needs have been identified and deemed appropriate, desirable, and feasible, they are ready to be recast into program objectives. As the culmination of an organized and efficient planning process, program objectives specify the ends or outcomes the whole educational program is intended to accomplish. As the most comprehensive type of objectives, program objectives should be stated at a level of generality broad enough to encompass the anticipated range and depth of learning sought, yet specific enough to indicate clearly whether the program has fulfilled its intended aims.

If the ultimate objective of an educational program is learning, and if learning is defined as the acquisition of new behaviors, then program objectives should indicate what new behaviors the learners will acquire as a result of their participation in the program. Because program objectives clarify what you intend to be the final outcomes of the instructional program, they need to be written as "terminal" objectives. Terminal or program objectives describe those behaviors that the learner should demonstrate at the end or termination of the program.

Terminal versus intermediate objectives. An educational program incorporates numerous intermediate component parts that taken together achieve the outcomes intended for the whole program. Unless these broad objectives are first identified, however, the intervening intermediate behaviors necessary to achieve them may not be readily identifiable.

Terminal behaviors are distinguished from intermediate behaviors in that one terminal behavior is obtained through learning a number of intermediate behaviors. For example, the terminal objective, "Without preceptor guidance, the participant will demonstrate how to care for a patient who requires mechanical ventilation," may be attained through some of the following intermediate objectives:

The participant will be able to do the following:
1. Identify the ventilator settings being used for peak pressure, tidal volume, and sigh frequency
2. Differentiate between whether the patient is on assisted or controlled ventilation

3. Assess the patient's tolerance of changes in ventilator settings
4. Demonstrate how to troubleshoot when the pressure alarm sounds

Because each of these intermediate behaviors can in turn be broken down into even finer specifications of behavior, it becomes obvious that there can be many levels in a hierarchy of educational objectives. In Chapter 5 these levels of objectives are discussed in greater detail. For the moment, however, attention will be paid to those general, broadly stated objectives that participants should attain by the end of the program.

Statement of program objectives

Behavioral component. As you formulate objectives in your mind, remember they will need to be stated so you will be able to recognize whether or not the objective was attained. Program objectives, then, should be stated behaviorally, that is, stated in relation to some discrete behavior that is observable or measurable by the persons responsible for judging if this learner behavior is present or not.

Concerning the category or type of behavioral change that may be achieved, behavioral change may occur in one of three categories: a change in what the participant or learner

1. Knows (cognitive learning)
2. Does (psychomotor learning)
3. Feels (affective learning)

Content and context component. A final characteristic of program objectives is that they are related to content and context. The content area or context delineates the specific situations about which or within which the behavior is demonstrated. From our earlier example, the care to be demonstrated was specifically that of "a patient who requires mechanical ventilation." The context or content area serves to distinguish the behavior sought from other occasions of demonstrated care.

Sample program objectives. The following will provide you with a sample of what terminal or program objectives should look like.

At the completion of the Critical Care Nursing Internship Program, participants will be able to do the following:

1. Use appropriate theoretical constructs in managing the psychosocial aspects of care for the critical care patient-family system
2. Describe how critical care nurses can successfully manage stressors present in the critical care work environment
3. Identify features of normal anatomy and physiology that influence the nursing management of critically ill patients
4. Perform an accurate, systematic assessment of patients who are critically ill, based on clinical and laboratory data
5. Describe the appropriate rationale underlying all aspects of care for patients who are critically ill
6. Provide the nursing interventions appropriate for management of patients who are critically ill
7. Appropriately use mechanical and electronic equipment required in the care of critically ill patients
8. Independently initiate life-saving procedures when a patient's condition warrants
9. Appropriately incorporate each step of the nursing process in developing a written plan of care for patients who are critically ill

Usefulness of program objectives

A clear statement of program objectives is useful both to the learner in the program and to the educator.

To the learner. Program objectives enable the learner to

1. Know what behaviors she can expect to learn in the program
2. Judge her present level of performance with respect to these objectives
3. Assess her own motivation toward meeting these objectives

4. Decide how closely the program objectives correspond to her personal and professional educational needs and objectives
5. Begin planning a course of activities designed to meet these objectives
6. Evaluate her individual progress in meeting each objective
7. Evaluate the overall effectiveness of the program from the learner perspective
8. Offer a critique of the program objectives to benefit future learners in the program

To the educator. Program objectives are useful to the educator in providing direction for all subsequent phases of the instructional process: instructional format selection, curriculum design and development, content selection and sequencing, instructional methods and techniques, program provision, and management and evaluation of all aspects of the program. More specifically, the educator uses program objectives as the basis for

1. Identifying what must be learned within the program
2. Defining more specific intermediate behavioral outcomes
3. Selecting, differentiating, and organizing didactic and clinical learning experiences
4. Identifying content areas and clinical situations relevant to meeting desired behavioral outcomes
5. Selecting instructional techniques and learning activities best suited to meeting these objectives
6. Specifying the appropriate participants for the program
7. Monitoring the overall effectiveness of the program
8. Evaluating whether or not participants have learned what was desired
9. Evaluating participants individually and collectively
10. Evaluating the effectiveness of selected learning activities
11. Designing tools to measure and evaluate learning in the program
12. Communicating and clarifying the thrust or intended outcomes of the program to others concerned with critical care education

Once terminal objectives have been formulated for an educational program, you need to select an instructional format that can lead program participants to these ends. The next chapter describes some available program formats.

REFERENCES

del Bueno, DJ: Need to know versus nice to know, J Nurs Admin 6:6, 1976.

Harris, HJ: The coming recession: how it will affect training—and what you can do to survive, Training HRD 16:26, 1979.

Knowles, MS: The modern practice of adult education, rev ed, Chicago, 1980, Follett Publishing Co.

PLANNING

Chapter 4

Selection of program format

Gathering all of the surviving educational needs in one hand and the summary of your educational and operational resources in the other, you are now ready to select an appropriate program format. The format selected should be consistent with the needs to be met and within the scope of resources available at the agency.

The most influential factors in determining program format are the degree of commonality that exists among the identified educational needs, the time frames available for instruction, and the amount of flexibility necessary in instruction. Based on these factors, educational program formats generally fall into one of two major categories:

1. Formats appropriate for group learning
2. Formats appropriate for individual learning

Although many educational programs require a mixture of the two to some degree, one type or the other usually predominates.

The following section describes formats available for group and individual learning and summarizes the resources required for each. As you consider each format, first decide whether the format is appropriate for meeting the identified educational needs. If you deem the format appropriate, decide whether it would serve as a primary or as a supplementary format. Remember that a learning format is simply a means with which to organize participants for learning; there are no hard and fast rules for selecting an appropriate format.

GROUP FORMATS FOR LEARNING
Traditional class or course
Educational feasibility

Range. The traditional approach to group learning is by means of a class or a course of learning activities. This may range from a single class, to a series of related classes (course), to a series of related courses (comprehensive program).

Depth. Depth is adaptable to all or any combination of levels: beginning, intermediate, or advanced.

Nature of learning need. Usual focus is on acquiring knowledge and attitudes rather than skills.

Learning style. Learning style is traditionally more formal, teacher-directed in classroom setting; learners are usually more familiar with this format.

Time frame. For a single class the time frame may involve minutes, hours, or days; for a course, hours, days, or weeks; and for a program, days, weeks, or months.

Educator as practitioner. The educator as practitioner is valuable for making pertinent illustrations and meaningful applications of theory to the reality of practice; generally there is less emphasis on clinical practice skills in the classroom setting.

Educator as educator. As range, depth, and time frame of educational needs increase, so does the need for experience and expertise in the educator role; depth and breadth of educational need determine how thorough and timely the educator's knowledge must be. The ability to apply principles of adult education will be necessary to promote active learner participation.

Educator as administrator. The educator's degree of proficiency as an administrator increases proportionately with the comprehensiveness of a program and the number of participants and faculty.

Operational feasibility

Time. Preparation and coordination time is usually linearly related to the range, depth, and time frame of a program. A single class on a single topic may take hours or days to prepare for, whereas a course on a limited number of topics may require days or weeks, and programs on numerous topics may require weeks or months.

Money. Greater expenditures of money will be necessary as the number of participants and the program's complexity increase. If instructors are from outside the hospital, you may need funds for honoraria.

Personnel. Need for faculty is largely a function of the program's complexity and the capabilities of the educator in required areas; need for additional faculty usually increases with more comprehensive programs. Need for support personnel may be unnecessary for single classes, desirable for a series of classes, and mandatory for large-scale programs.

Facilities. You need to secure adequate classroom space to seat comfortably the necessary number of participants. Satisfactory lighting, temperature control, visibility, and ventilation are necessary. Continued availability of space needs to be assured for comprehensive programs.

Instructional materials. Instructional materials used depend on the program's content, teacher preferences and experience, funds available, and the likelihood of their future reuse; ranges from no materials to a large variety.

Audiovisual equipment. Audiovisual equipment is chosen as appropriate to instructional software intended for use.

Supplies. There are greater needs for supplies with long-range programs involving substantial numbers of participants, faculty, administrative and support staff, and needs for information processing.

Conference

Educational feasibility

Range. The conference has a short range and is limited to specific problems of a particular patient or patient category.

Depth. Enough depth should be provided for comprehensive coverage of a limited topic.

Nature of learning need. Given the learning need, the typical focus is on a specific nursing problem, aspect of patient care, or the nursing care of a specific patient. The conference provides for problem solving related to common issues, interests, and aspects of patient management together with communicating an exchange of perspectives and alternative approaches to care.

Learning style. Learning style is usually informal. It may arise spontaneously or be scheduled, is usually unstructured, and is appropriate for adult learners seeking to solve common problems existing within the work situation.

Time frame. Time frame ranges from minutes to hours to 1 day, until there is a joint resolution of the problem.

Educator as practitioner. For the educator as practitioner, current clinical expertise and familiarity with content area are necessary because discussion focuses on examining actual nursing care, assessing results of that care, exploring approaches utilized, and making decisions on preferable alternative approaches to patient care.

Educator as educator. The educator as educator may share responsibility for designing conference segments with discussion participants and may determine problems and salient points that need coverage together with sequencing conference segments. This requires familiarity with the group problem-solving process.

Educator as administrator. The educator as administrator must coordinate topic sequence and participants, audiovisual support, and summary session. Administrative responsibilities expand to fiscal and management areas if formal or large group conferences are planned.

Operational feasibility

Time. Only minimal preparation time is necessary if the conference is informal and all participants are thoroughly familiar with the patient and with the problems to be discussed.

Money. Significant amounts of money required only when the conference is a lengthy formal one planned for large groups or if refreshments are provided.

Personnel. Discussants and the conference leader must know about patient problems and nursing care to be presented. Support personnel may be necessary during the planning stage and the operational stage for preparation and distribution of background materials and notices of conference time and place.

Facilities. Facilities should allow seating in circles or around a table for face-to-face contact and visibility of participants. Acoustics must be acceptable for maintaining discussion.

Instructional materials. Instructional materials are usually not necessary. A summary of salient points in patient problems to be discussed may be distributed to those unfamiliar with the patient.

Audiovisual equipment. Logistical and material support may not be necessary for small, informal groups. A chalkboard, overhead projector, or slide projector may be helpful for larger groups.

Supplies. No supplies are usually required.

Seminar

Educational feasibility

Range. Range is usually limited to examination of a single topic for a few hours to 1 or 2 days.

Depth. There should be a systematic investigation of a problem with conclusions and results formulated, basically an indepth study of a single topic or well-circumscribed area. Intermediate to advanced levels of instruction are probably most appropriate.

Nature of learning need. The seminar is an information exchange (knowledge, skills) and involves sharing experiences, knowledge, and problem-solving techniques. It is generally somewhat structured in a quasi-formal to formal format, directed by recognized experts in the area under investigation.

Learning style. Learning style usually actively involves participants. Participants assume responsibility in preparing for topics to be presented and discussed. The seminar requires self-directed or knowledgable participants. Its usefulness depends on audience participation and participant exchange following a lecture presentation.

Time frame. Time frame is typically short (a few hours to 1 day), and formal seminars meet at set intervals.

Educator as practitioner. The educator as practitioner performs as in class or course format.

Educator as educator. The educator as educator uses skills in leading and facilitating group discussions and in summarizing and reaching a group consensus. The educator may function largely in the wings, while participants actively provide both teaching and learning experiences.

Educator as administrator. The educator as administrator is responsible for selecting presentors, assigning roles, and distributing background materials. It may be necessary to keep discussions focused on the topic; assignments need to be coordinated and forwarded to participants in adequate time for their preparation.

Operational feasibility

Time. Time needed depends on duration and formality of seminar, number of sessions, background of participants, experience in coordinating seminars, ready availability of support personnel, and facilities.

Money. Expenses range from few if any for a small peer group, informal format to honoraria for an authority from outside the hospital. Funds may be necessary for renting a facility, providing meals and materials, or if more formal approaches are used.

Personnel. The seminar leader must be able to coordinate assignments, lead and focus discussions, and supplement, critique and summarize presentations and discussions. A panel of experts may be drawn from within the organization or secured from outside. Support personnel may be required for large or formal seminars.

Facilities. Necessary facilities include a room with a conference table around which all participants can be seated; smaller tables may be necessary if the members are to be divided into smaller work groups.

Instructional materials. Instructional materials include handouts and preparatory materials that may be useful for participants to review. Written time frames may assist in focusing discussion periods.

Audiovisual equipment. The leader may require audiovisual material for illustrations and summarizations; a chalkboard is often adequate for smaller groups.

Supplies. Few supplies are required, depending on the formality of the approach, the number of participants, and the use of handouts.

Workshops

Educational feasibility

Range. Workshops are generally short range projects; large group sessions may meet initially, followed by small group hands-on sessions.

Depth. An intensive, indepth study of a topic, skill, or problem is involved.

Nature of learning need. Learning needs include the acquisition, application, or refinement of clinical skills; competency in a defined area; improvement of individual proficiency; and hands-on experience.

Learning style. Learning style is designed to foster active participation by learners, using equipment and necessary procedures. This is typically provided in an informal, interactive atmosphere.

Time frame. Time frame ranges from less than 1 to a few days for multifaceted or complex skills.

Educator as practitioner. The educator as practitioner is essential for demonstrating how to perform skills and provide constructive feedback on participant performance.

Educator as educator. The educator as educator must be well versed in principles underlying skills demonstrated and be able to perform effectively all critical and intervening behaviors involved with those skills.

Educator as administrator. The educator as administrator must organize and sequence learning units by dividing the participant audience into smaller groups for practice. This requires coordination of speakers, facilities, equipment, accommodations, and meals.

Operational feasibility

Time. Increased preparation time is required for coordination of all facets of the program if workshop time is substantial. Time is required for preparation of teaching materials, for coordination of small and large group classes, and for practice sessions.

Money. Money is needed for supplementary instructional materials and equipment used for demonstration and practice. Vendors may be willing to underwrite equipment and supply costs.

Personnel. The number of instructors required increases according to the number of participants. Workshops require a low instructor:participant ratio. Support personnel may be required for setting up facilities, testing equipment, and providing teaching materials.

Facilities. Facilities must be adequate to

accommodate participant mobility, breaking off into large and small groups, and practice with equipment and procedures.

Instructional materials. All instructional materials necessary for demonstration and practice of the skill and its component parts will have to be provided.

Audiovisual equipment. Audiovisual equipment may be necessary for demonstration purposes to provide an overview or summary of skill sequences.

Supplies. Supplies necessary for hands-on experience sufficient for the number of participants

Club and study group
Educational feasibility
Range. The group is formed on the basis of some common and relatively circumscribed area of interest. The range of areas may be firmly restricted or open to change by consensus.

Depth. The group may focus on broad coverage of an area or indepth coverage of a single topic; it is flexible.

Nature of learning need. Learning needs include sharing and acquiring knowledge, broadening interests, and deepening cultural and professional appreciation.

Learning style. Learning style is generally informal with individual sessions structured around some aspect or subtopic to be explored. This is participant-centered, a social group.

Time frame. Time frame is decided by the group to meet its needs. Often ongoing, regularly scheduled meetings of a few hours or less are involved.

Educator as practitioner. The educator would act as practitioner if program is organized around nursing practice issues and topics.

Educator as educator. The educator as educator provides needed information, offers insights into the area of interest, and functions as a resource person.

Educator as administrator. Virtually no ad-ministrating is required; groups are self-sustaining entities.

Operational feasibility
Time. Time is mostly devoted to organizing general subtopics for each class within the available or desired time frame. Time for preparation for meetings might be included if the educator actively participates with other learners.

Money. There is probably minimal if any money needed unless the program is held during duty hours.

Personnel. Personnel need to know about the area under study. Usually no support personnel are necessary.

Facilities. Facilities need to be adequate for the size of the group and to accommodate informal discussion.

Instructional materials. Instructional materials are determined by the instructor for group needs; overall, there is probably a minimal need for them.

Audiovisual equipment. Probably no audiovisual equipment is needed, only as necessary or desired by participants.

Supplies. No supplies are needed.

INDIVIDUAL FORMAT FOR LEARNING
Self-directed learning activities
Educational feasibility
Self-directed learning activities incorporate formats and terms such as independent learning, modular instruction, programmed instruction, learning packages, and autotutorial instruction.

Range. Individual instructional units (lessons, modules, packages) are limited to a single concept or topic area together with component subtopics; multiple individual instructional units may be sequentially related into units or programs to provide a wider range of single topic coverage. Range may be infinitely varied to coincide with the range of educational needs. Subject matter must be capable of division into self-contained component segments.

Depth. These may have differentiated levels of depth (basic-intermediate-advanced) on same topic, and are readily adaptable to any desired depth. Greater depth requires that the program be systematically organized in a carefully ordered sequence.

Nature of learning need. Learning needs usually include acquiring cognitive learning through self-directed study and may be supplemented with media for affective and psychomotor learning. The individual format is directed toward attaining highly specific instructional objectives and can be used for remedial, initial, or review learning and reinforcement.

Learning style. Learning style is self-paced and learner directed with the teacher as a resource person. It involves self-directed inquiry that requires learners' commitment and pursuit of preferred learning style, and typically provides some form of immediate feedback on performance. It usually provides for pretesting performance to determine mastery of objectives, reduce unnecessary instruction, and facilitate rapid progression.

Time frame. Time frame is generally unlimited and lasts as long as necessary to meet objectives. Progress is determined by the learner and individual rate of learning. Development and pilot testing of self-instructional materials requires variable amounts of time, depending on the complexity of topic area and the educator's design experience.

Educator as practitioner. The educator is required to act as practitioner to assure relevance and accuracy of content to nursing practice and to evaluate the effectiveness of a specific instructional unit.

Educator as educator. The educator as educator develops prerequisites for units, topics, and subtopics, learning objectives, sequence of units, guidelines for use, instructional materials, pretests and posttests, media alternatives available for learning, handouts, bibliography, and worksheets. The educator should be skilled in the use of audiovisual material and equipment

and conducts pilot tests of instructional units. Familiarity with content, objectives, and resources existent to meet objectives is a must, as is the ability to evaluate learning. There is flexibility and expertise in supplementing requirements for meeting individual needs. The educator provides guidance, counseling, and evaluation of learning activities. Existing media may be used or adapted or original audiovisual supplements developed. The educator may need to teach learners how to use this format effectively if they are unfamiliar with it.

Educator as administrator. The educator as administrator makes audiovisual and teaching resources available when learners need them and is accessible to learners. The educator prepares each unit as a self-contained physical package, but may need to coordinate with other departments for scheduling use of hardware, software, facilities, or for developing new materials.

Operational feasibility

Time. Time is needed for introduction to this learning format at the initiation of the unit, to monitor progress, to provide assistance, to evaluate learning experience, and for developing and pilot testing instructional materials, media, objectives, pretests and posttests, study guides and packages, and the bibliography. This format eliminates spending time in providing repetitive lectures on same content, relearning areas already mastered, scheduling classes and classrooms and reduces time away from patient care areas.

Money. If resources and instructional materials are already available, this program may require minimal expenditures. Program design, development, and production could be costly if sophisticated media are used or if programs are complex. The planners need to determine policies regarding compensation of learners for off-duty study, learner versus agency purchase of materials, and whether instruction is mandatory or optional.

Personnel. This format can significantly reduce the number of instructor personnel necessary; minimal to no support personnel are necessary once materials have been developed. Instructors must be available to supervise the use of materials and supplement as necessary and to function as facilitators and validators of learning. Support personnel may be required to assist in coordinating audiovisual use with other agencies and departments as necessary and to assist with maintenance and scheduling of equipment and instructional materials.

Facilities. The educator may use existing audiovisual or learning center or nearby facilities as available and warranted. Depending on equipment and audiovisual materials, work may be done at the learner's home, on the clinical unit, in the learning center or in any other area offering the environmental features required by the specific format.

Instructional materials. The specific format dictates the necessary materials. A syllabus, guidelines and instructions, objectives, study guides, handouts, self-evaluation tools, bibliography, journals, supplementary readings, models, clinical laboratory facilities, and written or audiovisual media are some of the materials that may be required. Materials should be selected within the resource capability of the agency.

Audiovisual equipment. Audiovisual equipment requirements may be minimal or extensive, depending on the nature and sophistication of the program.

Supplies. The requirement for supplies varies extensively with specific format selected and program materials developed.

REFERENCES
Workshops

Clark, CC: The nurse as continuing educator, New York, 1979, Springer-Verlag.

Diers, D, and Johnson, JE: How workshops prepare nurses for the therapeutic role, Nurs Outlook 17:30, 1969.

Friedman, WH, Ganong, JM, and Ganong, WL: Workshopping, Nurs Educ 4:19, 1979.

Gerber, RM: The mini-workshop, Nurs Outlook 28:126, 1980.

How to plan and run off-site training meetings that work, Training HRD 16:95, 1979.

Murphy, J: The first hour: creating a learning environment, J Contin Educ Nurs 10:42, 1979.

Smyth, Sr K, and McMahon, J: A workshop approach to continuing education, Nurs Educ 1:16, 1976.

Stevens, B: The successful workshop: how to bring it off! Nurs Educ 2:16, 1977.

Self-instruction and independent learning

American Nurses' Association: Self-directed continuing education in nursing, Kansas City, 1978, American Nurses' Association.

Bell, J, and Miller, M: A new concept of teaching-learning experience in trauma nursing, J Contin Educ Nurs 8:22, 1977.

Brown, JW, Lewis, RB, and Harcleroad, FF: AV Instruction—technology, media and methods, New York, 1973, McGraw-Hill Book Co.

Clark, K, and Dickinson, G: Self-directed and other-directed continuing education, J Contin Educ Nurs 7:16, 1976.

Cooper, SS: Self-directed learning in nursing, Wakefield, Massachusetts, 1980, Nursing Resources.

Donohue, JD, Litz, KA, and Scott, SA: PSI: an innovative approach to teaching nursing technologies, JNE 15:7, 1976.

Gentine, M: Methods of teaching-revisited: self-learning packages, J Contin Educ Nurs 11:57, 1980.

Gudmundsen, A: Teaching psychomotor skills, JNE 14:23, 1975.

Hinthorne, R: Methods of teaching revisited: self-instructional modules, J Contin Educ Nurs 11:37, 1980.

Keeling, AW, and Noriega, L: Continuing education—independently! Superv Nurs 9:45, 1978.

Keller, FS: The Keller Plan handbook, Menlo Park, Calif., 1974, W. A. Benjamin Company.

Kellogg, CJ: Individualizing teaching of students, JNE 14:14, 1975.

Knowles, MS: Self-directed learning, a guide for learners and teachers, New York, 1975, Association Press.

Lange, CM: Adapting media for independent study, Nurs Outlook 24:546, 1976.

Lange, C: Autotutorial techniques in nursing education, Englewood Cliffs, N.J., 1972, Prentice-Hall, Inc.

Layton, J: Instructional packaging, JNE 14:26, 1975.

Lewis, L.: Independent-individualized learning, Nurs Forum 17:84, 1978.

Lewis, LC: Modules for independent-individual learning in nursing, Philadelphia, 1975, F.A. Davis Co.

Lindstrom, SR, and Archibald, EJ: A critical care teaching method, Superv Nurs 11:49, 1980.

Moran, V: Study of comparison of independent learning

activities vs. attendance at staff development by staff nurses, J Contin Educ Nurs **8**:14, 1977.

O'Connor, ME, and Jones, D: An innovative teaching strategy for nursing education, JNE **14**:9, 1975.

Paduano, MA: Introducing independent study into the nursing curriculum, JNE **18**:34, 1979.

Pensivy, BA: Traditional versus individualized nursing instruction: comparison of state board examination scores as a result of these two methods of nursing instruction, JNE **16**:14, 1977.

Puntillo, K, and Duncan, J: An alternative learning experience for intensive care unit nurses, J Contin Educ Nurs **11**;44, 1980.

Reinhart, E: Independent study: an option in continuing education, J Contin Educ Nurs **8**:38, 1977.

Sheahan, J: An evaluation of a workshop for teachers of nursing on an individualized teaching and learning strategy, J Adv Nurs **4**:647, 1979.

Smith, CE: Learning on your own for credit, Am J Nurs **80**:2013, 1980.

Sommerfeld, D, and Hughes, J: How independent should independent learning be? Nurs Outlook **28**:416, 1980.

Swanson, EA, and Dalsing, CW: Independent study: a curriculum expander, JNE **19**:11, 1980.

Thompson, MA: A systematic approach to module development, JNE **17**:20, 1978.

Wheeler, L: Designing and implementing modules: a guide for the educator, J Nurs Midwif **20**:19, 1975.

Chapter 5

Preparing instructional objectives

IDENTIFYING CONTENT AREAS

Chapter 3 described the process of formulating program objectives. Even these broadly stated terminal objectives should identify the outcome behavior sought in the learner as related to some specific content or context. The subject content of any learning experience is sampled from all that is known about a particular topic area, extracting only that content necessary to meet the stated objective(s). Using an earlier example, note how a properly stated program objective suggests the content areas necessary for the instructor to address for learners to meet that objective: "Without preceptor guidance, the participant will demonstrate how to care for a patient who requires mechanical ventilation." Content areas suggested by this objective include the following:

1. Oxygen therapy and toxicity
2. Tracheostomy care
3. Endotracheal suctioning
4. Responding to alarm systems on the mechanical ventilator
5. Weaning from the mechanical ventilation
6. Supplemental humidification of inspired air
7. Discontinuing mechanical ventilation

Objectives indicate the content areas relevant for inclusion within the program of instruction. When the scope of your program is more or less circumscribed, the range of content areas suggested will usually be similarly restricted. If your instructional designs encompass all major facets of critical care nursing, the range of relevant content areas will similarly expand.

In this latter situation, many critical care educators consult the American Association of Critical-Care Nurses' *Core Curriculum for Critical Care Nursing*. The *Core* provides a substantive outline for most of the major content areas related to this specialty. Because the expanse of critical care nursing practice is ever-widening, however, and because your institution may have patient populations and areas of critical care practice different from other critical care units, you may wish to supplement, amend, abridge, or otherwise modify the *Core* content areas to suit the educational needs of your own particular situation.

You need not feel restricted, however, to using such inclusive references. Look at your program objectives and see the content areas they indicate as necessary for inclusion. Publications such as the *Core* can be extremely useful or much too cumbersome for your purposes. Use your own program objectives to guide you in these decisions. It is very expensive and time-consuming to teach more than is really necessary.

Initially you may find it useful to delineate content areas for each related course. Divide the subcomponents or subdivisions of the curriculum into some natural or logical outline that covers all necessary subcomponent content areas.

For example, your curriculum may be composed of the following related courses:

Critical care nursing curriculum

Course I: Care of the critically ill patient in crisis
Course II: Care of the critically ill patient with pulmonary dysfunction
Course III: Care of the critically ill patient with cardiovascular dysfunction
Course IV: Care of the critically ill patient with renal dysfunction
Course V: Care of the critically ill patient with neurological dysfunction
Course VI: Care of the critically ill patient with endocrine dysfunction

Each course may then be logically subdivided into component units, each unit having its own subunit content areas:

Course II: Care of the critically ill patient with pulmonary dysfunction
  Unit 1: Functional anatomy of the pulmonary system
  Unit 2: Physiology of the pulmonary system
  Unit 3: Clinical assessment of the pulmonary system
  Unit 4: Management of care for patients with pulmonary system dysfunction

Each unit in turn may be subdivided into more specific units, each again having its corresponding levels of content:

Critical care nursing curriculum

Course II: Care of the critically ill patient with pulmonary dysfunction
  Unit 3: Clinical assessment of the pulmonary system
    a. Physical assessment techniques
    b. Laboratory assessment of the pulmonary system
    c. Radiological assessment of the pulmonary system
    d. Interpreting arterial blood gas levels
    e. Interpreting pulmonary function studies

As you may be envisioning, the process of subdividing the total content of the curriculum into its component content areas is seemingly endless. All you really need to strive toward is aiming at the level of specificity most useful for determining the content to be addressed during each instructional period.

SPECIFYING DESIRED OUTCOME BEHAVIORS

Learning is defined as a change in behavior. To identify the behavior desired and evaluate whether learning objectives have been achieved, it is necessary to identify the specific behavioral change sought in the learner.

Behavioral changes are traditionally categorized into three groups:
  1. Cognitive: change in what learner knows or understands
  2. Psychomotor: change in what learner is able to do
  3. Affective: change in how the learner feels

Within each of these categories are numerous and finely differentiated lists of action verbs available to denote the precise behavior intended in the objective. Educators such as Bloom, Krathwohl, and Gronlund have categorized many of these verbs into their appropriate sphere and level of complexity. A listing of such action verbs may be useful when writing the objectives for determining the precise behavior sought.

The important point here is that you clearly specify the behavior you will accept as evidence that learning objectives have been achieved. Well-stated behaviors are overt and explicit, observable, measurable, and subject to as few interpretations as possible for the learner or the learning evaluator. Mager suggests that you can judge that the performance has been correctly defined if it describes what the learner will be doing when demonstrating the achievement of the objective. If your stated behavior does not meet each of these criteria, greater precision is yet in order.

WRITING INSTRUCTIONAL OBJECTIVES

Now that you have outlined the necessary content areas and identified the performance behaviors to be demonstrated, you must link these two elements to form instructional objectives.

Instructional objectives may be thought of as the additive components of program objectives. Once all instructional objectives have been attained, the program objective these were derived from has been attained. Program or terminal objectives are broad in their scope and usually imply a number of subordinate behaviors that serve as evidence of their attainment. They represent the final outcome performances desired in the learner; in so doing, they infer one or more intermediate behaviors that will be recognized as evidence of achievement of the terminal behavior. Program objectives then only serve as the starting point of curriculum design, providing guides for determining subordinate objectives that lie at succeeding levels of specificity.

How many levels of specificity you use and the degree of specificity necessary at each level are determined by the depth, scope, and time frame of the program and the organizational format contemplated. In general you should write objectives that coincide with each major subcomponent or subdivision of the curriculum in such a way that the last objectives written are those you will use to prepare for each instructional class period.

Remember that you write objectives to know what kinds of learning experiences you have to provide for that, taken together, meet the program objectives. Aim at a level of specificity in the objectives that tells you what content and behaviors each class period is responsible for covering—no more or less. Your target is the individual instructional period, what is commonly referred to as "a class," whether its time frame is 15 minutes, 50 minutes, or 2 hours.

There is no practical use or value in composing books of erudite objectives that will be put to rest on some shelf in your office. Instructional objectives should be as useful to you as they are to the learner in knowing what any given instructional period is intended to achieve.

Objectives are the only pragmatic means for guiding both learners and instructors through a learning experience. They are worth the investment of time and energy required to make them meaningful and accurate. The nature and requirements of the desired performance will dictate whether an instructional objective can be called "well written" or "good." How instructional objectives are stated and what they must include are open to variable interpretation. Here two viewpoints on this issue are considered, and you can decide which is more useful for your purposes and experience right now. Just remember that objectives are not formulated to be written; they are written to be used by learners and teachers alike.

If the function of objectives is to give direction to the instructional process, the amount and nature of their form should be dictated by this standard. Mager suggests that useful instructional objectives have the following three characteristics:

1. Performance: describes what the learner is doing when demonstrating achievement of the objective
2. Conditions: describe the circumstances under which the performance must be demonstrated, including any restrictions warranted
3. Criterion: describes the qualitative or quantitative level of acceptable (satisfactory) performance

Whereas all objectives must specify the performance intended for the learner, conditions and explicit criteria or standards of performance are useful only to the extent that they serve to communicate more clearly the desired performance. At times, certain conditions or criteria of performance are critical to clarifying the desired performance. Consider the objective: "The nurse will be able to perform endotracheal suctioning." After reflecting on this objective, do any conditions or criteria for that performance seem in order? You might think that "acceptable" performance here would also need to include that this performance be carried out using strict aseptic technique, so you would rewrite the objective to clarify this additional condition: "Using strict aseptic technique, the nurse will be able to perform endotracheal suctioning." That sounds better. But if you were observing the learner's performance of the technique, would any other criteria seem warranted for your decision that this performance was indeed acceptable? Think about it a moment. Would it still be acceptable if the nurse were only able to perform the suctioning procedure if you gave her directions and guidance along the way? Would you still consider the performance "acceptable" if it required 5 minutes rather than 15 seconds to accomplish? If you expect the objective to be clearly understood and not subject to multiple interpretations, you should state and restate it until it incorporates all necessary conditions or standards that will be expected; the learner or other observers should not have to divine your intent; it should be clear to all: "Using strict aseptic technique, the nurse will be able to perform endotracheal suctioning without preceptor prompting and within a maximum of 15 seconds." Likewise, if "acceptable" performance necessitates any of the following criteria or conditions, they should be incorporated into the objective:

Criteria: desired levels of achievement

SPEED: The nurse will be able to record correctly a standard 12-lead ECG *within 5 minutes*.

ACCURACY: The nurse will be able to convert correctly a patient's body weight from pounds to kilograms *rounded off to the nearest whole number*.

QUALITY: The nurse will be able to administer all aspects of postmortem care *as described in the unit policy and procedures manual*.

QUANTITY: The nurse will correctly interpret 25 ECG tracings with no more than *two* errors.

Conditions: circumstances under which performance is demonstrated

1. *Given 10 sample ECG tracings from the workbook*, the nurse will be able to interpret correctly all tracings.
2. *Without the aid of a calculator*, the nurse will be able to calculate accurately the intravenous administration rate of dopamine hydrochloride (Intropin) as it appears on the order sheet.
3. *Using the neurological assessment form*, the nurse will record her assessment of the patient's neurological status.

Many who have attempted to follow Mager's format seem to get caught up in its potential intricacies. An element of rationality is indispensable in writing objectives; in the process of learning to write these beasties, however, it is easy for even a good thing to get out of hand:

Given a patient diagnosed as having acute renal failure, who has orders for peritoneal dialysis, a peritoneal trocar in place, and who has a signed permit for dialysis, the nurse will be able to administer peritoneal dialysis to the patient using Travenol infusion sets and dialysate without the assistance of the clinical preceptor, reference to text books or class notes, within the guidelines of established unit procedures, standards of care, and her 8-hour shift.

Only criteria and conditions truly pertinent to the learning behaviors warrant inclusion in the objective. Gronlund offers an alternative approach to writing objectives. Proceeding from the general to the specific, Gronlund suggests that objectives focus on two levels of learning outcomes: general instructional objectives and specific learning outcomes. His method involves enumerating adequate representative samples of specific learning outcomes that reflect attaining each general instructional objective. For example:

GENERAL INSTRUCTIONAL OBJECTIVE: Assesses the patient's cardiovascular status

SPECIFIC LEARNING OUTCOMES:

1. Identifies clinical parameters that indicate shock state
2. Correctly interprets ECG tracing
3. Identifies presence of ectopic beats on monitor
4. Correctly interprets cardiac enzyme test results
5. Determines need to titrate vasopressors
6. Auscultates heart sounds

For many objectives, a clear statement of the outcome performance will suffice to communicate your intent. After a while you will find you are able to differentiate which objectives require greater specificity and which do not warrant it. The participant objectives listed in Appendix A illustrate an adaption of Gronlund's approach for a 6-month critical care course.

REFERENCES
Writing instructional objectives

Bloom, BS, and Krathwohl, DR: Taxonomy of educational objectives. handbook I: cognitive domain, New York, 1977, Longman.

Curran, CL: Behavioral objectives: a necessity for nurse educators, J Contin Educ Nurs 8:3, 1977.

Dobles, RW, et al: If you're not doing it already, verify your training objectives, Training HRD 16:36, 1979.

Gronlund, NE: Stating behaviorial objectives for classroom instruction, ed 2, New York, 1978, Macmillan, Inc.

Krathwohl, DR, Bloom, BS, and Masia, BB: Taxonomy of educational objectives. handbook II: affective domain, New York, 1964, David McKay Co., Inc.

Mager, RF: Measuring instructional intent, Belmont, Calif., 1973, Fearon-Pitman Publishers, Inc.

Magner, M: Developing and evaluating inservice programs, Superv Nurs 9:10, 1978.

Nuttleman, D: Instructional objectives, Superv Nurs 8:35, 1977.

Reilly, DE: Behavioral objectives—evaluation in nursing, ed 2, New York, 1980, Appleton-Century-Crofts.

Reilly, DE: Preparation of objectives for continuing education programs, Occup Health Nurs 24:30, 1976.

Schweer, JE: Defining behavioral objectives for continuing education offerings in nursing: a four level taxonomy, Thorofare, N.J., 1980, Charles B. Slack, Inc.

Staropoli, CJ, and Waltz, CF: Developing and evaluating educational programs for health care providers, Philadelphia, 1978, F. A. Davis Co.

Sullivan, TJ: An experience with a systems approach to curriculum design, JNE 16:25, 1977.

Chapter 6

Administration of educational programs

Nurse educators who function in a hospital must recognize the need for collaboration in planning the details of educational programs. Chapter 1 described how educational programs affect the staff nurses, nursing care, and clinical units to emphasize the need for collaboration between nursing education and nursing practice. The present chapter considers areas in which collaborative decisions need to be reached between nursing education and the administration.

What kind of details need to be worked out with the administration? If the program is fairly substantive, you will need to consider at least the seven major issues discussed in this chapter.

NATURE AND PURPOSES OF THE PROGRAM

Scan your locale for programs similar in scope and purpose to your own. This will enable you to avoid inadvertent duplication of an already existent program and to investigate the possibility of pooling regional resources for common needs. When your proposal is to offer a program similar to one available elsewhere, be prepared to enumerate for the administration how you can justify this duplication of effort, how your program will be more attractive in recruiting and training nurses, or how you plan to coordinate local resources. Identify the critical features of your program that make it especially promising and worth the investment of your employer's funding and resources.

TYPE AND NUMBER OF PARTICIPANTS

In delimiting the program level, you must decide which group of critical care staff nurses will participate in the program: students gaining critical care experience, graduate nurses, registered nurses of various programs (diploma, ADN, BSN, MSN), head nurses, nurses with or without experience in critical care nursing, licensed practical nurses (LPNs), nursing assistants, aides, technicians, or a mixed group of orientees. For example, your program audience may be registered nurses with at least 2 years' experience in critical care nursing or it may be nurses with a bachelor of science degree who have little or no experience in critical care nursing. When appropriate, qualifying statements for any of these groups will be helpful in more clearly delineating the target audience you wish to address. The administration should be able to identify who the program intends to benefit.

Educational programs cannot realistically be designed to simultaneously meet the needs of many divergent groups of personnel. Because recruitment and selection of participants and the depth, scope, and nature of the learning experiences chosen are largely determined by the makeup and needs of program participants, crystalizing your intentions here is of central importance.

If minimum or maximum enrollments are appropriate, they should be delineated at this point. Minimum enrollments may be necessary to justify the cost of the program, whereas maximum enrollments may be necessary to accommodate clinical or classroom space restrictions or the required instructor-to-learner ratio.

PROGRAM DATES

You, the administration, and the participants need to be clear about the beginning and ending dates of a given program. Even if your proposal is for an ongoing schedule of classes, the time frames for the various component modules or units of the program should be specified. Administering, coordinating, financing, and evaluating the program may dictate that this timing be fairly circumscribed.

PARTICIPANT SELECTION PROCESS
Entry requirements of participants

Entry requirements necessary for participants should be clearly enumerated. Prerequisites for formal or informal education, work experience, grades (pretest, college, nursing school), time commitment, licensing, or health requirements need enumeration before recruitment and selection processes can be initiated. Essential and preferred characteristics should be differentiated. Example 6-1 illustrates how essential and preferred characteristics may be integrated into preparing an evaluation form used to process applications for a hospital-based educational program. Preentrance examinations to be used should be developed and validated at this point.

Processing applications

A mechanism for efficiently processing all applications is necessary. This mechanism should specify where applications are to be received, who will be responsible for processing and responding to application requests, what "processing" will consist of, how applications are to be completed and submitted, how scheduling and conducting interviews will be put into operation, how participants will be selected, who will answer inquiries related to participation in the program, and how applicants will be notified of selection results.

Selection of participants

In the selection of participants, decisions need to be made in the following areas:
1. What criteria will be used to evaluate and select the applicants for participation?
2. Who should comprise the selection committee?
3. What selection techniques will be used? Some available techniques include preentrance questionnaires, pretests, and interviews. A pre-entrance questionnaire (Example 6-2) may be used:
   a. For screening potential problem areas
   b. To identify areas needing further discussion during an interview
   c. To verify applicant's understanding of program objectives and requirements
   d. To elicit a fuller description of the quality and nature of the applicant's expectations, motivation, and experience
   e. To verify the degree to which prerequisites and preferred characteristics are possessed
4. Pretest: The pretest may be used:
   a. To identify present level of understanding, performance, and experience with respect to the program objectives
   b. To identify areas that will require remedial work
   c. To compare with the posttest at end of program
5. Interview: The interview allows the interviewer:
   a. To meet the applicant personally
   b. To elicit more fully the applicant's needs, background, and experience
   c. To verify concordance between the applicant's and the program's goals
   d. To elicit information about intangible areas: motivation, interest, attitudes

Text continued on p. 64.

Example 6-1. Applicant evaluation form

Applicant: _____ Interview date: _____
Address: _____ Notified of decision by: _____
_____ Notified of decision on: _____
Telephone: (_____) _____ Notified via ☐ telephone ☐ letter
AC

Part I: Essential prerequisites

Prerequisite	Has	Does not have	Comments
1. Current RN license	☐	☐	Number: _____ Expires: _____
2. Ability to work day shift	☐	☐	
3. Ability to rotate shifts	☐	☐	
4. Willingness to fulfill 1-year work commitment	☐	☐	
5. Willingness to devote adequate time to studying, reading, homework, and preparation for examinations	☐	☐	
6. Physical capability to perform duties required of a critical care nurse	☐	☐	
7. Capability of administering basic bedside care	☐	☐	
8. Concordance between career goals and program objectives	☐	☐	
9. Realistic understanding of advantages and disadvantages of critical care nursing practice	☐	☐	
10. Realistic expectations of program goals	☐	☐	
11. Favorable recommendation of present supervisor/head nurse (if currently employed)	☐	☐	

Example 6-1. Applicant evaluation form—cont'd

Applicant: _____

Part II: Characteristics preferred in applicants

Characteristic	Evaluation of degree possessed				Comments
	Fully	Par-tially	Mini-mally	Not at all	
1. High degree of *positive* motivation for participating in program	☐	☐	☐	☐	
2. Demonstrated potential for successful completion of academic and clinical requirements	☐	☐	☐	☐	School references GPA _____ Clinical _____
3. Clinical experience in critical care nursing within the past 5 years	☐	☐	☐	☐	Student experience _____
4. Clinical experience in medical-surgical nursing within the past 5 years	☐	☐	☐	☐	
5. Experience in clinical nursing within the past 5 years	☐	☐	☐	☐	
6. Successful completion of formal courses in critical care nursing	☐	☐	☐	☐	Date(s): _____
7. Evidence of participation in continuing education in nursing	☐	☐	☐	☐	
8. Demonstrated stability in previous nursing positions	☐	☐	☐	☐	
Other employment	☐	☐	☐	☐	
9. Demonstrated evidence of progression in clinical and managerial proficiency in previous nursing positions	☐	☐	☐	☐	
10. Relating well with peers and co-workers	☐	☐	☐	☐	
11. Maintaining interpersonal and peer relationships conducive to team effort	☐	☐	☐	☐	
12. References recommending participation in program	☐	☐	☐	☐	

Continued.

Example 6-1. Applicant evaluation form—cont'd

Applicant: _____

Part III: Summary

1. Factors *favoring* suitability for selection: _____
_____
_____
_____
_____

2. Factors *limiting* suitability for selection: _____
_____
_____
_____
_____
_____

3. Additional considerations: _____
_____
_____
_____
_____

4. Recommendations: _____
_____
_____

5. Decision made: Decision made by: (signatures)
   ☐ Accepted   _____
   ☐ Alternate list   _____
   ☐ Not accepted   _____
6. Reasons for nonacceptance: _____

Example 6-2. Preentrance questionnaire

Applicant: _____   Interview date: _____
Address: _____   Basic nursing program: ☐ Diploma ☐ ADN
_____   ☐ BSN
                              ZIP
Telephone: (_____) _____   School of nursing: _____
           AC
Social Security no.: _____ ____ _____   Location: _____
Date of birth: _____   Graduation date: _____
If GN, date of state board examination: _____   If RN, license no. _____ State: _____
Grade point average in nursing school: _____
Scale used: _____

1. How did you find out about this program? _____
_____

2. Why do you wish to participate in this program? _____
_____
_____
_____

3. What do you expect this training program to provide for you? _____
_____
_____
_____
_____
_____

Example 6-2. Preentrance questionnaire—cont'd

4. What areas of critical care nursing are you most interested in learning about? _____
_____
_____

5. Do you have any specific objectives to achieve through the program? _____
_____
_____

6. While in nursing school, what subjects/courses did you find:

Most difficult	Most liked	Least liked
_____	_____	_____
_____	_____	_____

7. Problems anticipated during the training program: _____
_____
_____

How will you attempt to resolve these? _____
_____

8. Problems anticipated in year of employment following training program: _____
_____
_____

How will you attempt to resolve these? _____
_____

9. What would you say are your:

Greatest strengths	Areas most in need of improvement
_____	_____
_____	_____
_____	_____

10. Previous education or training in critical care nursing: _____
_____

11. Previous experience in critical care nursing (units, position, dates): _____
_____

12. Previous experience in nursing (position, dates): _____
_____

13. Why do you want to be a critical care nurse? _____
_____

14. Unit you hope to work on: ☐ ER ☐ CCU ☐ SICU ☐ MICU ☐ PCU ☐ No preference

Please supply three references (e.g., nursing school instructors, dean of school of nursing, previous supervisors, employers) who can attest to your character and professional/student performance:

1. Name: _____
   Title: _____
   Address: _____
   _____
   _____ ZIP

   Capacity in which reference knows you:
   _____
   Telephone: (_____) _____
                AC

2. Name: _____
   Title: _____
   Address: _____
   _____
   _____ ZIP

   Capacity in which reference knows you:
   _____
   Telephone: (_____) _____
                AC

3. Name: _____
   Title: _____
   Address: _____
   _____
   _____ ZIP

   Capacity in which reference knows you:
   _____
   Telephone: (_____) _____
                AC

6. Will references or grades be required of applicants?
7. What procedure or tool will be used to select participants for the program?
8. How will participants be notified of selection results?
9. How will the hospital know if those who were selected will actually accept their participation in the program?

POLICIES AND PROCEDURES GOVERNING PROGRAM ADMINISTRATION

The agency's organizational chart should identify the location of this program, its administration, and providers within the existent structure. Lines of authority, responsibility, and accountability should be readily identifiable and more fully described in job descriptions and statements of policy and procedure related to the program and its administration.

Among the areas to reach consensus on here are the role of hospital and nursing administration with respect to the program, the selection and role of the program's director or coordinator and support staff, and any requirements for participation in the program.

Role of hospital and nursing administration

The role of the administration in the program needs to be spelled out more fully than merely placing it atop the communication pattern on organizational charts. Developing an effective working relationship between the program and the hospital administrators will require that:

1. The organizational structure of the program be firm enough to provide clear sets of mutual expectations, yet flexible enough to reflect the setting, goals, and constituence involved.
2. Lines of communication between the program and top administration remain open and sensitive to keeping each other informed of the other's activities and needs.
3. Mutual sets of expectations between these

two parties be realistic and feasible with respect to each other and the whole organization.
4. The administration recognizes the educator's need to be involved in program planning and be granted the prerogatives to select, plan, implement, and update her own ideas.
5. The educator recognizes the administrator's needs to be responsive to the composite needs of the department of nursing and the hospital in addition to those of the program.
6. Financial, operational, and professional support systems are readily allocated to assure that the program objectives are achieved within the established timeframe.

Selection and role of program director and support staff

The individual with direct responsibility for the administration of an educational program should be competent to fulfill this charge. Hospital-based educational programs in critical care nursing require that the program director be competent in the following areas: hospital-based critical care nursing practice, application of traditional principles of teaching and learning, application of principles of adult education, and service-based educational administration. Competence in critical care nursing practice alone does not imply competence as a nurse educator, an adult educator, or an educational administrator. No more than "A nurse is a nurse" holds does "A nurse is an educator" follow.

The selection of an educational program director should be based on the expertise to develop, implement, coordinate, and evaluate the educational offering as defined in the program objectives. The program director should also possess a finely tuned liaison capability. Throughout the educational program, the program director serves as a continual link between administrators, educators, practitioners, and program participants. Without the ability to establish and maintain cooperative working relationships with each of these groups, the program director will not likely be successful in the educational endeavor. Without administrative and practice underpinnings, hospital-based nurse educational endeavors do not survive.

If you are contemplating becoming an educational program director, be careful not to seize this position blindly. Review the program objectives carefully to determine how well your capabilities match the program goals. Find out who you would be responsible to and for, both formally and informally. Talk to your immediate supervisor or the director of nursing to hear their perspectives and responses to your inquiries. Find out where all bottom line decisions are made. Inquire about budgetary and personnel allocations for the program, employee educational benefits, and monetary and other forms of compensation to staff nurses for participation in agency, outside agency, and self-directed educational offerings. Peruse staffing schedules, staff:patient ratios, and patient care hours. Scrutinize all relevant job descriptions related to the educational offering and, if necessary, request clarification of the clause, "and other duties as necessary." Determine who peers and co-workers would be and try to meet these individuals. Assess the prior nature and adequacy of staff educational programs to identify pinnacles and pitfalls. Tour the educational facilities to estimate clinical, laboratory, classroom space, and the amount and availability of audiovisual hardware and software. Tour the clinical units and meet the staff nurses you would be working with. Be sure you have a clearly defined position description that includes administrative support for your continuing education.

If all these criteria and customary personnel policies meet with your satisfaction, the program director position may be a good one for you. No position is ever assumed without unknowns, but looking and listening beforehand will help to diminish these for you.

When appropriate, job descriptions for assistants, instructors, and preceptors involved with providing for the program may need to be formally developed and administratively ratified.

One extremely important issue to clarify is how clerical support will be provided for the program. It is essential to know who will be responsible for such assistance as typing, xeroxing, collating, telephoning, scheduling, processing forms, and sundry other related duties. It is both wasteful and inefficient to use nurse educators in this capacity.

Whichever positions are developed to provide for the program, the delineation and interrelationship of each within the local and departmental organization should be as unambiguous as possible. Smooth operations require an adequate number of qualified personnel who know how they interrelate with each other to reach program goals.

Requirements of program participants

When a substantial amount of money, time, and other resources is invested in an educational endeavor, administrative policies pertaining to the entry, continuation, and successful completion of the program by participants may be necessary. Even for less inclusive programs, apportioning continuing education units for attendance at the offering may dictate that some requirements be set for participants to receive these. Your experience in providing such offerings may also suggest that some general or specific administrative guidelines would be helpful in clarifying your expectations of the participants and in avoiding problems that could arise.

Some problems you may wish to consider in developing requirements or guidelines for participants include the following:

1. Absence and tardiness. If necessary, policies related to reporting absence time, recording time made up, the acceptability of reasons for absence or tardiness, and mechanisms for resolving these kinds of

problems may be developed. For continuing education units to be granted, records verifying participants' attendance may be necessary.

2. Class decorum. This may initially seem an unnecessary area of concern, but experience may indicate a need for becoming concerned if abuses such as disruptive behavior, late arrivals, unnecessary noise, smoking during classes, and side conversations become bothersome and disruptive to the group.

3. Dress code. When classes are held within the hospital or participants learn in clinical areas during part or all of a day's instruction, it may be helpful to remind participants to wear the appropriate attire.

4. Criteria for successful completion of the program. If the educational experience requires that participants successfully complete written or performance evaluations (tests, examinations, quizzes, return demonstration), the criteria and policies related to these should be outlined. Criteria should be specific enough so that participants understand what constitutes successful completion of the program. When possible, it is often helpful to include a description of the format or mechanism that will be used for the evaluation process. So that expectations are mutually understood, passing grades and acceptable levels of performance should be unambiguously defined.

Example 6-3 illustrates how such requirements may be delineated.

Example 6-3. Requirements of participants

---

1. Attendance and absences

Attendance at scheduled classes and clinical sessions is required for participants to remain in the program and to receive continuing education units (CEUs) for their participation. For this reason, participants may have no more than 32 accumulated hours of absence from classroom sessions or no more than 24 accumulated hours of absence from clinical sessions at the end of the program.

Absence from class sessions: Requires that the participant:
1. Submit, in writing, the date, hours, and reasons for the absence
2. Provide this information directly to the Program Director or her designate on the first day the nurse returns to work following the absence

In addition, the participant remains responsible for all materials and topics discussed during her absence.

Absence from clinical sessions: Requires that the participant:
1. Submit, in writing, the date, hours, and reasons for the absence
2. Provide this information directly to the Program Director or her designate on the first day the nurse returns to work following the absence
3. Make up all clinical hours in excess of the maximum (24 hours) on the participant's own time to fulfill the requisite amount of clinical experience time
   a. Makeup hours are to be fulfilled on the ICU, CCU, or PCU units. The ER may be utilized to fulfill these hours only with the approval of the Program Director.
   b. Submit in writing, the date, hours, and units in which absence from clinical sessions was made up. **This form is to be signed and dated by the participant and cosigned and dated by the charge nurse or head nurse on duty in the unit worked.** This record of clinical hours made up for absence is to be submitted directly to the Program Director or her designate on the first weekday following the makeup time.

Absences in excess of those stated above, unless approved in writing by the Program Director, are sufficient cause for termination of the nurse as a participant in the program or for the participant not to receive continuing education units.

Example 6-3. Requirements of participants—cont'd

PLEASE NOTE: It is the responsibility of the nurse participant to be certain that all necessary documentation is forwarded to the Program Director. Neither the Program Director nor the clinical preceptor will actively solicit this information from the participant.

2. Tardiness

Tardiness will be considered as absence in calculating attendance records. Frequent or habitual tardiness for classes or clinical sessions may lead to termination of the nurse as a participant.

Out of respect for your colleagues and the instructor who has prepared the class for your benefit, we request that you be ready for classes to begin at their scheduled times.

3. Class decorum

For everyone to gain as much as possible from the classes, we will attempt to structure classes as informally as possible. Please remember, however, that side conversations, tardiness, sleeping during classes, and late arrivals all tend to be disruptive to the class and annoying to others around you. During classes *no smoking* is allowed as a courtesy to our nonsmokers. While smoking is allowed at breaks and after classes, please remember not everyone enjoys sharing this habit with you.

4. Dress

On days when *any* time is spent on the clinical units (clinical class or clinical experience), all participants must wear a complete nursing uniform as described in the dress code.

On days where no time is scheduled for the clinical units, please remember that you will be entering the hospital cafeteria and should, therefore, be dressed in street clothes appropriate for your position at the hospital. Jeans and sandals are not presently considered appropriate attire.

5. Written examinations·

A satisfactory passing score must be attained on each written test. In the event a passing score is not attained, one retake examination by a comparable examination will be allowed. Failure to obtain a passing score on the retake examination constitutes sufficient cause for academic termination of the nurse from the program.

6. Clinical skills

Participants must complete all "required" clinical skills (marked by an asterisk) by _____(date)_____, when the Clinical Skills Inventory Series booklets are due for submission. **Any participant who has not completed these skills and submitted the skills booklet to the Program Director by the date specified will not receive CEUs for the program.**

These booklets must be brought to each clinical experience, as they will be periodically reviewed and used to evaluate your progress. Participants are not allowed to sign off skill booklets of their peers.

7. Clinical evaluation

Each nurse participant must demonstrate satisfactory progression in clinical performance as determined by appraisal of the:
   a. Mastery of all "required" clinical skills
   b. Co-worker assigned as her "buddy"
   c. Staff nurses familiar with her performance
   d. Head nurses of the critical care units
   e. Program Director, clinical preceptor, and Coordinator of Critical Care Units

Unsatisfactory progression in clinical performance is sufficient cause for termination of the nurse from the program.

Critical care training program nurses are subject to all other hospital personnel policies in force at the time of their participation in the program.

FINANCING THE PROGRAM
Why prepare a budget?

To assure that the resources necessary to fulfill program objectives are allocated, a budget must be prepared with sufficient foresight and frequency to keep it current and reflective of program needs. A budget also provides a basis for financial planning and for the orderly control of expenses and income realized within the program. A well-planned budget allows one to measure the cost-effectiveness of a program and its financial impact in related administrative areas, enabling the analysis and comparison of trends in budgetary needs for continuing education in nursing with local, regional, and national costs of these programs. Because educational programs inevitably entail some expenditure of funds, the program's budget is a financial goal complementing its educational goals.

Who prepares a budget?

Depending on the critical care educator's position within the hospital, the educator may be wholly or minimally responsible for preparing the budget. Under decentralized forms of administration, the director of nursing or the director of continuing education will likely prepare the departmental budget, allocating a certain amount of funding toward critical care nursing education programs. With more fully decentralized organizational structures, the critical care educator may be vested with full responsibility for budget preparation, using the bottom line figure allocated by the nursing department budget.

How often should a budget be prepared?

A budget should be prepared as often as necessary to keep it current and reflective of program needs. In most cases, this requires at least an annual fiscal year review. If a program is new, a proposed annual budget inclusive of operational costs will need to be projected together with estimated expenses and incomes. If the educa-

tional program is ongoing or repeated in a similar form throughout the year, budget preparation may occur annually, based on previous budgetary history or on a per program basis.

What considerations enter into budget preparation?

A number of divergent considerations influence budget preparation and outcome. Briefly, they include the following:

1. Independence of the program's budget. The expenses incurred for an educational program may be assigned to single or multiple units or departments within the hospital. Program funding may be a fixed or variable percentage of the total unit or departmental budget. Depending on where your budget belongs within the hospital organization, this has the potential to provide more or less revenue than if the program's budget existed as a solitary entity. When costs are incorporated within another, larger department, the actual costs and cost-effectiveness of the program often become obscured and difficult to retrieve and substantiate. If the program's costs will be underwritten by another, larger department, you should determine precisely what your budgetary ceiling is.

2. Whether employee participants will be paid salary or benefits during their attendance in the program. Participants who are employees of the hospital may be paid their usual rate of work pay, a reduced rate of pay, overtime, or compensation time during their participation in an educational program. Especially when the program lasts more than a few hours, compensation during attendance at educational programs becomes significant in determining how costly the program will be. Programs that require a substantial amount of time may even necessitate decisions on whether such customary employee benefits as sick time, vacation and holiday time, and life and health insurance will be provided for participants. When participants are paid for their attendance, consideration must be given to

how the hospital's return on its potential double investment (program costs and salary and benefits to employee participants) will be protected if employees fail to continue their employment after the program, do not complete the program, or are academically or administratively released from the program.

3. Whether instructors will be paid. When a program requires professional consultants, outside faculty, or other experts to supplement or totally provide the instruction, decisions will need to be made concerning the following:

   a. Whether some form of compensation is appropriate
   b. What that form of compensation should be: honorarium or fee for services
   c. How these payments should be dispensed
   d. Whether all instructors will be given the same type and amount of compensation; what the basis for determining the amount of compensation received will be—teaching hours, per unit or course, or flat salary amount

If all instructors will be paid their customary rate of pay as educators or if all instruction is given voluntarily, then only the customary rate of pay is necessary to include in calculating program costs. If the unit nursing staff and other professionals are teaching during their regular work hours or being paid overtime or extra pay for their teaching, these salary costs in excess of normal staffing costs should be calculated as such into the program's budget. In actuality, all salaries paid for teaching time should be included in calculating total budgetary costs for personnel. In paying nonemployee instructors, one should take account local practices and standards for this service in comparable agencies within the community. Be mindful of the stature of the individual sought, and the tuition rates participants can reasonably afford when considering these persons as instructors. Instructional expertise costs money, but can prove a worth-

while investment. Before allocating funds for outside expertise, however, be certain that the reputations of these individuals as educators are as highly regarded as their supposed stature.

4. The costs offset by the program. In viewing a budget realistically, one should not address only the debit side of the ledger. In addition to considering the use of outside sources for program funding, one should do some accounting of the program's anticipated effect on reducing costs in other sectors of the hospital. Looking at other administrative objectives for the program may suggest where to start. The program's actual or potential effect on such tangible and intangible variables as staff recruitment to critical care areas, retention rates, reduced turnover, morale, job satisfaction, public relations image of the hospital locally and regionally, and other such factors should be assessed in light of budgetary credits. The effect of the program on reducing hospital-paid educational benefits for outside educational programing and its reduction of duplicated expenditures for coexisting programs should also be considered.

5. Amount and nature of bookkeeping required. Accurate records of all financial transactions should be maintained and reported at least annually. The more complex the financial scheme is, the greater the necessary amount and complexity of accounting. Unless someone else will assume this responsibility, the program director will be responsible and must have the time, expertise, and ability to accomplish this. These tabulations may be important for determining the cost effectiveness of the program and in providing data for evaluation of the program. Attention to sound accounting principles and practices is therefore necessary. Your administrative supervisor should be able to assist you.

Sources of program funding

Three major sources are available to finance a hospital-based educational program. Programs may use more than one of these sources, but typically one predominates. The major sources are internal, participant, and external funding.

Internal funding. Internal funding involves using the general or departmental funds of the hospital to underwrite program costs. Program costs may be incorporated within the operational budget of the hospital, or within one of the following departments: nursing, nursing in-service, staff development, or critical care. Highly specialized programs may have their costs borne by the individual unit or department they are associated with or be included under the umbrella of a more ir.clusive department or division within the hospital.

One benefit of internal funding is that it minimizes expenditures for expensive outside services or personnel that may require higher rates of pay. Internal funding may also assist in minimizing the financial impact of the program on the overall departmental or hospital budget. Internal funding may be immediately accessible, thereby reducing processing, recording, and bookkeeping time.

A disadvantage of internal funding is that generating a new educational program may require large initial start-up costs that can take a long time to recover. When using internal funding, an associated tendency is to reduce or reallocate expenditures from other areas that may truly be in need of this funding.

Internal funding may provide for all the major costs incurred in developing and operating a program, or it can be supplemented by either participant or external funding.

Participant funding. Participant funding involves charging those individuals who directly benefit from the program a tuition fee or other form of assessment that makes the program partially or totally self-supporting. Costs may be borne entirely by the participant as an employee of the hospital or may be shared between the employer and the employee. Some shared costs are tuition fees, laboratory fees, and charges for textbooks and instructional materials.

If you anticipate using participant funding, remember that the tuition costs cannot be prohibitive to prospective participants. Surging costs of materials and services may obliterate the potential market for the program. Educational programs have traditionally been evaluated by other than cost-effectiveness yardsticks because of their tendency to affect costs in more indirect (job satisfaction, improved job performance, improved morale, increased quality of staff) than direct ways. Simply dividing the costs by the number of participants may be a neat and clean approach to budgeting, but is not very realistic. Other considerations must often be accounted for or you may find your audience cannot afford your programs.

Some advantages of participant funding are that it assists in making programs self-supportive and self-sustaining, it shares costs only among direct beneficiaries rather than all beneficiaries of the program, and it minimizes the tendency to redirect funds from other areas where they may be needed. Participant funding is a direct approach to managing budgetary responsibility for educational programs. It may motivate participants to value more highly their educational experiences and to gain the maximum benefit from them.

One obvious disadvantage of participant funding is that participants may not be able to afford costly educational programs. Participant funding may convey a more business than educational overtone to the participants involved. Participant funding may require more record keeping, accounting, and record maintenance by the program director or support staff nurses, especially if flexible payment schedules are offered. For a newly developed program in need of further refinement, participants may not feel they "got their money's worth" of education. Finally the program may not be able to generate a market sufficient to sustain it without establishing a minimum number of participants needed to balance fully the costs involved. If minimum enrollments are not attained, much time and effort may go to waste.

External funding. External funding may provide full or partial revenues for hospital-based educational programs. Money may be secured from a wide variety of sources, such as the following:

1. Donations from community or volunteer services, foundations, or organizations
2. Tuition fees charged to outside agencies or organizations wishing to send their employees to participate in the program
3. Outright grants from pharmaceutical or hospital supply companies to sponsor participants
4. Federal, regional, or local government grants
5. Gifts from patients, families of patients, or medical staff members
6. Scholarships or awards to cover tuition costs
7. Local fund-raising drives

Relying on external funding for program costs is a less reliable mechanism than other sources for guaranteeing that funds will be available when needed, but may be well worth the necessary investment of time and energy.

As you can readily see, numerous administrative details need to be worked out in definitively planning an educational program of any substantial size. Many of these decisions ultimately have a direct effect on the specific characteristics of and the mode of providing for a program.

Cost-effectiveness in educational programming

Cost-effectiveness in educational programming is important to consider because the trend toward mandatory continuing education for nurse relicensure coupled with acute relative shortages of critical care nurses have combined to escalate the costs of hospital-based nurse educational programs. To recruit and retain staff nurses, some hospitals have found it necessary to offer numerous educational incentives for ini-

tial and continuing employment. When balanced against the costs of high staff attrition and turnover rates, soaring recruitment costs, closed hospital beds or units, and the necessity for using private nurse personnel agencies, the price of hospital-based staff nursing education appears somewhat less awesome. Nonetheless, as long as economic sobriety resulting from inflation and budget trimming is prevalent, hospitals may need to seek alternative ways to improve the cost-effectiveness of nurse educational programming.

Two obvious approaches to improving the cost-effectiveness of a service-based educational program are to reconsider the educational offering as a budgetary cost center or to trim all programs to essentials only.

Staff education as a cost-revenue center. When staff education is considered as a functional cost-revenue center, all factors that affect financial gain and loss are enumerated. In so doing, both covert and subtle debits and credits can be identified in addition to the more obvious costs incurred. Unfortunately, most hospital educational budgets are recorded more as *cost* centers than *revenue* centers. Often even readily calculable financial gains (dollar effects on recruitment, advertising, turnover, orientation, duration of employment, reliance on private nursing personnel agencies, reopened beds) are overlooked, producing a narrowly defined budget for staff education. Intangible gains in such areas as staff morale, job satisfaction, standards of nursing practice, and time spent making staffing ends meet are barely taken into account, yet have a significant impact on overall operating costs. When conceived of in this light, hospital nursing educational endeavors frequently result in notable credits that more than offset their costs. As a hospital-based educator, you have a responsibility to your employer to weigh the full financial ramifications of your activities. Reconsidering educational programs as cost-revenue centers is one way to fulfill this responsibility.

Educational trimming. Trimming off all the nonessentials and providing only the absolute essentials is a second means of improving the cost-effectiveness of hospital-based educational programs. In general this approach is quite feasible for orientation and in-service programs, which focus on the minimum necessary learning essentials. If your nursing staff is undergoing rapid turnover and has a high proportion of newcomers, the educational emphasis is more properly placed on the minimum essentials necessary for job performance. When most of the nursing staff are thoroughly experienced in their clinical specialty, however, their needs for continued educational development are less likely to be met by a no frills approach. Improved staff retention, morale, clinical advancement, and job satisfaction may warrant educational offerings that extend well beyond the basics.

Contractual agreements. Contractual agreements are used by some hospitals to better assure that the employer's investment in educational offerings is offset by some reciprocal obligations of the program's participants. The purpose of a contractual agreement is to state the conditions under which the program will operate and attendees participate. A clear description of these conditions or terms of the contract specifies the obligations and responsibilities of both the provider and the recipient of the program, so that rights and obligations are mutually observed and understood.

Some elements that can be incorporated into a contractual agreement include the following:

1. Beginning and ending dates of the program
2. Salary provisions and other forms of compensation for the participants
3. The effect of the program, if any, on such employee benefits as vacation time, sick time, health insurance, and seniority
4. Fees charged or conditions under which fees are assessed
5. Conditions under which participants enter, continue, and successfully complete the program
6. Payment for books and supplies used by participants
7. Work agreements incurred by participating in the program: conditions, duration, unit assignment, seniority, shift, and salary
8. Conditions under which participants may be released from or discontinue their participation in the program
9. Differentiation between employee and nonemployee participants in these considerations

Some educational offerings necessitate changes in personnel policies, procedures, salaries, or employee fringe benefits. Your personnel department and legal counsel should be able to offer guidance in preparing contract terms and in verifying the contract's consistency with federal and local labor laws. Nursing and hospital administrators will also need to review and approve these conditions.

Do not be misled into thinking that what appears to be a legitimate contract is in fact a binding agreement. Employing agencies cannot dictate that many unforeseen events such as illness, spouse relocation, and pregnancy will not surface and void even well-formulated agreements. Employment contracts are often more friendly agreements than legally binding documents, and hospitals typically will not pursue the costs of litigation for contract violations. In some instances, however, these quasi-formal written agreements may be useful vehicles to effect some assurances of financial balancing.

Pooled educational resources. Pooling common educational needs into providing multi-sponsored educational offerings is a fourth approach to enhancing educational cost-effectiveness. Rather than each hospital providing comparable educational offerings independently, needs and resources may be merged into joint program sponsorship. Typically, agencies and institutions within the same geographic locale participate as providers and participants in the offering. Hospitals, community colleges, university schools of nursing, and voluntary and private agencies may variously converge in cooperative efforts that result in reduced costs for all.

The collaborative spirit can be extinguished rather readily if numerous groups are involved in a joint endeavor or if the program focus strays from common areas of need. Frequently, only didactic courses are offered in this manner, with each participating agency assuming responsibility for clinical follow-up. Issues of professional liability, hospital liability, and policy are difficult to address from a multi-sponsor perspective and are frequently best relegated to each agency's separate sphere of responsibility and supervision.

MARKETING EDUCATIONAL PROGRAMS

Unless educational programs are mandatory for staff nurses, you will need to advertise and sell them to the intended audience. Brief informal programs may only require posting a notice or relying on word-of-mouth to attract an audience. Longer, costly programs or offerings open to nurses outside your agency may justify a sizable advertising and promotional campaign that assures enough participants to make the program cost-effective.

Knowles divides program marketing into the following four steps:

1. Defining the clientele
2. Planning the promotional campaign
3. Preparing and distributing promotional material
4. Evaluating results

The initial stage of marketing involves analyzing the need for a given program. If the proposed program is sufficiently grounded in an assessment of valid educational needs, the first step in marketing is well under way. The program plan to meet these needs is transformed, in marketing terms, into the product. Just as the scope and depth of the program level were set to meet the needs of a given category of nursing personnel, so marketing the program is also designed to meet the needs of a specific audience or clientele. For purposes of advertising and promoting the program to recruit this audience, the public relations department may request a detailed definition of the intended clientele: their age, sex, marital status, education, work or other relevant experience, economic status, interests, desired attributes, and career goals. The public relations department will be better able to develop promotional materials for the program if you can supply them with this detailed information.

For the public relations department to assist in preparing promotional materials for the program, you will need to set maximum and minimum enrollments, anticipated fees, and necessary time frames.

In addition to using customary promotional media such as posters, notices, and word-of-mouth advertising, you may also wish to consider using the following:

1. Newspaper advertising in your own agency's publications, or in community and regional papers.
2. Press releases to local and regional newspapers
3. Radio and television announcements
4. Advertising in professional journals and publications of professional organizations
5. Direct mail advertising (letters, announcements)
6. Brochures for distribution on inquiry about program
7. Materials used for staff recruitment

The materials chosen for promoting and advertising the program should reflect the primary selling points you wish to communicate to your potential audience. The quality of the program should be highlighted with emphasis on the features that make it unique, timely, and meaningful to the intended participants. If neighboring institutions have offerings similar to yours, you should consider distinguishing your offering to recruit the audience from their programs to yours. Consumers of educational programing will do comparison shopping; being able to attract an audience to your offering is more often a result of an astute business sense than of educational expertise alone. In many ways, hospital-based educational programming could learn a great deal from marketing techniques and selling in the face of competition. The public relations department should be able to help you distill the most valuable aspects of the program into summary form.

Any printed material to be distributed should contain a common core of information that may include the following:

1. Title and objectives of the program
2. The program's sponsor or provider
3. Characteristics of the intended audience
4. Program content and activities
5. Names and qualifications of faculty and providers
6. Date, time, and location of the offering
7. How and when to apply (including any necessary deadlines)
8. Fees and other costs (parking, meals)
9. Telephone contact for further inquiry
10. Continuing education units or accreditations awarded
11. Miscellaneous information such as directions to the facility, parking facilities, provision for meals, telephone numbers for messages, processing and notifying applicants, receipts, and notes on the cancellation of a registration

Artwork, layout design, and lettering of the promotional materials may be provided as a service of the art department or the public relations department or be subcontracted to an outside printer. You will need to review carefully the drafts of these proposed materials to be certain they are accurate and are esthetically appealing to the appropriate audience.

As promotion and advertising of the program begins, the public relations department should also be able to monitor the results of various kinds of advertising. To limit future marketing costs, it is always helpful to know which advertising vehicles were successful and which were not.

GAINING ADMINISTRATIVE APPROVAL: SOME HELPFUL HINTS
Maybe you don't need these hints . . .

Take a moment to peruse the following story. If you can identify closely with it, you need not read the remainder of this section.

Once upon a time, there was a critical care instructor named Sally Supernurse. Sally developed an endless multitude of outstanding and thoroughly effective teaching programs that the critical care nurses demanded admission to. The hospital's administration willingly lavished unlimited financial, clerical, classroom, and personnel support without question. Other departments within the hospital begged to be allowed to participate in the program, and the physician, staff, and patients pleaded that only nurses trained by Sally be responsible for patient care. Scores of critical care nurses from other hospitals in the area sought employment at this hospital just to have the opportunity to participate in this unprecedented educational experience. And everyone, especially Sally, lived happily ever after.

Maybe you do need these hints . . .

The less you and Sally Supernurse have in common, the more you will probably benefit from some administrative savvy you likely did not acquire in your basic or even advanced nursing education program. These are issues central ultimately to realizing your educational proposals rather than lamenting that the "hospital administration doesn't support us."

If you would prefer not having all of your proposed efforts negated by an administrative veto, you must prepare the presentation of your proposal so that it reflects the party you will find on the other side of the negotiating table. Remember that the impact of and response to your proposal will be colored not only by how effectively you communicate your ideas, but also by the frame of reference of those who are listening to what you say.

The yardstick used by the administration to support and evaluate educational programs for nurses may be at variance with your criteria. Unless you can transpose your intentions into the concerns and issues the administration confronts, you may find the administration has little interest in listening to well-intentioned rhetoric. Your sincerity and commitment to an educational project has little to do with your ability to market it effectively to the administration. The hospital administration—especially in these days of cost containment, government and other regulatory controls, litigation and labor disputes—cannot afford to invest in the ethereal. Ivory tower approaches to health care education only work well within such structures. Health care institutions in general and hospitals in particular are not ivory towers.

How can you best present your program proposal to the administration? Although no one can guarantee you a full measure of success in this endeavor, you can take some steps to minimize the risk of failure.

Step 1: appraise your credibility with the hospital administration. Determine what the administration's perceptions are of the value of your work within the hospital organization. Does the administration know you exist? If so, what do they think of staff nursing education and your role in it? You can accomplish this by an honest appraisal of the following factors:

1. The priority given to critical care nursing education programs in the past and present
2. The overall value placed on staff nursing education at your institution
3. Whether staff nursing education is generally viewed as a valuable service that contributes to health care or only as a JCAH requirement or necessary employee fringe benefit

4. Whether the hospital and nursing administration know you exist
5. Your past performance evaluations
6. Your reputation within the hospital

By acquainting yourself with the administration's concept of staff nursing education in general and your performance in particular, you can prepare for one of three possible receptions: adamant resistance, noncommitted toleration, or willingness to listen and consider your ideas. Even if you anticipate a brief encounter with seemingly little interest in listening to you, it is always best to know this ahead of time so you can prepare for it. If your findings are less than encouraging here, you might consider closing the credibility gap before approaching the administration.

Step 2: appraise your credibility with the nursing administration. It is important to know who in the nursing administration you will be meeting with to discuss your proposal. If you will need to depend on the support of successively higher levels of administrators between you and the director of nursing, you will want to be sure they are aware and supportive of your intentions. Because the director of nursing may solicit the opinions of these people to help in judging the proposal, knowing what these individuals need clarified, what they support, object to, and find problematic in the proposal will help to better prepare you to respond to their comments.

At some point you will likely meet with the director of nursing to clarify and promote your ideas. Before this meeting, review the philosophy, goals, and policies of the department of nursing and those of the in-service or staff development department. In your review, identify how your program's goals and objectives assist in fulfilling, in more fully realizing, or in complementing these larger departmental goals. If the statement of your proposal does not make these correlations obvious, you should be able to make them explicit when you confer with the director of nursing. Concern for and loyalty to the organization and its mission are important in attaining departmental credibility. You cannot reasonably expect the administration to support proposals that are self-seeking or not in the best interests of the entry hospital. Find out about other current administrative issues and problems within the nursing department. Try to relate how your proposal positively affects these problems, that is, how it alleviates, minimizes, or resolves these problems.

Be sure the presentation of your proposal reflects your concern and your assumption of the responsibility for both fiscal and administrative matters. Try to point out how your program assists in the following:

1. Stimulating and enhancing job satisfaction, staff morale, and employee motivation.
2. Reducing staff turnover, attrition, and job dissatisfaction
3. Reducing costs involved with orienting graduate nurses, training programs, and high staff attrition and turnover rates
4. Promoting further continuing education
5. Recruiting and retaining qualified staff
6. Resolving staffing problems
7. Fostering improved quality of patient care

The contemporary hospital is a complex business organization besieged by federal, state, regional, and local guidelines and restraints. These regulating bodies form a minutely subspecialized maze where "accountability," "liability," "cost-effectiveness," "balanced budget," and "long-term planning" are the recurring obstacles along the way. Proposing educational programs that do not result in demonstrated effectiveness for some aspect of health care services, that will not likely facilitate administrative, budgetary, or patient care services, or that work to the eventual detriment of other departments within the hospital are bound to encounter a rocky and uphill course in obtaining administrative approval. Such proposals often construct impermeable walls of protest and indignation—not support.

If the director of nursing will intercede with the hospital administrator on your behalf, be certain she clearly understands all details and ramifications of the proposal. Try to evaluate her degree of understanding and support of your intentions. Listen closely to her comments to better understand her perspective. The director of nursing may be able to enlighten you about issues and interdepartmental effects you had not previously identified. Because her frame of reference is more broadly based than yours, she may be able to assist you in addressing those issues and identifying possible alternatives to deal with them.

If you and the director of nursing will jointly approach the hospital administrator with your proposal, try to elicit suggestions from the director of nursing on how this may best be accomplished. Directors of nursing are ordinarily quite familiar with how the hospital administrator usually perceives and reacts to issues raised; this knowledge may prove invaluable to you in structuring the presentation to place it in the most favorable light. The director of nursing may also be helpful in selecting the best time to make the presentation. Knowing how to present your ideas and when the most opportune time to do so is an art cultivated by those with real know-how in administration. Timing often makes the difference in whether the proposal will be seriously considered at all by the hospital administrator.

In preparing to present your proposal to the director of nursing, succinctly summarize:

1. Overall goal of the program
2. A forecast of the advantages of the program to the unit, department, physicians, patients, and the hospital
3. Disadvantages and anticipated problems of the program
4. Alternative courses of action to resolve any identified disadvantages or potential problems
5. Anticipated cost of the program together

with various alternatives for modifying or reducing this cost

6. What attendant costs if any would be off-set or reduced by the program
7. Amount and nature of resources necessitated by the program and any options available here to improve cost-effectiveness
8. How your program is related to the hospital's primary mission
9. Public relations value of the program for the hospital's image to the patient, hospital, and surrounding academic community
10. Intended participants and the duration of the program
11. How you are planning to evaluate the program

If you can prepare for the presentation of your proposal in this manner, your credibility will be greatly enhanced. Insofar as possible, try to convert your ideas into tangible and measurable indications of success that translate into dollars saved or quality provided. You may even find it helpful to translate your proposal into a listing of long-and short-term administrative goals that could be achieved through your ideas. The following illustration will serve to demonstrate how you might accomplish this.

Critical care nursing internship program

GOAL OF THE PROGRAM. The goal of the critical care nursing internship program is to prepare professional nurses with the knowledge, attitudes, and skills deemed essential for competent nursing practice in acute and post-acute patient care settings.

SHORT-TERM ADMINISTRATIVE OBJECTIVES

1. To provide educational benefits to critical care nurses that are competitive with those of adjacent hospitals
2. To provide a sufficiently unique educational program that serves as an incentive for staff nurse recruitment and retention in the critical care units

3. To reduce the attrition rate of critical care nurses that can reasonably be attributed to limited continuing education offerings
4. To facilitate and reduce the time required for developing the clinical competencies of graduate nurses who are to practice in the critical care units
5. To assist newly graduated professional nurses in the transition from students to staff nurses
6. To expand the continuing education offerings currently available for critical care nurses

LONG-TERM ADMINISTRATIVE OBJECTIVES

1. To provide a mechanism for facilitating communication and collaboration among all members of the critical care health care delivery team
2. To provide a more consistent level of preparation and clinical expertise among the critical care nursing staff
3. To develop a more comprehensive and integrated program for the continuing education of critical care nurses
4. To heighten staff awareness of the need actively and continuously to pursue continuing education for maintaining current competence in critical care nursing practice
5. To provide the theory and clinical base necessary to prepare staff nurses to complete successfully the national certifying examination in critical care nursing (CCRN) offered by the AACN Certification Corporation or to pursue a baccalaureate or masters degree in nursing
6. To provide the educational means for improving the quality of nursing care provided for patients in the critical care units
7. To improve the hospital's standards of critical care nursing practice
8. To enhance the public relations and community service image of the hospital

Step 3: "Please knock before entering"

As you ready yourself to approach hospital administrators, strive at being:

1. Clear in your own mind about what you intend to do
2. Capable of expressing your ideas in administrative terminology
3. Business-like in your approach, manner, and dress
4. Straightforward, clear, and organized in your discussions
5. Concerned with issues and facts rather than with a clutter of feelings and innuendos
6. Ready for any possible reaction
7. Reasonable and open to negotiation and renegotiation of issues
8. Organization-minded rather than departmentally myopic
9. Supplied with facts and figures to support your viewpoints

The culmination of your efforts will have a better chance of success if your homework has been thoroughly conceived and completed. In short, do your homework well!

REFERENCES

The administrative perspective

Alspach, J: A critical care nursing internship program: gripping versus griping, Superv Nurs 9:31, 1978.

Bitgood, G: Critical care nurse-intern program, Superv Nurs 7:42, 1976.

Boyer, CM: The answer doesn't always come prepackaged, Nurs Educ 3:17, 1978.

Cohen, HA: The fine art of negotiating, Leadership 1:27, 1980.

Feener, EL: A regional cardiac care program: planning and development, J Nurs Admin 9:27, 1979.

Fiorenza, LA: Area inservice educators unite, J Contin Educ Nurs 8:37, 1977.

Gibbons, LK, and Lewison, D: Nursing internships: a tristate survey and model for evaluation, J Nurs Admin 10:31, 1980.

Haymes, H: Running a CE program: administrative strategies, Nurs Outlook 28:183, 1980.

Hoover, JJ: Record keeping, J Contin Educ Nurs 9:25, 1978.

Lancour, J, and Reinders, AA: A pilot project in continuing education for critical care nursing, J Nurs Admin 5:38, 1975.

Magner, M: Developing and evaluating inservice programs, Superv Nurs 9:10, 1978.

Prescott, PA: Cost-effectiveness: tool or trap? Nurs Outlook 27:722, 1979.

Rosentreter, G: Evaluating training by four economic indices, Adult Educ 29:4, 1979.

Simonds, SK: Quality, accountability, and professional responsibility: new tasks for inservice education directors, J Contin Educ Nurs 6:5, 1975.

Staropoli, CJ, and Waltz, CF: Developing and evaluating programs for health care providers, Philadelphia, 1978, F. A. Davis Co.

Role of program director in continuing education

Marenco, E: Continuing education in nursing as an enterprise, J Contin Educ Nurs 9:16, 1978.

Poole, D: Roles and functions of staff development directors, J Contin Educ Nurs 8:31, 1977.

Popiel, ES: The director of continuing education in perspective. In Popiel, ES, editor: Nursing and the process of continuing education, ed 2, St. Louis, 1977, The C.V. Mosby Co.

Tobin, HM: Staff development: a vital component of continuing education, J Contin Educ Nurs 7:33, 1976.

Woske, M: Role of a hospital based health educator, Crit Care Update 5:28, 1978.

Budget preparation

Becker, SP: How to prove—and report—return on training investment, Training HRD 13:39, 1976.

Coye, C: Budget, J Contin Educ Nurs 8:42, 1977.

Coye, D: Organizational structures: considerations which facilitate effectiveness, J Contin Educ Nurs 8:42, 1977.

del Bueno, DJ: The cost of competency, J Nurs Admin 5:16, 1975.

del Bueno, DJ: How to get your money's worth out of continuing education, RN 41:37, 1978.

del Bueno, DJ, and Kelly, KJ: How cost-effective is your staff development program? Nurs Educ 5:12, 1980.

Donovan, L: Who's going to pay for all that continuing education? RN 41:48, 1978.

How to buy furniture and furnishings that enhance classroom comfort—and learning, Training HRD 17:45, 1980.

Marenco, E: Accounting concepts and techniques for managing continuing education and inservice, Nurs Admin Q 3:75, 1978.

Poole, D: Roles and functions of staff development directors, J Contin Educ Nurs 8:31, 1977.

Popiel, ES: Providing a financial base for continuing education programs. In Popiel, ES, editor: Nursing and the process of staff development, ed 2, St. Louis, 1977, The C.V. Mosby Co.

Porter-O'Grady, T: Financial planning: budgeting for nursing—part II, Superv Nurs **10:**25, 1979.

Prescott, PA: Cost-effectiveness: tool or trap? Nurs Outlook **27:**722, 1979.

Sovie, MD: The role of staff development in hospital cost control, Nurs Educ **5:**25, 1980.

Stevens, BJ: Cost accounting in inservice education, Superv Nurs **6:**23, 1975.

Tobin, H: Process of developing a budget, J Contin Educ Nurs **8:**27, 1977.

Wise, PSY: Preparing budgets for inservice educators, J Contin Educ Nurs **10:**17, 1979.

Continuing education program marketing

Calderon, JR: Marketing your program, J Contin Educ Nurs **9:**12, 1978.

Knowles, MS: The modern practice of adult education, rev ed, New York, 1980, Follett Publishing Co.

Lenz, E: Continuing education goes to market, Adult Leadership **24:**163, 1976.

Chapter 7

Curriculum design for critical care nursing

ORGANIZING THE CURRICULUM

Regardless of the time available for your curriculum, you obviously cannot teach and learners obviously cannot learn everything all at the same time. Some things will have to be learned first, some later, and some at the end. Part of your responsibility as an educator is to decide the order of learning experiences. This process of chronological organization is called sequencing.

How important is the order in which material is presented and learned? At one time or another, each of us has wrestled with a concept we found "impossible to understand." Much later, after discovering the missing links we needed, we finally understood it. For example, nurses who attempt to interpret a patient's arterial blood gas (ABG) results immediately after learning the four categories of acid-base disturbances usually find to their dismay that they still cannot make sense of the values. Until they have first learned prerequisite concepts such as gas tensions, partial pressures, oxygen transport, and the oxyhemoglobin dissociation curve, the ABG results are meaningless numbers. The order in which material is presented and learned, then, is of paramount importance for understanding, integrating, retaining, and transferring learning.

When sequencing is well planned for a particular group of learners, facts and concepts are gradually introduced and related. This creates a comfortable and meaningful flow of learning that provides continuity and integration over time. The effect of appropriate sequencing in a 6-month curriculum is no less significant than it is in a 60-minute class. Learning from a speaker whose presentation is totally disorganized can be virtually impossible, whereas even very complex material can be readily learned if presented in a logical, orderly fashion of concept development—what students usually refer to as "painless learning."

As you attempt to decide on the best order for presenting material, try to remember the following:

1. The optimal sequence pattern is the one that most facilitates learning. No one "right" sequence exists for any curriculum.

2. As the composition and the characteristics of the learner group vary, the composition and the order of the sequence are also likely to vary. A sequence for planning learning experiences must reflect the learner's background, prior education and experience, knowledge, and ability. The same sequence is not applicable to all groups of learners. A meaningful way to learn for one group of learners may not be at all meaningful to another group of learners.

3. The ultimate purpose of sequencing is in its cumulative effect; that is, attaining smaller elements of learning at the appropriate times and in the appropriate sequence forms a meaningful whole that is

reflected in attaining the program objectives.

4. The ability to sequence learning requires that the educator be familiar with both the material to be learned and the characteristics of the intended learners. Unless you understand the material and know what your learners know now and what they need to know in relation to that material, your sequence will likely both begin and end in inappropriate locations.

5. Experience and experimentation with various sequencing patterns provide a wealth of valuable insight into what is best for each particular group of learners.

Armed with a knowledge of the material, the instructional objectives of the program, and an understanding of your particular group of learners, you have the raw materials for deciding how to put the components of the curriculum into the most appropriate sequence.

A wide variety of approaches is available for planning a curriculum sequence. The best sequence is whichever most facilitates meeting the course objectives. Some alternatives available for sequencing include ordering learning on the basis of the following:

1. General to specific
2. Known to unknown
3. Concrete to abstract
4. Simple to complex or complex to simple
5. Facts to principles to the application of each
6. Most important to least important
7. Most interesting to least interesting
8. Part to whole or whole to part
9. Chronological order
10. The inherent and natural logic of the subject matter
11. The established order of steps in a procedure
12. The customary or traditional way of learning the subject

Although the overall sequence typically incorporates one or two major approaches, sequencing is usually determined by using a variable combination of these approaches. Even the approach of presenting the material in "the way it has always been presented" is acceptable and valid if this is truly the approach that most facilitates reaching the instructional objectives.

Nursing has usually followed the medical model when presenting material related to patient care: defining the disorder, pathogenesis, signs and symptoms, medical treatment, and nursing care. The best idea is not to get locked into any approach so rigidly that optimal learning is bypassed in favor of rigid approaches to teaching. Adapt, modify, and be open to new and alternative approaches to sequencing. Experimentation, experience, and learner feedback will help you more closely approximate the best approach. You will know your sequencing is appropriate when learners report that learning complex material was relatively painless and that they can readily infer and deduce practical applications of the material in daily practice.

ALLOTTING INSTRUCTIONAL HOURS

You must allot various amounts of time to specific content components once content areas and behavioral outcomes have been arranged in a meaningful sequence. That the time available for instruction is usually limited must be taken into account in deciding how much time will be devoted to each division and subdivision of the material within the total curriculum.

Just as no magical formula for sequencing the curriculum nor any one "right" sequence exists, no foolproof approach exists to allot instructional time. One guideline to keep in mind is that time is a valuable resource available in a limited supply; it is a resource you will want to use in the most efficient way possible.

One way to approach allotting instructional time is by first considering the total amount of time available for instruction as 100% and then allotting decremental percentages of time to each program objective, based on the priority assigned to it earlier in program planning. The amount of time apportioned to each program objective is then in turn considered as 100% and decremental percentages of this time are assigned to each set of instructional objectives that follow from that program objective.

The usefulness of this approach varies somewhat with the length of the program. In long programs it may be useful only for the initial breakdown of curriculum hours, whereas for short programs it may be entirely adequate. Moderate or long programs usually require that you consider a number of other factors that may influence how instructional time allotments are apportioned. Some of these factors include the following:

1. Total time available for instruction
2. Priority of importance assigned to each objective
3. Specific nature and complexity of objectives
4. Total number of objectives
5. Learners' present knowledge, skills, and experience in relation to the objectives
6. Nature of teaching methods used for instruction
7. Resource availability (facilities, personnel, media)
8. Nature and complexity of subject matter
9. Instructor's experience in teaching this subject matter to comparable audiences
10. Instructor's familiarity with this subject matter

In attempting to allot instructional hours, remember that your purpose is to distribute the time available in a manner most efficient for assisting learners meet the program objectives. Because the teaching-learning process is largely human social interaction, it is not readily amenable to rigid scheduling. Be certain to build in the flexibility necessary for humans to be human.

A final reminder: no matter how exacting your approach to time allotments, you will rarely encounter *the* way to do it. Your own experience in this process will serve you better than a stopwatch or any exacting formulas. All educators miscalculate now and then—just keep your mind and eyes open for necessary adjustments and you will develop a more valid basis for knowing how to proceed.

SELECTING APPROPRIATE INSTRUCTIONAL MEDIA
Rationale for using instructional media

Instructional media such as slides, films, and tape recordings serve a number of useful purposes in the teaching-learning process. Media are generally thought to enhance the effectiveness and retention of learning by recruiting alternative and multiple sensory avenues to receive instruction. If it is true that we can only retain 10% of what we read, 20% of what we hear, and 30% of what we see, whereas we retain 50% of what we both see and hear, 80% of what we say, and 90% of what we say as we do something, then it should be apparent that listening to a lecture or reading a textbook may not be the most efficient mode of learning.

Individuals differ in the pace or rate with which they can learn and in the sensory learning style they prefer: whereas some may learn best by hearing, others may learn more efficiently by seeing or doing what is to be learned.

Media are generally used to complement or supplement other teaching activities. They can be used to stimulate and control learner attention; to introduce creativity, variety, and flexibility in approaches to learning; to provide cues or stimuli for learning; to stimulate recall of previous learning; to allow for repetition, expansion, reinforcement, and new applications of learned material; and to evaluate feedback or the extent of learning.

Considered practically, instructional media allow for greater flexibility and adaptability to time constraints placed on both learners and instructors in hospital-based settings. They offer a pragmatic approach for providing a means of self-instruction for nurses on all shifts. Media can accommodate the limited amount of time that nurses can be away from the bedside or can more effectively use those rare quiet periods when patient care demands are temporarily diminished.

Media offer the flexibility of making instruction available at any hour it would be helpful, needed, or desired and, for many media forms, also make such instruction available in the most desirable location. They potentially offer both static visual and continuous motion illustrations required for learning the complex skills needed by critical care nurses. Audiovisuals may also be useful for illustration while teaching fine auditory or visual skills of discrimination, such as heart sounds, skin color changes, or neurological assessments.

From the instructor's vantage point, using media may provide additional time for expanding on the material covered or for working individually with learners who are encountering learning problems. It can reduce repetition of frequently needed instruction and extend the capabilities of the single instructor for reaching a larger audience. When staff nurses with widely varying capabilities and backgrounds join the critical care staff, the instructor responsible for in-service education can provide a "core course" of essentials to be learned through a multimedia program rather than repeating the same information each month as new staff nurses enter the unit. This gives the instructor more time to reinforce the material, to follow through with its transferred application in the clinical setting, and to validate that the essentials have indeed been learned.

Criteria for evaluating and selecting instructional media

If possible, media should always be previewed before purchase to avoid an outlay of funds for materials later found to be inadequate, unsuitable, or inappropriate for the purposes they were intended. When dealing with audiovisual companies that do not offer free previewing services, renting the material or paying preview charges may prove to be worthwhile.

The primary criterion for judging the usefulness of any media resource is that medium's ability to help meet learning objectives. Predetermined instructional objectives should dictate the appropriate media; learning objectives should not be modified on the basis of what is available in audiovisual support. Media should be selected or rejected on the basis of whether they can be helpful in meeting these predetermined objectives.

A number of other considerations, however, should be taken into account in evaluating media for use or purchase. Some preliminary considerations include determining the following:

1. What media are currently available to you for the content area?
2. What areas most need supplementation by audiovisual media?
3. What hardware will be required to use the media? Is it presently available to you? Is it feasible and cost-effective to make this equipment available? Is the hardware easy to operate and maintain?
4. Could you develop your own media that would more closely meet your needs? Are resources available to accomplish this? What would be the projected cost?
5. What funds are available to you for purchasing commercially prepared media or for media development and design?
6. Would purchasing the media be cost-effective given the frequency of their use, the audience size, and the amount of learning they would provide? Would any cost be incurred by the learners themselves?
7. Are special facilities (studio, auditorium,

soundproof rooms, audiovisual laboratory) or personnel (audiovisual technician, secretary, room monitor, librarian) required to use the media? Would these facilities be readily available to you as needed or have to be obtained for use?

8. Are the media adaptable for both large and small group instruction or individualized instruction? Will they limit instruction to classroom or laboratory use?

9. How familiar are you with the use of the media?

10. With respect to the instructional media themselves, are their contents accurate, up to date, and appropriate to use with these learning objectives? Are they relevant, unbiased, and ethically acceptable?

11. Are any references provided to validate the accuracy of the content?

12. Is the content likely to become obsolete soon?

13. Is the level of instruction appropriate to the intended audience at your institution?

14. Do the media provide the features (visual, motor, auditory) deemed essential for effective instruction in this content?

15. Are the media useful for providing review, overview, reinforcement, evaluation, or supplementation? Do they offer basic or advanced instruction?

16. Will learners need to be able to operate the equipment themselves to optimally use the media? Is this within their present capabilities and time availability?

17. Have these media ever been used for the intended audience before and, if so, with what degree of success?

18. Are the technical features of the media (photography, text, soundtrack, color, clarity, and organization of presentation) of satisfactory quality?

19. How much supplementation by the instructor would be necessary if these media were used? Would their use save instructor time for other teaching responsibilities, clinical follow-up, or expanding content?

20. What other audiences, uses, and applications could benefit from these media?

If using instructional media has a logical place in your educational program, and if you can justify the use or purchase of a given item, you should follow some general guidelines in the actual use of these materials.

Guidelines for using instructional media

Because instructional media may be inappropriately, inadequately, underused or overused, their proper utilization warrants some mention. Especially if they are to be employed for self-paced, independent learning, media resources should be used efficiently and appropriately. The following guidelines will be helpful in assuring their optimal use:

1. Be certain the resources are consistent with and form an integrated part of meeting the predetermined learning objectives.

2. Ensure that the level and scope of instruction provided in the media are compatible with the background, knowledge, and skills of the intended audience.

3. If necessary, demonstrate to learners how to operate and repair the equipment.

4. Prepare the audience or users for the presentation by discussing the purpose, content outline, significance, and objectives of the program before its showing.

5. Anticipate the need for clarification, application, supplementation, or correction before the presentation; provide these as necessary and feasible during and following the presentation.

6. Make every effort to relate concepts and facts from the media's theoretical or hypo-

thetical consideration to their application in your unit, patient population, or to specific patients with whom the audience is acquainted.

7. Give the learners responsibility for actively participating in the learning experience by noting points for them to watch or listen for, noting the purpose of their viewing the media, and noting the accuracy or consistency of the presentation with their own experience.

8. Review and summarize major points made in the presentation with open discussion of areas of disagreement and clarification, and validate the audience's understanding of the material.

9. Provide a period following the presentation for audience and instructor to critique the media—the content, format, pace, accuracy, and technical quality.

Remember that the more complex and sophisticated the media, equipment, and system, the more likely you will need the assistance of audiovisual experts to make the right decisions. You may find individuals with this expertise located at local college or university audiovisual centers, in learning libraries, or in the audiovisual departments of large teaching hospitals.

This section has reviewed the potential value of using instructional media, outlined criteria for evaluating and selecting media, and listed some guidelines for their use. The following section summarizes the characteristics of various categories of media currently available.

Characteristics of instructional media

Audiotapes (reel, cassette, or cartridge)
Usefulness
1. An alternative to printed media; readily available, highly mobile; can stop or advance at any point; can coordinate easily with other media; hardware easy to operate; precludes repetition by instructor; consistency of content in presentation

2. To present brief vignettes for analysis and for learning communication skills
3. Can preserve expert presentations
4. Can use for independent or group study
5. To teach cognitive or affective domains
6. For sharing verbatim programs with those unable to attend
7. For self-evaluation of communication skills
8. Inexpensive; can reuse indefinitely; hardware relatively inexpensive
9. Inexperienced personnel can learn to record and edit with relative ease

Limiting factors
1. Can be boring if lengthy, if use only a single speaker, or if delivered in a monotone
2. Lack of a visual focus often results in audience losing attention
3. May be confining if acoustics or amplification distorts quality
4. May be frustrating or confusing if visuals are not available for illustration, reinforcement, and clarification of content discussed
5. Are often used too long after content becomes obsolete
6. Inappropriate and generally ineffective for teaching most psychomotor skills and procedures
7. Quality of locally produced tapes may vary widely
8. Some sounds (heart sounds, breath sounds) become distorted in recording process—result is product does not sound true or lifelike

Chalkboard (see also markerboard)
Usefulness
1. A familiar medium to most people
2. Readily available
3. Relatively inexpensive
4. Indefinitely reusable
5. Colored chalk can enhance visual effects

6. Can modify information written while teaching

Limiting factors

1. Space limited; only serves as static display
2. Chalk dust may be bothersome; need for frequent erasure
3. Special features such as color or texture will increase cost
4. Visibility may be restricted for some class members
5. Instructor must turn away from students to use
6. Time will be lost while writing data
7. Difficult to teach while writing or erasing
8. Instructor's handwriting may be illegible
9. Instructor may be a poor artist
10. May be distracting with students copying rather than listening

Charts (flipboards, maps, posters, pictures, photographs)

Usefulness

1. Can use professional artwork and illustrations
2. Can alter sequence of presentation
3. Reusable, portable
4. Relatively inexpensive

Limiting factors

1. Restricted visibility with distance from object
2. Require instructor to operate and to teach with
3. May be large, bulky, and difficult to stabilize while using

Film (8 or 16 mm motion picture, reel or cartridge)

Usefulness

1. Particularly useful in teaching skills or procedures that require motion for understanding or in developing observational skills
2. Action can be slowed to demonstrate more clearly sequence of motions to be learned

3. Can teach with visual and auditory sensory avenues reinforced simultaneously
4. Simultaneous use of color, motion, and sound commands attention and stimulates interest
5. May be poignant and effective in teaching affective material and in patient teaching
6. Readily available for rental or purchase with wide variety of subject matter
7. Cartridge easy to use for staff learners, patient, and patient's family
8. More readily adaptable for self-instruction than many other media
9. Can present unique and rare phenomena not commonly observed
10. Versatile for heightened discussion, reinforcement, illustration, or application of learning

Limiting factors

1. Use requires projectionist familiar with troubleshooting equipment; many instructors are limited in ability to operate reel equipment
2. May be difficult to procure when needed if rented
3. Reels usually require darkened room for best viewing; audience often unable to take notes; instructor may be unable to halt film for asking or responding to questions as they arise
4. Sequences may progress too rapidly for audience to integrate new material
5. Subject matter portrayed may become obsolete and updating may not be possible; limited versatility for editing and updating
6. Film breakage disrupts further use of any portion of program
7. Rental and purchase relatively expensive
8. Production requires skilled professionals in media and education, appropriate equipment in setting; is very expensive

Filmstrips (35 mm sequential frames of film, usually with accompanying record or tape narration)

Usefulness

1. Can be used with silent projection, while teacher narrates at each frame, or with sound projection through synchronous record or tape narrations
2. Sequence of frames is always in correct order, reducing instructor preparation time
3. Equipment is easy to use, relatively inexpensive, and portable, with automatic or manual film advances
4. Can convert to slides by mounting individual frames
5. May be produced by relative amateurs
6. Commercially available filmstrips are relatively inexpensive
7. Can produce a filmstrip to visually augment a good audiotape

Limiting factors

1. Film and narration must advance at proper times or audience attention is misdirected toward lack of synchrony
2. Fixed order of frames limits flexibility, versatility, and ability to update, transpose order, or add or delete frames
3. Manual film advance signals (beeping) may be annoying or distracting to audience
4. Film is subject to breakage with handling required for each use
5. May only be available for purchase or preview of only some representative segment of program rather than in its entirety
6. Less useful for patient and family use or for self-instruction because of more complicated equipment and operation

Markerboard

Usefulness

1. Same general features as a chalkboard except that surface is white, melamine, or porcelain

2. Bright, vivid, and erasable marker colors are more eye-catching and visible than powdered chalk
3. Liquid chalk markers are dust free and washable
4. Nonglare surfaces enhance visibility even in sunlit rooms
5. Nonreflecting matte finishes enable using board as projection screen
6. Can be mounted on wall or movable frame, single or double surfaced with magnetic surface feature; available in a variety of sizes

Limiting factors

1. Board and markers are more expensive than standard chalkboard and chalk
2. Board surface requires more care in cleaning and maintenance

Models (simulated replicas of real objects)

Usefulness

1. Provide fuller dimension of reality for learners to manipulate, and to observe how parts are related and function
2. Can provide hands-on simulation for experience and practice in learning procedures and psychomotor skills, especially when repeated practice is necessary
3. Provide three-dimensional illustrations of objects
4. May be scaled to reality for illustration, larger than reality for clarification, or smaller than reality for seeing the whole object
5. Usually portable and infinitely reusable

Limiting factors

1. May be wholly inappropriate for large group use when model is small
2. Need to repeat presentations and explanations as each group views model
3. Frequently lack true feel of real object
4. Often break down
5. Some very fragile
6. May be large and bulky to manipulate and transport

Opaque projector

Usefulness

1. Projects image of flattened objects (usually books or photographs) or small opaque objects for group viewing
2. Magnifies and projects in natural color and appearance of materials
3. Some models have built-in pointers

Limiting factors

1. Limited to use with relatively small, flattened objects a few inches thick
2. Often generate heat quickly, causing distortion of or damage to objects
3. May distort image at periphery of viewing screen
4. Some materials require special mounting for projection
5. Projector is bulky; use usually confined to classroom
6. Requires presence of operator to feed materials onto platen
7. May need to darken room fully for optimal viewing
8. Time is wasted in exchanging materials to be viewed

Overhead projector (images taken from transparent acetate sheets)

Usefulness

1. More dynamic than slides; preserves color features and versatility
2. More readily visible to larger group than chalkboard or models
3. Can limit learner attention to desired amount of information and maintain that attention while adding to as desired and only when desired
4. Can prepare materials ahead of time or during presentation
5. Can heighten impact and reduce time by using multiple overlays and diagrams
6. Relatively inexpensive equipment and materials
7. Easy to produce with felt pen, wax pencil, photocopier, typewriter, or diazo copy
8. Instructor able to maintain face-to-face contact with learners and maintain attention while writing
9. Can preserve materials for reuse or use temporarily and reuse
10. Can use in lighted room
11. Projector easy to operate
12. Professionally prepared transparencies are available commercially

Limiting factors

1. Require instructor's presence
2. Time wasted while changing sheets may be annoying or distracting to audience
3. Instructor may be poor illustrator
4. Necessary to take precautions while handling acetate sheets

Printed materials (books, journals, handouts, reprints)

Usefulness

1. Readily available in virtually all topic areas and incorporates multiple perspectives
2. Learners may refer back to as often as necessary for reinforcement and clarification
3. Most familiar medium of learning
4. Often easy to obtain

Limiting factors

1. Information may be outdated relatively soon or may be incomplete
2. Learners' reading abilities, comprehension, and reading speeds will vary
3. May provide too much or too little information on a given topic
4. Often require verbal supplementation, demonstration, or both
5. Limited ability for learners to retain what is read over time

Slides (2 × 2 inches, 35 mm)

Usefulness

1. Versatile and flexible: can arrange in any sequence; can alter sequence readily, update, and alter for various topics; can

combine locally made slides with those commercially available; can pace to any rate desired

2. Attractive and eye-catching in multicolor or with special effects
3. Readily loaded and stored with minimal maintenance
4. Can remotely control rate of viewing and focusing
5. Can be synchronized with tapes or other recordings
6. Satisfactory slides can be produced even by amateurs after some experience, although they usually lack professional quality
7. Relatively inexpensive to produce or purchase
8. Projector and its attachments are easy to operate

Limiting factors

1. Substantial time may be spent in arranging in sequence and in inserting correctly
2. May be out of order, improperly positioned, or contain too much material
3. May distract audience from listening
4. Usually need to darken room for viewing
5. Slides can be damaged by misuse, exposure to heat, bending, or humidity

Slide-tape (cassette, cartridge, record)

Usefulness

1. Combines usefulness and features of each separate medium into one, overcoming disadvantages of verbal message alone and enhancing effective learning through simultaneous multisensory perception
2. Can be produced by amateurs at nominal costs
3. Readily adaptable for self-paced instruction at any hour and location
4. Can alter, edit, and update either medium without reducing value of the entire program

Limiting factors

1. Must arrange slides in proper sequence

2. Pacing must be well timed
3. Limitations similar to those for filmstrips except for ability to alter and update frames
4. Shares general limitations of audiotapes and individual slides

Television (closed circuit, videotape, videocassette, videodisc)

Usefulness

1. Extremely versatile and sophisticated medium for reaching large audiences in multiple localities simultaneously
2. Can be used to teach both content and skills, to evaluate and test performance and knowledge, and to learn from vignettes, peer teaching, and critiquing performance
3. Equipment can be portable or stationary
4. Relatively easy to use and amenable to self-paced instruction
5. Can preserve and disseminate information presented by experts for viewing by many who would not otherwise have access to it
6. Flexibility of viewing times, individual or group use

Limiting factors

1. Significantly more complex media form
2. Equipment for viewing and production is elaborate and expensive, frequently requiring extensive facility construction
3. The number of programs available for meeting specific needs is limited
4. Production requires expert consultation with educators and technical assistants, and is expensive
5. Most hospitals lack equipment for producing and viewing video programs already commercially available

SELECTING AND MANAGING PROGRAM FACULTY

As soon as the level and scope of a program are defined, the program director should initiate at least a mental search for qualified faculty to teach the behaviors and material desired. Especially in hospital settings, "qualified" is usually equated with the practitioner's professional status in such a way that "good teacher" is assumed to be synonymous with the higher status or position of practitioners. Physicians, assumed to be the most knowledgable and prestigious of professional practitioners, are usually recruited as faculty for all categories of health care personnel. Whereas many physicians are exceedingly good teachers, it remains true both that most professional practitioners lack any formal preparation for the teaching role and that "good practitioner" and "good teacher" are not interchangeable terms.

The criteria for selecting a good instructor should include more than being well versed and current in the subject matter and the practice to be taught. Effective teaching, especially teaching adult learners, requires a number of teacher capabilities judged even more pertinent than these most basic prerequisites. Whereas these traits are surely not the only elements of effective teaching, they are thought to exert some positive and discernible influence on learners and the learning process.

Selecting and securing qualified faculty

Some teacher characteristics are thought to facilitate the learning process. Look for these traits when categorizing a potential teacher as a "good instructor" for adult learners. The following is a list of facilitative traits compiled from personal experience and from the experience of others:

1. Enthusiasm for the subject matter
2. Enthusiasm for teaching
3. Clarity, audibility, and organization of thought and expression
4. Interest, concern, and respect for learners and their experiences
5. Fairness and impartiality toward learners

6. Flexibility and openness to others' opinions and new ideas
7. Sense of humor, friendliness, and permissiveness toward others
8. Ability to admit mistakes and listen to learners
9. Ability to use positive reinforcement and to reward creativity and individuality
10. Understanding and ability to adapt knowledge and expertise to intended audience
11. Facility in correlating theory with practice
12. Principle- and problem-oriented approaches
13. Ability to stimulate learner participation
14. Ability to provide instruction consonant with established objectives
15. Innovative and creative in teaching methods
16. Broadly experienced and formally prepared in the subject matter

Conversely, individuals who exhibit teacher traits thought to inhibit the learning process should be deleted from your resource pool. Some of these undesirable traits have been identified, as follows:

1. Little toleration of disagreement with own views
2. Disinterest in learners
3. Disorganized, inaudible, boring, or too rapid in presentations
4. Discounting or critical of students; talks down to learners
5. Disseminates facts to be memorized
6. "Reads" lecture notes
7. Inability to respond effectively to questions or requests for clarification
8. Marked insecurity, anxiety, and inexperience with teaching role

Many educational programs in nursing use not only classroom instructors, but also clinical instructors. Sometimes the classroom and clinical instructors are the same individuals, but they may function more in one setting than the other. Given preparation and experience, these individuals may be more educator than practitioner, approximately expert as both educator and practitioner, or more practitioner than educator.

When the well-grounded educator is also an expert practitioner, she will likely function very efficiently in the clinical preceptor role. If she is more of an educator than a practitioner, however, she may function far more effectively in the classroom than in the clinical setting. If her primary interest is in learners learning, then the nurse educator's ego must, at times, be willing to accept the notion that someone else may be better able to demonstrate clinical nursing practice. In this instance, a highly competent staff nurse from the critical care unit may function as a clinical preceptor.

A number of benefits can accrue by having a staff nurse participate as a clinical preceptor. These include the following:

1. Adds a differing perspective on nursing practice: how it is and *can be* practiced in addition to how it *should be* practiced
2. Eases the transition of student to nurse or nurse to critical care nurse
3. Adds reality-based dimension to learning that minimizes reality shock and burnout
4. Promotes climate conducive to learning for all staff
5. Actively involves a staff member in educational activities, facilitating better rapport between nursing service and education on the unit
6. Motivates staff members to participate actively in clinical teaching
7. Facilitates learners' identities as staff nurses
8. Provides more effective mechanism for staff nurses to communicate their reactions, evaluations, problems, concerns, and suggestions related to educational activities in the unit

Whether this clinical instructor or preceptor is a full-time clinical educator, clinical specialist, or staff member functioning as a clinical preceptor, a number of traits are highly desirable to seek in potential clinical preceptors, as follows:

1. Is able to orient newcomers to unit, its policies, and its procedures
2. Shows enthusiasm for teaching the art of clinical nursing practice
3. Is readily available and approachable to learners
4. Explains and demonstrates procedures clearly, precisely and adeptly
5. Relates theory to practice
6. Identifies and provides timely, meaningful, and challenging learning experiences
7. Acknowledges progress in skill attainment
8. Differentiates among learners' needs for direction, guidance, and freedom to learn from mistakes
9. Encourages learners to solve problems for themselves
10. Acts as exemplary nurse and professional role model
11. Fosters independence in problem solving
12. Provides constructive and immediate feedback on performance
13. Demonstrates good judgment and sensitivity to both patient needs and learner abilities
14. Has a good working relationship with all members of the health care team

Managing and coordinating program faculty

Communication between educator and program faculty. For the program instructors to be prepared adequately for the role they are to assume, the educator must be prepared to provide them with certain information. Experience suggests that faculty members are more able to fulfill your expectations of them if they know the following beforehand:

1. The topic and major subtopics they are to speak to
2. The specific instructional objectives for that class
3. The time, date, and location of the presentation
4. The composition, number, and characteristics of the audience they are to address
5. The topics already covered and yet to be covered in that unit, module, or course
6. The handouts available for their subject
7. The references or bibliography provided for that subject
8. Any audiovisual material and hardware available
9. How to secure audiovisual equipment or other types of support assistance related to their presentation

Although some of these items may only need to be mentioned verbally, it is usually a better idea to provide faculty with a written letter or form with this information. Especially if you schedule speakers far in advance or use multiple instructional locations, getting the right instructor to appear at the right time in the right place for the right subject can be a major undertaking. Example 7-1 illustrates a sample of such a confirmation notice.

A useful approach to dealing with this logistical problem is to initially schedule over the telephone or through personal conversation, and then follow this with a letter that confirms the information as you recorded it. If necessary, you may wish to have the instructors return signed confirmation notices or cards, indicating their concurrence with and understanding of the information provided.

If you decide to have instructors return confirmation notices, you may also request that they indicate on the confirmation whether they will need any audiovisual equipment or other types of assistance from you. You may then plan accordingly to assure in advance that all support services will be available when needed. Example 7-2 illustrates the type of notice you may wish to use.

Monitoring and evaluating program instructors. Even after expending much effort in selecting only individuals who meet the criteria of a "good instructor," you may later realize your judgment did not serve you well in all instances.

Remember that scheduling other instructors to teach certain topic areas does not necessarily assure the instruction provided was in fact effective. The program director has a responsibility to the learners not only to provide instructors, but also to monitor the effectiveness and quality of instruction they provide.

To verify your selection of instructors, it may be useful for you to attend classes taught by instructors you have never personally observed before. It will not take much listening to determine if the instructor is either very good or very poor. If the class seems to be deteriorating rapidly, getting off on tangents, or not focusing on the target objectives, you may be able subtly to reconstruct, reorganize, or refocus the discussion or fill in the gaps and avoid a total waste of the learners' time.

Even when using instructors with established teaching reputations or those you have observed many times before, intermittent monitoring is a good way to provide for assured quality in your programs and a starting point for clinical follow-through.

If class members will be evaluating instructors, it is courteous to show instructors any evaluation forms used or describe how you will request evaluations of their instruction. Instructors may request knowing the results of learner evaluation; you may provide the results in written or verbal form, as the situation dictates.

Counseling and developing program instructors. A program director's responsibility for monitoring the effectiveness of individual facul-

Example 7-1. Critical care nursing training program

FACULTY CONFIRMATION

This is to confirm your agreement to lecture for approximately 50 RNs enrolled in the Critical Care Nursing Training Program:

Lecturer: _____ Date: _____ Time: _____ AM PM

Major topic(s): _____ Location: _____

Subtopic(s): _____

If you need any audiovisual equipment for your presentation or if you have any questions regarding your participation, please call me at x0000

Attached please find an outline of the major content areas we would like you to cover. If we do not currently have your curriculum vitae on file, please complete the enclosed "Professional Biography" form and return this (or a copy of your own CV) to me. The latter is necessary for our obtaining CEUs for this program.

Before your presentation, the nurses will have already had classes covering: _____

_____

Related areas to be covered in future presentations include: _____

_____

Objectives: At the end of your presentation, the participants should be able to: _____

_____

_____

_____

_____

Copies of the handouts, bibliographies, and reading assignments are attached for your reference. Please complete, sign, and return the "Faculty RSVP form" at your convenience.

Many thanks for your willingness to participate in this program. We appreciate your sharing both your time and expertise with our nursing staff. If you have any suggestions or comments regarding your participation, please convey these to me.

Sincerely,

Grif Alspach, RN, MSN, CCRN
Director, Critical Care Nursing Training Programs

Example 7-2. Critical care nursing training program

FACULTY RSVP FORM

This is to confirm my agreement to provide instruction for registered nurses participating in the Critical Care Training Program:

Assigned topic: _____

Designated time: _____ AM PM

Designated date: _____

Designated location: _____

Signature: _____
(typed name)

Date: _____

I will need the following audiovisual aids for my presentation (check as appropriate):

☐ Carousel projector
☐ Overhead projector
☐ Cassette player
☐ Videocassette player
☐ Videodisc player
☐ Videotape player

☐ Lantern projector
☐ Filmstrip with record player
☐ Filmstrip with cassette player
☐ Chalkboard
☐ Electric pointer
☐ Classroom pointer (wood)

☐ Classroom calipers
☐ Markerboard
☐ Podium
☐ Microphone
  ☐ Remote
  ☐ Stationary

ty members does not end with the monitoring process. Besides evaluating the instruction provided in various learning settings, the program director should be somewhat accountable for counseling and developing program instructors. Furthering the development of course instructors is important for two reasons. First, this instructor guidance should produce a larger cadre of proficient teachers for the program director to draw on. Second, instructor counseling should ultimately improve learners' abilities to meet program objectives.

To further the development of program instructors, you need to identify both the strengths and the weaknesses each brings to the teaching role. You need to be aware of the strengths to reinforce them. You need to be aware of the weaknesses to improve them. Few instructors are so expert that they cannot improve in at least some aspects of their teaching role. Even professionals who have taught for many years could more finely tune their capabilities. Especially if you employ staff nurses as clinical preceptors or as classroom instructors, your ability to assist in their development as teachers is important for the program's overall success. The more you can assist these individuals in fulfilling their teaching roles, the more effective their teaching is likely to be.

The process used to develop instructors and preceptors should be a systematic and balanced effort that maximizes strengths and minimizes weaknesses in the educational process. A positive feedback system that reinforces effective teaching and offers suggestions for improvement, or that corrects ineffective teaching usually produces the best results. The need for a balanced approach toward evaluating instructors and clinical preceptors is perhaps less often acknowledged. On the basis of hearsay, you may decide an instructor is very good or very poor and fail to distinguish your impressions more finely. This is not fair to either the learners or the instructors.

Reinforcing effective teaching is a relatively easy task. Well-seasoned instructors are sensitive to the feedback cues learners give when they are successful in integrating learned material. Your compliments and expressions of gratitude will confirm the adequacy of an instructor's instructional methods and approaches. This is typically a pleasant circumstance for the learners, instructors, and program director.

Correcting or minimizing deficiencies in instructor performance can be a fairly easy or a fairly awesome task. Depending on the nature and extent of instructional weaknesses and the availability of other competent faculty, you may need to pay nominal or extensive attention to this problem. Because correcting ineffective teaching is difficult to accomplish, this section focuses on teaching areas that commonly need improvement in neophyte instructors, and offers some approaches for you to use in eliciting these improvements. Only counseling instructors for classroom and clinical learning settings is considered here. Skillful teaching in the laboratory setting primarily involves the effective use of simulation, instructional media, and other teaching methods discussed elsewhere.

Problems in instructor performance emanate from shortcomings in either preparing for or providing instruction. Once a teaching deficiency can be defined and then related to one of these two areas, the approaches necessary to resolve this deficit become more clearly apparent. After identifying an instructor's teaching strengths, devote an equal amount of attention to identifying weaker areas. For each instructional area needing improvement, formulate a plan on how you might be able to assist the instructor's development. The following outline offers some areas for you to consider and suggests ways in which you may be able to augment the teaching prowess of classroom or clinical instructors.

Classroom instruction

A. Preparation for instruction: areas in need of improvement

1. *Variation in teaching method*
   Suggested approaches for improving: Locate media and other instructional aids that would enhance presentation. Describe alternative teaching methods appropriate for content and setting. Provide guidance and demonstration in using alternative teaching methods, emphasizing advantages and disadvantages of each.

2. *Expertise and preparation in content area (general comprehension, currency of information)*
   Suggested approaches for improving: Direct instructor to available learning resources such as references, self-instructional materials, or bibliography. If knowledge or skills are lacking in a limited area, provided supplementary tutoring as needed and feasible.

3. *Use of appropriate level of instruction*
   Suggested approaches for improving: Provide faculty with descriptions of what audience has already mastered in knowledge, skills, and related topics previously presented. Share any required or suggested readings, assignments, or other forms of information that indicate what the appropriate level of instruction should be. Describe to instructor audience characteristics that specify the participants' present cognitive, affective, and psychomotor competencies relative to the topic area. Suggest questions (direct or rhetorical) or cues the instructor might use spontaneously to adapt the level of instruction as deemed necessary. For nonnurse instructors, delineate the scope and nature of the content usually covered in basic nursing programs. Suggest careful review of instructional objectives as indicators of the appropriate instructional level.

4. *Organization of presentation*
   Suggested approaches for improving: Provide or strongly suggest using a content outline to guide instructional flow and direction for both instructor and audience. For neophyte instructors, be certain they comprehend how concepts are related to one another in some logical fashion. Assist instructor in identifying an organizing system that would be appropriate by use of practice worksheets.

5. *Clarity in presentation*
   Suggested approaches for improving: Verify that the instructor's level of instruction and understanding of concepts are adequate. Assist instructor in attempting to conceptualize and to explain major concepts in alternative ways that more lucidly describe and illustrate the concept. Guide instructor in citing concrete illustrations and applications of abstract ideas that the audience will find meaningful. Provide practice for the instructor in restating explanations, locating examples, and reformulating alternative explanations for key concepts. Use simulated situations, videotaping, or role-playing to achieve greater proficiency. Emphasize objectives to be attained and how major points relate to these.

6. *Consistency between learning objectives and presented learning experiences. Failure to relate learning experiences to instructional objectives.*
   Suggested approaches for improving: Provide faculty with copies of instructional objectives and evaluation tools to reinforce how each class segment coincides with evaluation items and course goals. Assist instructor in process of correlating method and content of presentation with specific learning objectives. Guide instructor in decisions related to selecting appropriate teaching methods and instructional materials. Provide practice in these determinations through written simulation worksheets and verbal reinforcement.

7. *Ability to adhere to time restrictions; pacing of presentation*
   Suggested approaches for improving: Review content depth and scope for feasibility of coverage within stated amount of time. Suggest ways to apportion time allotments in content outline based on the complexity and importance of various concepts. Might suggest marking specific time segments for each subtopic or using markers in notes to signal time limits. Supply room clocks that face instructor or stopwatch at podium. When confirming plans with faculty, be certain to define total amounts of available instructional time.

8. *Ability to emphasize major points*

Suggested approaches for improving: Points of emphasis can be highlighted in notes, written on chalkboard or other media, and summarized in separate handout. Verify that instructor can identify accurately major points as they are portrayed in instructional objectives and evaluation items. Might suggest instructor prepare subtopic summaries and succinct overall summary for presentation ending.

9. *Correlating theory to clinical practice*
   Suggested approaches for improving: Emphasize necessity for relating abstract concepts and scientific principles to bedside patient care. Guide instructor in identifying correlates in nursing practice for all major concepts to be presented. Review principles of adult education related to meaningfulness and immediacy of application to work setting. Provide practice in illustrating theoretical or scientific notions to everyday practice situations with written simulations and practice worksheets.

10. *Learning environment*
    Suggested approaches for improving: Review various aspects of environment that should be readied before class (i.e., seating, lighting, equipment, media software, room temperature) so that needless interruptions and delays are avoided.

B. Providing instruction: areas in need of improvement

1. *Technical qualities of verbal presentations*
   Suggested approaches for improving: Try role-playing in deficient area, with instructor assuming role of audience. Assist instructor in gaining insight into how vocal qualities and visibility of instructor affect communication with participants. Offer suggestions on how better to project voice, vary modulation, improve enunciation, and enhance visibility as appropriate. May use videotape or simulations to reinforce alternative approaches and to improve or diminish distracting habits or mannerisms.

2. *Ability to motivate learning and learner participation*
   Suggested approaches for improving: Briefly review principles of adult education if these appear to be neglected. Might suggest introducing class with a clinical situation or problem that learners can closely relate content to while developing the presentation as a strategy for problem solving. Assist instructor in retaining practice-oriented focus throughout presentation. Assist instructor in formulating review points, case studies, and questions that generate class participation. Guide instructor in how to differentiate among various sources for nonparticipation such as boredom, preoccupation, fatigue, inappropriate instructional level, or inability to relate content to practice.

3. *Instructional atmosphere*
   Suggested approaches for improving: Create a classroom atmosphere that facilitates openness and participation by audience. Role-play or simulate problem area so instructor can experience its effects and cite approaches toward resolving these. Suggest ways to elicit and manage frank discussions on controversial issues and how to respond to challenges and questions without becoming defensive, dogmatic, or intimidating.

4. *Providing positive reinforcement to learners*
   Suggested approaches for improving: Inquire about instructor's experiences in gaining motivation and positive feedback on past performance. Suggest how various techniques can be used to further enhance learning process. Design written worksheets that require instructor to formulate positive and facilitative responses to a full spectrum of learner comments. Review these and offer appropriate alternative reinforcements.

5. *Ability to demonstrate a sense of humor appropriate to the situation*
   Suggested approaches for improving: Emphasize importance a therapeutic sense of humor plays in human affairs and how this is especially important in adult learning situations. Demonstrate how humorous incidents and anecdotes can be used to reinforce learning and make adult learning more meaningful. Attempt to have instructors relate examples of this from their own past experience and suggest ways humor can be used to enliven even relatively dry content.

Clinical instruction

A. Preparation for instruction: areas in need of improvement

1. *Quality of performance as role model*
Suggested approaches for improving: Distinguish between instructor's deficits in knowing how to perform and faulty demonstration. Review performance elements or demonstration techniques as warranted. In either case, verify instructor's recognition of critical procedural elements to emphasize together with elements essential to teaching practice skills. Practice in learning laboratory until instructor's proficiency is maximized.

2. *Ability to demonstrate concepts and principles underlying nursing practice*
Suggested approaches for improving: Determine if instructor can readily identify principles of specific nursing practices; if not, review these with instructor. Explore various means by which principles could be illustrated and made meaningful to learners in patient care situations instructor may encounter. Verify that instructor can portray each accurately and can describe these succinctly for learners. Role-play with instructor until this can be readily performed.

3. *Providing meaningful and relevant learning experiences for participants*
Suggested approaches for improving: Review learning objectives for clinical area with instructor and have instructor prepare outline of approaches used to meet these objectives for each cinical session. If necessary, set aside brief conference time at beginning of each clinical session to reemphasize objectives serving as focus for that session. Work collaboratively with instructor in practicing how to translate instructional objectives into appropriate patient assignments. Written simulations can also be used. Demonstrate how instructor conveys these same instructional objectives to learners so learners understand how their patient assignments will serve as learning experiences and as means for evaluating attainment of objectives. Assist instructor in conducting group conferences that highlight and underscore how objectives can be reached in various patient care situations.

4. *Equitable availability of instructor to learners*
Suggested approaches for improving: Emphasize importance of preceptor availability to learners. Inquire about how instructor provides for availability and discuss effectiveness of these mechanisms. May be helpful to have instructor prepare a schedule for time allocated to each learner based on a realistic appraisal of total time available and the instructor to learner ratio. Suggest alternative means for efficiently using time and emphasize importance of quality rather than quantity of apportioned time. Provide practice for instructor in how to manage extraneous, time-consuming distractions and how to manipulate learning situations to derive the greatest amount of learning in the shortest amounts of time.

5. *Structuring the learning environment*
Suggested approaches for improving: Demonstrate for instructor how to minimize distracting and irrelevant elements of the learning environment that disrupt, interrupt, or blur the learning focus. Provide role-playing situations where instructor can practice how to reduce or eliminate extraneous noise, personnel, and other situational variables so that the goals of clinical learning experiences are not diminished. Practice in this skill should be provided until instructor can perform with proficiency and tact. Videotaping actual performances over time may be useful in refining this ability.

6. *Ability to use effectively spontaneous learning situations*
Suggested approaches for improving: Elicit instructor's past experience in deriving learning benefits from everyday clinical situations. Emphasize immediate relevance of these learning situations and how this relates to principles of adult learning. Assist instructor in identifying common occurrences of incidental learning typical of critical care and in tentatively planning to take advantage of these when they next occur.

7. *Consistency in evaluating learner performance*
Suggested approaches for improving: Ask

instructor to identify potential pitfalls in subjectively evaluating clinical performance.
Might assist instructor in developing criteria
for clinical performance evaluations that
denote critical versus nonessential performance elements. Emphasize benefits of such
a tool for learning and evaluating competent
performance.

8. *Using attainable and reasonable expectations
   in judging learner performance*
   Suggested approaches for improving: If learner group is fairly homogeneous in capabilities,
   review appropriate expectations for the group
   with the instructor. If learner group is quite
   heterogeneous in capabilities, review appropriate expectations of individuals instructor is
   responsible for supervising. Assist instructor
   in identifying various levels of competency
   ranging from the minimum competencies of a
   beginning practitioner to the maximum competencies of an experienced nurse. Provide
   practice for instructor in determining and
   adjusting the appropriate level of evaluative
   expectations through written, verbal, or
   filmed simulations.

9. *Reinforcement and transfer of classroom
   learning to clinical situations*
   Suggested approaches for improving: Share
   copies of classroom instructional objectives
   and content outlines with clinical instructors.
   Review these and provide fuller explanations
   of concepts and principles suitable for transfer
   to clinical practice. If program is long, assist
   instructor in planning an orderly sequence of
   clinical reinforcement that coincides with the
   classroom material. Demonstrate how to provide for natural transfer of learning in common patient care situations.

10. *Providing clear, succinct instructions to guide
    learner performance*
    Suggested approaches for improving: Verify
    that instructor is well versed in procedural
    details of nursing practice. Provide practice
    through verbal simulations or role-playing in
    formulating concise directives and guidance
    for learners. Could have instructor judge the
    relative helpfulness of various instructor
    explanations appearing as alternative re-

sponses in written simulations, indicating
which response is most helpful and why.

B. Providing instruction
   1. *Instructor-learner rapport*
      Suggested approaches for improving: Exam-
      ine how instructor views relationship with
      learners. Determine if relationship is peda-
      gogical (teacher is source of all knowledge) or
      "andragogical" (facilitator of fellow adult
      learners) and explore learner responses to
      each of these. Describe how to work with
      learners as other adults who have valuable
      life and professional perspectives to offer in
      learning situations. Demonstrate for
      and assist instructor in using principles of
      adult education when working with learn-
      ers and in avoiding dogmatic and rigid ap-
      proaches.

   2. *Promoting independence and autonomy in
      clinical decision making*
      Suggested approaches for improving: Assist
      instructor in identifying clinical situations
      that provide opportunities for learners to
      exercise decision-making skills. Have instruc-
      tor describe learning benefits derived from
      facilitating independence versus interceding
      on behalf of learner. Role-playing may be use-
      ful in having instructor learn hands-off
      approaches to guiding learning process rather
      than hands-on doing for learners. Have
      instructor cite examples of patient situations
      when this is the appropriate teaching meth-
      od.

   3. *Direct intervention when patient situation
      warrants*
      Suggested approaches for improving: Have
      instructor differentiate between situations
      warranting direct and immediate intervention
      by instructor and those when indirectly facil-
      itating learning is feasible. Verify that instruc-
      tor is very clear in criteria wherein direct
      intervention is necessary and how to accom-
      plish this without compromising learners'
      self-confidence.

   4. *Frequency and nature of feedback on learner
      performance*
      Suggested approaches for improving: Review
      with instructor the various forms of feedback

and how learners typically respond to each. Provide written or verbal simulations for instructors to formulate appropriate responses to and obtain practice in offering constructive feedback on learners' deficient performance. Collaboratively assist instructor in determining how frequent evaluations of learner performance should be. Assist instructor in preparing a schedule for planned evaluations that may be supplemented by spontaneous feedback.

PREPARING CLASS SCHEDULES

The final phase in curriculum design is the practical outcome of all preceding phases. A class schedule reflects the established instructional and program objectives set into a timely and orderly sequence of planned instructional activities. Class schedules may also incorporate the faculty who will provide the instruction and the instructional media that will supplement the presentations (see Appendix B).

In formal academic settings, the class schedule is incorporated into a course or program syllabus that includes a course description, an outline of course content, specific dates, times, and locations of various learning experiences (classes, clinical, laboratory experiences) and perhaps an enumeration of due dates for assignments, required and suggested bibliography, and evaluation periods.

Even if your program is only a few hours long and certainly if it spans many weeks or months, you and the program participants will find it helpful when both the instructors and the learners are mutually informed about how the teaching-learning process will proceed. Participants will find the class schedule useful in organizing their preparation and work time, in seeing when the objectives will be attained and when the assignments will be retrieved. A clearly delineated class schedule informs faculty and participants of the right place to be at the right time for the right class. Instructors responsible for providing these learning experiences will find the schedule useful in the final planning of all facets of obtaining resources and arranging learning experiences.

The amount of information that needs to appear on a class schedule should be dictated by what is necessary and most helpful for both instructors and participants. Overly detailed schedules are often more confusing than helpful, whereas those with inadequate detail fail to provide direction to either instructors or learners. Think of the class schedule as a map with the established learning objectives as your final destination. Include in it only what is most useful and necessary for everyone to know to get from the learners' present situation to where they need to be at the end of the unit, course, or program.

First devise a rough draft of your class schedule. Before the rough draft can be transformed into a final draft for distribution, it needs to meet the following necessary criteria:

1. Validity and clarity: plans learning activities that directly reflect learning objectives

2. Intelligibility: anyone reading it can easily understand it

3. Feasibility: faculty are confirmed for times scheduled; media, facilities, and other resources are reserved and available; time allotments are realistic; flexibility is evident in scheduling

4. Continuity: flow and sequence of learning activities, assignments, and evaluation sessions are in proper order

5. Utility: both instructors and learners find it useful as a map of planned learning activities

6. Variety: learning experiences and teaching methods and approaches are not sustained for prolonged periods, but vary to promote interest, attention, and continued motivation; variety of learning experiences are incorporated over time

Appendix B (Sample Class Schedule) illustrates how these criteria may be incorporated into a published class schedule.

Curriculum design is not a mystical process. If anything, it is a rather methodical art form that blends and matches desired and necessary instruction with the resources available for providing it. It is more nearly a logical outflow of the objectives established for instruction together with the learners' present capabilities in relation to these objectives. When designed well, a curriculum is successful in bringing to fruition the planned learning activities necessary for participants to meet the program's objectives. As such, it is rooted in the reality of what can be provided in relation to what is desired and available. Curriculum design, in short, makes instruction operable. Actualizing these plans is the subject of the next chapter.

REFERENCES
Curriculum organization

Knopke, HJ, and Diekelmann, N.: Approaches to teaching in the health sciences, Reading, Mass., 1978, Addison-Wesley Publishing Co.

Packer, J: Curriculum consistency, JNE 18:47, 1979.

Posner, GJ, and Strike, KA: A categorization scheme for principles of sequencing content, Rev Educ Res 46:665, 1976.

Selecting and using instructional media

Bell, DL, and Bell, DF: The medium helps the message, CE Focus 3:3, 1980.

Blactchley, M: Media center: it's great, but, JNE 17:24, 1978.

Brown, JW, Lewis, RB, and Harcleroad, FF: AV instruction: technology, media, and methods, ed 5, New York, 1977, McGraw-Hill Book Co.

Coburn, E: Developing or expanding a multimedia instructional program for continuing education for nurses. In Popiel, ES, editor. Nursing and the process of continuing education, ed 2, St. Louis, 1977, The C.V. Mosby Co.

Davis, LL, and Hayes, WS: Media for an integrated nursing curriculum, JNE 16:12, 1977.

Koch, H: The instructional media: an overview, Nurs Outlook 23:29, 1975.

Lange, CM: Availability and cost of media, Nurs Outlook 25:164, 1977.

Lange, CM: Determining cognitive styles, Nurs Outook 24:734, 1976.

Lange, CM: Developing low-cost teaching materials, Nurs Outlook 24:614, 1976.

Lange, CM: Matching media to learning styles, Nurs Outlook 25:18, 1977.

Lange, CM: Media and learning styles, Nurs Outlook 24:672, 1976.

National Medical Audiovisual Center: Catalogue of audiovisuals for the health scientist, Bethesda, Md., 1980, US Department of Health and Human Services.

Olson, GR: The instructional media service framework: a user-oriented organizational structure for instructional media operations, JNE 16:36, 1977.

Peters, JM, and Ulmer, C: How to make successful use of the learning laboratory, Englewood Cliffs, N.J., 1972, Prentice-Hall, Inc.

Podratz, RO: Audio-visual project: an alternative learning experience in pediatrics, JNE 15:33, 1976.

Price, AW: The effective use of the multimedia approach in staff development. In Popiel, ES, editor: Nursing and the process of continuing education, ed 2, St. Louis, 1977, The C.V. Mosby Co.

Sherer, BK, and Thompson, MA: The process of developing a learning center in an acute care setting, J Contin Educ Nurs 9:36, 1978.

Skalnik, RJ: Emphasizing audio/visuals, Life Support Nursing 2:40, 1979.

Sparks, SM, and Kudrick, LW: Avline: An audiovisual information retrieval system, JNE 18:47, 1979.

Sparks, SM, and Mitchell, G: National medical audiovisual center, JNE 17:29, 1978.

Wittich, WA: Instructional technology: its nature and use, ed 6, New York, 1979, Harper and Row, Inc.

Overhead projectors and transparencies

Cooper, SS: Methods of teaching—revisited: the overhead projector, J Contin Educ Nurs 11:56, 1980.

Reed, S: The overhead projector and transparencies, JNE 7:9, 1968.

Smith, J: Choosing and using transparencies and overhead projectors, Training HRD 17:35, 1980.

Telephone teaching

Cooper, SS: Teaching by telephone, Nurs Educ 4:10, 1979.

Lutze, RS: The telephone as a teaching medium, J Contin Educ Nurs 11:58, 1980.

Rost, MA, Barber, GM, and Frank, T: Evaluation of Maine's telelecture continuing education program: part I, J Contin Educ Nurs 12:34, 1981.

Videotapes

Cooper, SS: Methods of teaching—revisited: films and videotapes, J Contin Educ Nurs 12:34, 1981.

Fenn, J, and Fassel, B: Research in critical care education:

production of videotapes for in-hospital use, Heart Lung **8**:313, 1979.

Holland, JAS: Videotaping clinical experience, Nurs Outlook **25**:337, 1977.

Rynerson, BC: Using videotapes to teach therapeutic interaction, Nurs Educ **5**:10, 1980.

Shaffer, MK, and Pfeiffer, IL: Videotape as a method for staff development of nurses, J Contin Educ Nurs **9**:19, 1978.

Shaffer, MK, and Pfeiffer, IL: You too can prepare videotapes for instruction, JNE **19**:23, 1980.

Slomka, S: Want more effective video-based training? Try writing media specs, Training HRD **16**:58, 1979.

Valentine, NM, and Saito, Y: Videotaping as a viable teaching strategy in nursing education, Nurse Educ **5**:8, 1980.

Vogt, RB: Enhancing students' experience through the use of tape recording, JNE **19**:51, 1980.

Television

Falotico, JB: Staff development via television, Nurs Educ **5**:21, 1980.

Memmer, MK: Television replay: a tool for students to learn to evaluate their own proficiency in using sterile technique, JNE **18**:35, 1979.

O'Conner, RJJ: Evaluation of an interactive instructional television program in Hansen's Disease, J Contin Educ Nurs **11**:47, 1980.

Shaffer, MK, and Pfeiffer, IL: Television can improve instruction, JNE **15**:3, 1976.

Audiotapes: speech compression

Evans, AD, Ullom-Morse, AT, and Engle, CM: Speech compression: options for speeding nursing education, JNE **19**:20, 1980.

Smith, J: Speech compression units cut training time and fatigue and boost learning, Training HRD **17**:14, 1980.

Slides

Cooper, SS: Methods of teaching—revisited: slides and slide-sound presentations, J Contin Educ Nurs **11**:52, 1980.

Forsyth, DM: Assisting in the development of a slide tape: a learning experience, JNE **19**:42, 1980.

Computer-assisted instruction

Bitzer, M: Clinical nursing instruction via the PLATO simulated laboratory, Nurs Res **15**:144, 1966.

Bitzer, MD, and Boudreaux, MC: Using a computer to teach nursing, Nurs Forum **8**:234, 1969.

Buchholz, LM: Computer-assisted instruction for the self-directed professional learner? J Contin Educ Nurs **10**:12, 1979.

Collart, M: Computer assisted instruction and the teaching learning process, Nurs Outlook **21**:527, 1973.

Davis, JH, and Williams, DD: Learning for mastery: individualized testing through computer-managed evaluation, Nurs Educ **5**:9, 1980.

de Tornyay, R: Strategies for teaching nursing, New York, 1971, John Wiley and Sons.

Dyer, CA: Preparing for computer assisted instruction, Englewood Cliffs, N.J., 1972, Educational Technology Publications.

Frantz, RF: Computers in nursing education: implications for the future, Image **8**:23, 1976.

Hoffer, EP, et al: Use of computer-aided instruction in graduate nursing education: a controlled trial, J Emer Nurs **1**:27, 1975.

Huckabay, L, et al: Cognitive, affective, and transfer of learning consequences of computer-assisted instruction, Nurs Res **28**:228, 1979.

Kirchoff, K, and Holzermer, W: Student learning and a computer-assisted instructional program, JNE **18**:22, 1979.

Levine, D, and Weimer, E: Let the computer teach it, Am J Nurs **75**:1300, 1975.

Meadows, LS: Nursing education in crisis: a computer alternative, JNE **16**:13, 1977.

Nievergelt, J: A pragmatic introduction to courseware design, Computer **13**:7, 1980.

Olivieri, P, and Sweeney, MA: Evaluation of clinical learning: by computer, Nurs Educ **5**:26, 1980.

Porter, SF: Application of computer-assisted instruction to continuing education in nursing, J Contin Educ Nurs **9**:5, 1978.

Rees, RL: Understanding computers, J Nurs Admin **8**:4, 1978.

Stolurow, LM, Peterson, TI, and Cunningham, AM, editors: Computer assisted instruction in the health professions, Newburyport, Mass., 1970, Entelek.

Sugarman, R: A second chance for computer-aided instruction, Spectrum **15**:29, 1978.

Sumida, SW: A computerized test for clinical decision making, Nurs Outlook **20**:458, 1972.

Valish, AU, and Boyd, NJ: The role of computer assisted instruction in continuing education of registered nurses: an experimental study, J Contin Educ Nurs **6**:13, 1975.

Ward, JA, and Griffin, JM: Improving instruction through computer–graded examinations, Nurs Outlook **25**:525, 1977.

Managing program faculty

Feldman, KA: Grades and college students' evaluations of their courses and teachers, Res Higher Educ **4**:60, 1976.

Fry, MS: An analysis of the role of a nurse-educator, JNE **14**:5, 1975.

Ketefian, S: A paradigm for faculty evaluation, Nurs Outlook **25**:718, 1977.

Knowles, MS: The modern practice of adult education, rev.

ed., New York, 1980, Follett Publishing Co.

National League for Nursing: Concepts and components of effective teaching, New York, 1978, National League for Nursing.

National League for Nursing: Evaluation of teaching effectiveness, New York, 1977, National League for Nursing.

Niemi, JA, and Davison, CV: The adult basic education teacher: a model in the analysis of training. In Popiel, ES, editor: Nursing and the process of continuing education, ed 2, St. Louis, 1977, The C.V. Mosby Co.

Norman, EM, and Haumann, L: A model for judging teaching effectiveness, Nurs Educ 3:29, 1978.

Page, S, and Loeper, J: Peer review of the nurse educator, JNE 17:21, 1978.

Stuebbe, B: Student and faculty perspective on the role of a nursing instructor, JNE 19:4, 1980.

IMPLEMENTATION

Chapter 8

Principles of curriculum implementation

ATTENDING TO SOME GUIDING PRINCIPLES

Designing a curriculum and actually providing the learning experiences are two distinct processes. An exemplary program design does not guarantee that the program will be of comparable quality. To increase the likelihood that the program is as good as its design, keep some guiding principles in mind: general principles of the teaching-learning process and of the principles of adult education. The more you teach the more you will recognize the truism that problems encountered in the teaching-learning process are typically caused by violating one or more of these principles.

PRINCIPLES OF THE TEACHING-LEARNING PROCESS

As you prepare to participate in the teaching-learning process, remember that your primary mission as an educator is to facilitate learning. Teaching is only a means to this end; it is neither *an* end nor *the* end in itself. Teaching activities are valid, effective, and successful only to the extent that they contribute to learning. If you can keep your sight focused on learning, your teaching activities are not likely to waver too far off course.

Certain principles of learning constitute the mainstay of the teaching-learning process. Regardless of your setting, clientele, or content area, these principles hold true and provide direction for all major facets of curriculum implementation.

The following section delineates these generally accepted principles of learning and describes their implications for the teaching-learning process.

Learning is a self activity of the learner

Even high-quality teaching does not assure that learning will occur. The learner's willingness to attend, listen, reflect, recall, associate, visualize, memorize, reason, judge, and assimilate what is to be learned will determine the amount and extent of learning. Unless the learner is willing and able to engage in these activities, there will be no learning. The learner who invests energy toward learning is likely to learn more, to learn faster, and to better retain what is learned.

As an instructor, you must recognize that to learn the learner must actively participate in the teaching-learning process. Your responsibility as an educator includes eliciting and incorporating learners' participation in determining instructional objectives, planning and organizing learning activities, implementing these activities, and evaluating their success in meeting the program objectives. Reminding learners of their responsibility in the teaching-learning process and providing opportunities for their participation at various points in the program will assist in transforming passive listeners into active participants in the teaching-learning process.

Learning is intentional

Learning is intentional, not passive or accidental. The extent of learning is determined by learners' perceptions of their own unique learning needs. Learning is, therefore, a purposive goal-directed activity of learners, aimed at meeting learners' perceived needs for learning.

Learning is most effective when directed toward goals learners can personally identify with; that is, toward goals they perceive as meaningful and worthwhile. Without a knowledge of and a sharing in these goals, little energy will be expended in learning activities to meet them. The goals for learning may originate with learners or be acquired by them, but energies invested toward reaching the goals are always both active and willed. Unless learners already want to learn or unless you can catalyze this desire, they will not learn.

To enlist the active participation of learners, you need to consider learners' goals in relation to the program objectives and determine the degree of concordance between them. You can facilitate learners' intentions to learn by indicating the value of the material to the learners' present or future situation. Explaining the overall purpose of the course, the terminal objectives, and what will be expected of learners assists in clarifying goals so they know what they are striving for.

The teacher's responsibility is to promote learners' intentions to learn by making learning tasks meaningful, by supplementing or providing learners with the knowledge, skills, or attitudes required for learning, and by providing the resources necessary for learners to achieve their intended aims.

Unless learners intend to learn, no amount of coercion will produce the desired result. Requiring adults to attend mandatory classes often alienates their interest and obviates the likelihood that they will learn.

Learning is an active and interactive process

If learning requires active participation and a desire to learn, then the degree to which learners participate in learning experiences will largely determine what and how much they learn. Learning is dynamic; it does not take place without the activity of the learner. Dewey's maxim that "we learn by doing" underscores the importance of actively involving the learner in the learning experience.

Learning experiences such as simulation exercises or return demonstration of techniques provide a proportionally greater amount of interaction in the learning experience and increase the probability that learning will be effective. Learning experiences that are primarily passive such as the lecture usually minimize the extent of learner interaction in the learning experience. Providing experiences in applying what is learned or, better yet, setting up learning experiences whereby learners come upon learning by their own realization (discovery learning) maximizes learner involvement and improves the ability to acquire, retain, and transfer learning to similar situations.

When learners need to know how to operate new equipment or develop assessment skills, you should provide hands-on learning experiences with the actual equipment or with real or simulated patients; do not assume a lecture alone will be a meaningful learning experience.

Learning is a unitary process

Learning is a unitary process: the learner responds to the teaching-learning process and to the learning situation as a whole. The composite of features that distinguish one individual from another—those physiological, psychological, emotional, intellectual, hereditary, experiential, and maturational aspects of the learner—all function simultaneously in influencing the learner's interaction with and response to the learning experience. Learning requires and has its physical basis in the adequate functioning of physical structures, inclusive of the sensory apparatus and the intellect. Also operative in the learning situation is the wholeness of the learning situation itself: the psychological climate, the physical comfort of the learning environment, the subject matter being addressed, and the instructor's influence.

All of these factors are operative in the teaching-learning process at any given time and influence the outcome of learning. Because learning occurs in relation to the collective effect of these many disparate features, the outcome of the teaching-learning process is characterized as a functional unity.

Insofar as possible, individual differences should be taken into account in planning learning experiences. You may accomplish this by doing such things as varying the focus of teaching on differing perspectives and interests of learners, adjusting the level of teaching for varying audiences, relating material to varying areas of applicability or experience, or varying the teaching pace to learning speed.

Learners' weaknesses or physical impairments may be accommodated by offering multiple avenues for learning similar information. Providing comparable material in lectures supplemented with suggested readings, cassette modules, programmed instruction, or film strips results in multiple learning vehicles. Amplifying visual and auditory media assists learners with sensory deficits. Using concrete simulations rather than abstractions for illustrating principles and concepts assists learners who have difficulty conceptualizing ideas.

Ensure that the learning setting is comfortable, informal, relaxed, and nonjudgmental. These environmental features facilitate creating a climate conducive to the learner's active participation in learning, and will complement making the subject matter relevant, interesting,

and digestible for learners. When learning is viewed as a functional trilogy of the learner, the teacher, and the learning situation, the influence of these many variables becomes readily apparent.

Learning is influenced by the motivation of learners

Learning is more easily acquired and retained when learners have a strong desire to learn; when they genuinely want to learn, they will put forth the effort required. Assuming learners have the intrinsic capability to learn, their degree of commitment to participate actively in the learning process will largely depend on their levels of learning aspiration. In its most basic terms, the motivation for learning is generated by the incompleteness learners acknowledge in attaining their learning needs or goals; once learners have attained their goals, the learning need is satisfied and continued motivation wanes unless additional needs for learning are perceived by the learners.

When a person truly wants to learn something, extrinsic motivators such as threat, grades, salary incentives, and awards are unnecessary. In this situation, intrinsic motivators such as feelings of adequacy, competence, prestige, and self-satisfaction are more than adequate to assure that the learner will attend and follow through with programs. Motivation primes and fosters receptiveness to the learning experience. Only in the least desirable situation, that is, when learning is necessary but not desired by the learner, should external forms of motivation be entertained.

In the ideal situation, the educator can simply devote attention to facilitating learning among learners already highly motivated to learn. In reality, however, aspirations for learning certain things wax and wane; even if learners are highly motivated for the terminal outcomes of learning, they may not be equally motivated to work through all of the prerequisite stages that culminate at that end.

To perpetuate continued motivation, the educator can attempt to stimulate the learner's attention, activate intrigue, and provide intermittent incentives for learning by emphasizing the relevance and applicability of the material and the importance and value of the learning outcomes. Rekindle interest in the subject matter by inspiring and exemplifying your own appreciation of its usefulness and merit. Point out specific and realistic clinical applications of the principles learned. Demonstrate how to apply learning in the clinical practice area.

Insofar as possible, always attempt to generate intrinsic motivation in the learner and resort to the negative extrinsic motivation only under duress and lack of all other alternatives.

One of the single most important motivating forces by far is the experience of success in learning. Especially with learners who may appear unable to develop intrinsic motivation, the basis for this is often a history of perceived or real failure in past learning experiences. If you can demonstrate that learning is not only possible, but brings with it success and self-satisfaction, you will encounter fewer problems with motivating learners to learn. If and when negative motivators such as censure become necessary, use them judiciously, hesitantly, and sparsely, for they rarely create lasting results.

Learning is influenced by the readiness of the learner

Learning readiness denotes a complex state of physical, psychological, and intellectual preparedness for acquiring some particular knowledge, skills, or attitudinal change. It seems to require the aggregate presence of physical and emotional maturity, mastery of prerequisite learning and—most important of all—a perception that the material to be learned is somehow necessary, important, desirable, or otherwise worthwhile. The learner who demonstrates readiness is in short primed for learning: learning is now both timely and meaningful.

A number of ways exist to determine learner readiness. Individuals who voluntarily participate in educational offerings and others who notify educators of subjects they would like to learn about openly exhibit their readiness for learning. New staff nurses who want to learn all that is necessary to function competently or experienced staff nurses who would like to extend or broaden their roles are all indicating readiness for certain types of learning.

The most direct way to determine readiness is by asking potential learners what they feel they would like to learn more about. The expressed educational needs point up their readiness for learning. As discussed in Chapter 2, however, educational needs are arrived at by many means other than learners' perceived needs for learning.

Keep in mind that readiness is an attribute of the learner, not the instructor; you may be ready to teach, but if learners are not ready to learn, they are not likely to learn.

Readiness is a complex functional state that depends primarily on the learner's perception of how useful, meaningful, or worthwhile the material presently is. You may be able to enlighten, encourage, threaten, or sustain the need for learning, but readiness remains the learner's prerogative.

Learning is social

Earlier it was noted that learning is an active process engaging the learner in interaction with others. Co-participants and instructors all interact collectively with the learning environment and the subject matter itself. If the teacher is viewed as a facilitator in the learning process, even employing teaching machines and multimedia developed by instructors can yet be seen to involve social interactions at some point in the learning process. Learning, then, is a mutually shared responsibility of teachers and learners.

The climate for learning is largely dependent on the nature and attributes of the social relationship between instructors and learners.

If learning depends on the active participation of the learner, and if this interaction between instructor and learner forms the essence of the teaching-learning process, then social interaction that facilitates the learner's participation will promote learning.

An instructor's nonjudgmental and democratic leadership style promotes learner participation by supporting the learner's right to disagree openly, to vary in stated opinions, and to make mistakes. Authoritarian learning climates characterized by a teacher's dogmatic, caustic, or belittling tone, a rigid adherence to rules, or a teacher who criticizes, discounts, or defends against inquiry inhibits participation and discourages learning.

Educators can enhance the social elements of the teaching-learning process in numerous ways. Getting to know learners as individuals, engaging in frequent informal discussions, communicating clearly, critiquing constructively, and being available when needed are especially good initiatives. Maintaining and sharing enthusiasm for their interests, acting on learners' suggestions, being prompt, organized, and prepared for classes, providing adequate time for discussion and questions, practicing the art of effective listening, exercising patience, and accepting individual differences among learners will also be helpful. When this social interaction has been managed effectively, the instructor and the learners become co-learners, each sharing and gaining insight from having encountered one another in this highly social process.

Learning is influenced by the learning environment

In addition to the psychological climate of a learning situation, learning may also be influenced by the physical environment. To foster active participation by learners, you must provide such things as adequate lighting and acoustics, comfortable temperature control, clarity of projected images, and adequate seating arrangements and workspaces.

Learning proceeds best when it is organized and clearly communicated

Regardless of the method selected to sequence instructional units, you should pay attention to assuring that smaller component pieces of information are woven into some meaningful whole so that learners are able to integrate the material with past, present, and future experiences. Learning unrelated bits of information out of their meaningful context reduces the chances that learning is acquired, retained, or transferred to new situations. Depending on the subject matter and on the background of the learners, the educator is free to select the organizing principle that seems most appropriate and conducive to learning. Well-organized learning experiences enable learners to experience a gradually developed professional maturation.

Good organization also requires that learning resources, materials, and physical settings are all well prepared. Learners should not waste their time while media are readied, equipment is delivered, or locations for class are decided on. Writing out a schedule of learning activities and then adhering to it are important logistical aspects of the educator's responsibility.

Clear and unambiguous communication lies at the heart of the educational process. Learners and instructors should have a clear and mutual understanding of the program objectives, the subject matter to be addressed, the location and schedule of learning activities, their performance expectations, and how the evaluation process will be proceed. The more all involved parties understand these things, the more cohesive, organized, and effective learning experiences will be.

The level of instruction must be predicated on

the experimental and knowledge base of the learners. You should avoid overly abstract discourses that result in learner frustration or overly concrete or simplistic summaries that lead to boredom. If solicited, learners can often provide useful suggestions on how they can best be assisted in learning certain kinds of subject matter.

Learning is facilitated by positive and immediate feedback

The positive and immediate reinforcement of a new behavior will usually make it recur. Reinforcement given shortly after learning leads to a lasting association between the learned behavior and its approval. In general, the closer the reinforcement occurs to the behavior itself, the greater its potential effect on influencing that behavior.

Positive learning reinforcement enables the learner to be successful in the learning experience by rewarding the desired, correct, or appropriate behavior. If learning is defined as a change in behavior and if the educator's responsibility is to foster these behavioral changes, then imbuing reward systems into the learning situation will usually enhance acquiring desired behavioral changes. The learner's feelings of success in the learning situation are a strong motivating force for continuing to pursue learning as an enjoyable and self-satisfying endeavor.

Positive feedback can take many forms. Recognition, attention, approval, encouragement, and praise are extrinsic social rewards, whereas good grades, increased pay, or career advancement are more tangible extrinsic reinforcers. Each of these is based on an appraisal of performance by others.

All learners, however, have their own standards for self-appraisal of performance; the perception of success in learning situations, especially for mature learners, is not wholly dependent on outside evaluation.

Instructors can motivate learners by guiding early attempts at learning, providing an abundance of opportunities for success at learning, offering approval freely and frequently, communicating anticipated success in attempts at learning, being patient with slower learners, evaluating constructively, being realistic in expectations of performance, and being genuinely empathetic in relationships with learners.

Retention and transfer of learning can be facilitated

Retention of learning is facilitated by proximal recall and distributed practice. Early review and summary combined with feedback on performance favors the solidification of new learning. Repetition without feedback has virtually no effect. Spaced practice reinforces and refines previous learning, appreciably adding to its meaningfulness and applicability.

Retention of learning is useful insofar as it enables the learner to transfer what was learned to subsequent situations. Before learning can be transferred it must first be retained. As mentioned earlier, retention is enhanced when learning is meaningful and desired by the learner, when it is communicated in a systematic, organized, and comprehensible fashion, and when it is reviewed periodically. Other factors that promote learning transfer include emphasizing principles and general concepts rather than specific details, providing adequate time for learners to integrate new material into their bank of experience, and providing for numerous applications of learning in decreasingly similar situations to the one in which initial learning occurred. An example of this would be teaching the skill of tracheal suctioning. Following a review of the objectives and principles involved in this skill, one acceptable technique could be provided to illustrate the steps involved. Learners could then have ample time to practice this and other approaches to performing the skill, provided that they adhere to principles of asepsis. Once the procedure can be performed satisfactorily on patients with nasotracheal tubes, it can then be transferred to related clinical situations such as nasotracheal suctioning of the secretions from nonintubated patients, and suctioning secretions from patients with endotracheal tubes, with tracheostomy tubes, and with permanent tracheal stomas. The wider the variety of experiences with this technique, the greater its transferability to each situation. The learner acquires the ability to identify the commonalities of the situation among a wide variety of circumstances and influences.

Learning is creative

Learning is creative, a sum of successively acquired behaviors. Learners engage in a continual process of integrating new learning with their past experience, and in so doing, modify, delete, or add to what was previously known. This process of integration results in a reorganization of understanding that is distinctively rewoven and new rather than merely being an addition to what was previously perceived to be true. The degree of significance and applicability of the learned material is highly specific to each learner; learning has different meanings for different people.

Learning is inferred rather than observed

Learning is not directly observable, but is inferred on the basis of some behavioral change that can be demonstrated as a result of a learning experience. Whenever evaluation of learning is warranted, therefore, it is necessary to remember that the evaluation process is only indirectly related to the learning process. The methods, tools, and procedures used in evaluation will be the topic of Unit IV.

Learning is influenced by the nature and variability of the learning experience

Learning activities should be planned on the basis of instructional objectives, subject matter, and the learner's level of ability and knowledge. As in the earlier discussion of program formats, a logical correlation is needed between the method of instruction, the setting for instruction, and the learning objectives. In general, classroom learning experiences are appropriate for didactic learning, whereas experiential learning situations are more appropriate for acquiring skills and attitudes.

Once the nature of each instructional objective has been determined, the educator is responsible for assigning that objective to its most appropriate learning setting (classroom, laboratory, clinic) and determining the teaching method most likely to be successful. During this process, educators need not feel restricted in the kinds of learning experiences they select. Many kinds of learning are amenable to multiple possible teaching methods. Both of these responsibilities are discussed later in this unit.

As in the use of media for instructional purposes, teaching methods also need to be tailored to different learning styles. Some learners seem to learn adequately when the lecture method is used, whereas others require concrete experiences, and still others prefer to learn through group discussion.

A final factor to consider here is the need to introduce novelty into planning learning experiences. Persistent use of the same kind of learning experience inevitably produces boredom, the stifling of learner interests, and a diminished ability to profit from the experience. Novelty not only stimulates and motivates learning, but exemplifies an openness toward multiple avenues to attain learning and introduces learners to new ways of participating in this process.

PRINCIPLES OF ADULT EDUCATION

There was a time, at the beginning of this century and before, when education was a largely single event in one's life; what one learned while young was generally adequate for a lifetime's work. What is learned in formal education today, however, becomes obsolete in an exceedingly brief time, often by the time it is available in published form.

As in other spheres of science and technology, theories and practices in health care are modified frequently and replaced by newer ideas, more advanced techniques, and fuller understandings. Educational programs designed for adult professionals therefore cannot consist merely in transmitting presently held beliefs, but must of necessity focus on improving one's ability to continue learning in a lifelong process. Health care professionals in general and critical care practitioners in particular cannot afford to acquire only dated half-truths; as adults, they must be adequately prepared for their professional roles and the full spectrum of their responsibility for the well-being of their patients.

How can we best approach this responsibility for teaching adult learners? Unfortunately, many educators approach curriculum implementation in much the same way as they themselves were taught. For a moment, reflect on your previous educational experiences. If your memories include desks bolted to the floor, a vacuous silence that never questioned a teacher's authority, rigid discipline, and a feeling of passively ingesting large volumes of useless information, you will likely find these even less palatable now than you did as a child. Just because you are sitting on the other side of the desk do not be misled into perceiving your audience as academic adolescents in need of your parenting. If you hope to be successful in educating critical care nurses, one fundamental factor that must be incorporated into your planning and implementation is that these nurses are first and foremost adults. They will respond to being treated as a child in the same way you would.

Adult learners are not merely aging replicas of their juvenile counterparts. They are a distinct and qualitatively different group of learners who perceive and respond to the teaching-learning process very differently than they did as children. You as an adult educator have the attendant responsibility of acknowledging these differences as you conduct learning experiences for adults. The following section describes some of the distinguishing characteristics of adult learners and considers the implications of each characteristic for the adult educator.

Distinguishing characteristics of adult learners: their implications for educators

1. Adults form a heterogeneous group of learners, highly differentiated and commanding of the respect that is due them as mature individuals.
   Implications for educators
   a. Treat learners as mature adults by involving them in decision-making processes of curriculum design and implementation.
   b. Assiduously avoid talking down to learners in all your interactions, both formal and informal; avoid imposing disciplinarian rules or policies.
   c. Respect and encourage the unique perspective each learner conveys and resist attempts to pressure them into group conformity and passive recipience in learning situations.
   d. Expect and encourage differences of opinion and interpretations; learn to learn from learners entrusted to your teaching rather than becoming defensive.
2. Adult learners are often married and have multiple responsibilities for children, spouses, homes, careers, and civic obligations.
   Implications for educators
   a. Recognize adults' needs to assume the same degree of responsibility for their own learning and to be actively involved in all phases of the learning process.
   b. Insofar as feasible, have adults share in the responsibility for determining what they need to learn, how they learn it

best, when they learn it best, and which options they prefer for learning.

c. Respect adults' time and energies as valuable commodities by not wasting them on irrelevant, repetitious, or ineffective learning experiences, and by delineating objectives and expectations as early as possible.

d. Provide for maximum flexibility in scheduling learning activities so that afternoon, evening, night, or weekend class hours would be available if learners deemed these most suitable.

e. Insofar as possible, provide alternative means to learn either at work or outside of work situations so that other time commitments of adult learners are acknowledged.

f. Be sensitive to the fact that concurrent responsibilities of adult learners may affect learning readiness and the quality of their participation in learning activities. Sick children and dental appointments do not go away merely because no one planned for them.

3. Adults possess a large reservoir of life and work experiences as they enter any learning experience; they value highly both their own experiences and those of others. Adults are often very familiar with issues related to the current learning situation.

Implications for educators

a. In some manner (formally, by pretest or questionnaire, or informally) attempt to determine the background of knowledge, skills, and experiences of learners.

b. Use sharing learners' experience in planning learning activities to avert needless repetition with a resultant loss of motivation for learning.

c. Frequently recognize already gained competencies.

d. Draw out and use learners' experiences by selecting teaching methods that are

enriched by this information (group discussion, role playing, open seminars).

e. Guide participants in the art of learning from their personal experiences; practice deriving principles learned, generalizing, and reflecting on experiences as they occur.

f. Emphasize experience-centered learning by relating current learning to adults' past experiences, by incorporating learning into the present situation, and by projecting current learning into its future applications.

4. Adult learners are usually older participants in the learning process; their learning speed may be slow.

Implications for educators

a. Plan for a learning environment suitable or appropriately adapted for the older learner that includes attention to decor, comfortable seating arrangements, temperature and humidity controls, adequate ventilation and lighting, and good acoustical quality.

b. Verify that media used can be heard and viewed by persons with diminished auditory or visual acuity; use microphones if necessary.

c. Be sensitive to the pace of presenting learning activities; be certain to provide adequate time for learners to integrate information before proceeding to subsequent learning activities and to performing learning tasks.

d. Plan for adequate rest periods between learning experiences to minimize mental and physical fatigue.

5. Adults may be less flexible as learners; adult habits, attitudes, and perspectives are more rigidly adhered to, whereas new ideas and approaches are resisted, challenged, discarded, or discounted.

Implications for educators

a. Be open-minded and flexible in planning and conducting learning activities.

b. Assess readiness for learning and provide remedial learning as necessary before instituting learning activities for which participants have not been adequately prepared.

c. Emphasize the gray areas of learning rather than attempting to be black and white in your approach; reinforce the reality that frequently no one right answer or right way of doing something exists.

d. Attempt to integrate new concepts and ideas with learners' previous beliefs, values, and attitudes rather than challenging their validity.

e. Be mindful that new ideas inconsistent or contrary to learners' perspectives may diminish your credibility as an educator; learners need time to accept and verify new concepts.

f. Ease and guide adults in acquiring new or modified attitudes and approaches to learning.

g. Provide clear and adequate instruction for the use of audiovisual media technologies if you are contemplating using independent study and media; facilitate rather than threaten adults in acquiring new skills.

6. Adults frequently have had negative past experiences as learners, producing feelings of inadequacy, fear of failure, and diminished self-confidence.

Implications for educators

a. Provide positive reinforcement for learning frequently and in large doses, while avoiding placing learners in situations where failure or feelings of inadequacy are probable.

b. Provide a physical and psychological learning environment conducive to positive learning experiences:
   (1) Physically comfortable and informal
   (2) Nonjudgmental in its mutuality of trust and respect

(3) Characterized by a sense of humor
(4) Focused on realities rather than ideals
(5) Accepting of differences and supportive of learning
(6) Devoid of ridicule, belittling remarks, censure, or embarrassment for learners

c. Convey your confidence in learners' abilities to acquire necessary knowledge and skills.

d. Plan and coordinate learning experiences to ensure that participants will perform adequately in the learning situation; provide sufficient resources for learning skills so that participants do not feel stranded when they are required to perform.

e. Be sure comments concerning performance are constructive and helpful to learners rather than demeaning.

f. Clarify any misconceptions that others around them "already know everything."

g. Be overt in demonstrating that the instructor is always a co-learner with the participants in a learning situation.

7. Adults are usually voluntary learners who engage in learning activities for a variety of reasons.

Implications for educators

a. Recognize that motives for participating in continuing education are widely variable (to update previous learnings, acquire new skills, change jobs, advance careers, attain relicensure, do something constructive and stimulating, get out of the house) and will not likely be uniform within a given class. Keep your expectations of participants realistic.

b. Attempt to determine the specific motivations learners have for participating to better meet needs; determine how participants intend to use what they learn.

c. If attendance falters in early stages, re-evaluate your approach and assumptions about meeting learning needs, content relevance, or methods of providing learning experiences to determine why learners are failing to attend.

d. Avoid "captured audience" and "soapbox" approaches to learning experiences. Adults are likely to exercise their option to leave experiences that threaten, bore, or offend them personally or professionally.

8. Adults typically engage in learning activities with the intention of immediately applying what they learn to solve problems in their present roles and responsibilites. Adults' readiness for learning is dependent on demands already present or impending in their current situations.

Implications for educators

a. Manage adults' impatience in pursuit of their learning goals by attempting to determine and meet their highest priority needs first.

b. Focus instruction on concrete and immediate realities rather than on theory or idealism.

c. Use a problem-centered approach to subject matter, relating usefulness of learning the material in light of current or anticipated problems.

d. Remember that learners' own acknowledgments of problems faced in work situations are strong, self-sustaining, and self-motivating factors in choosing to pursue learning aimed at solving them.

e. Insofar as possible, sequence and time learning experiences to coincide with learners' present needs to know and avoid extensions far beyond that (e.g., focus on orientation to new position without incorporating all of staff development or career ladder advancement experiences). Concentrate on providing learning experiences most meaningful to learners at that time.

9. Adults work best with teachers who interact with them as knowledgable colleagues, who facilitate learning, and who are subject to the same human shortcomings as they are. Adults can readily detect pretenses, shams, and façades.

Implications for educators

a. Be yourself and be real in interactions with learners rather than be the "all-knowing expert" stereotype; admit areas of uncertainty or lack of understanding, rather than pretending to always know all the answers.

b. Focus on principles governing decision making and problem solving rather than on supplying a list of right answers.

c. Admit mistakes and be able to laugh at yourself.

d. Be available when needed rather than overbearing with learners; allow learners freedom to learn from their own mistakes and experiment without doing for them or taking over.

e. Function more as a role model than as a paradigm.

10. Adults expect to be given the opportunity to evaluate learning experiences in terms of their own goals and expected outcomes of the experience.

Implications for educators

a. Use learners' evaluations of the learning experience as a primary tool for evaluating the program and making modifications for subsequent programs.

b. In soliciting learners' evaluations, attempt to differentiate between individual and collective learning needs that were addressed by the program to obtain both perspectives and the extent to which these were met; incorporate learners' self-assessment of learning into evaluation tools.

c. Be certain to provide both adequate time and a valid vehicle for learners to indicate their evaluations.

• • •

Critical care nurses seem to comprise a special category of adult learners who have some distinguishing features of their own that critical care educators should be aware of.

1. Critical care nurses often place a high premium on their advanced knowledge and clinical skills; their self-concepts and the respect of peers and colleagues are closely tied to their knowledge and skills.

    Implications for educators
    a. Provide professionally stimulating and meaningful learning experiences that supplement previously attained learning, challenge and motivate continued learning, and finely tune skills.
    b. Provide for increasingly advanced levels of learning once the basics have been learned to challenge even the most experienced staff nurses.
    c. Keep communication lines open among all members of the health care team to readily disseminate learning.

2. Because of the nature of their work, critical care nurses cannot afford to function on the basis of outdated or erroneous information.

    Implications for educators
    a. Convey findings of research and professional literature to staff nurses.
    b. Assist in translating research findings into improved patient care practices.
    c. Keep yourself up to date in theory and clinical practice so that your own expertise is maintained and assured.
    d. Work with and learn from staff nurses in your area of practice.

3. As a group, critical care nurses may be amenable to making changes or modifications in their practice.

    Implications for educators
    a. Foster open-mindedness to new ideas, interpretations, and practices.
    b. Attempt to make learning and change for improvement an integral part of the work situation rather than a disquieting interjected element.
    c. Solicit staff nurses' perceptions of necessary changes in policy or procedure and their participation in making these changes.

4. As a group, critical care nurses may be especially direct, vocally assertive, no-nonsense individuals who dispense respect for peers somewhat judiciously after it is earned.

    Implications for educators
    a. Know your subject matter and clinical skills thoroughly.
    b. Expect challenges to your credibility and be prepared to substantiate your assertions and opinions.
    c. Be open, honest, and pragmatic in interactions with staff nurses.

REFERENCES
Teaching and learning in adult education

Applegate, M: Adult education: a simulation game. In National League for Nursing: The community college and continuing education for health personnel, New York, 1978, National League for Nursing.

Bille, DA: Successful educational programming: increasing learner motivation through involvement, J Nurs Admin 9:36, 1979.

Broschart, JR: Lifelong learning in the nation's third century, Washington, D.C., 1977, Department of Health, Education, and Welfare.

Clark, CC: The nurse as continuing educator, New York, 1979, Springer-Verlag New York, Inc.

Clark, KM and Dickinson, G: Self-directed and other-directed continuing education: a study of nurses' participation, J Contin Educ Nurs 7:16, 1976.

Dubin, SS, and Olsum, M: Implications of learning theories for adult instruction, Adult Educ 24:3, 1973.

Harrington, FH: The future of adult education, San Francisco, 1977, Jossey-Bass, Inc.

Jones, MC: A continuing eduation dilemma: luring the adult learner, Occup Health Nurs 27:17, 1979.

Kidd, JR: How adults learn, New York, 1973, Association Press.

Knowles, MS: The adult learner: a neglected species, ed 2, Houston, 1978, Gulf Publishing Co.

Knowles, MS: Gearing adult education for the seventies. In Popiel, ES, editor: Nursing and the process of continuing education, ed 2, St. Louis, 1977, The C.V. Mosby Co.

Knowles, MS: The modern practice of adult education, rev ed, New York, 1980, Follett Publishing Co.

Knox, AB: Adult development and learning, San Francisco, 1977, Jossey-Bass, Inc.

Malarkey, L: The older student—stress or success on campus, JNE 18:15, 1979.

Miller, HG, and Verduin, JR: The adult educator—a handbook for staff development, Houston, 1979, Gulf Publishing Co.

Norris, CG: Characteristics of the adult learner and extended higher education for registered nurses, Nurs and Health Care 1:87, 1980.

Popiel, ES, editor: Nursing and the process of continuing education, ed 2, St. Louis, 1977, The C.V. Mosby Co.

Richardson, JA, and Matheney, KB: Teaching effectiveness: the science of the art. In Concepts and components of effective teaching, New York, 1978, National League for Nursing.

Sanford, ND: Teaching strategies for inservice and staff development educators, J Contin Educ Nurs 10:5, 1979.

Schoen, DC: Lifelong learning: how some participants see it, J Contin Educ Nurs 10:3, 1979.

Smith, CE: Planning, implementing and evaluating learning experiences for adults, Nurs Educ 3:31, 1978.

Stevens, BJ: The teaching-learning process, Nurs Educ 1:9, 1976.

Tarnow, KG: Working with adult learners, Nurs Educ 4:34, 1979.

Tibbles, L: Theories of adult education: implications for the development of a philosophy for continuing education in nursing, J Contin Educ Nurs 8:25, 1977.

Verduin, J, Miller, H, and Greer, C: Adults teaching adults, Austin, Texas, 1979, Learning Concepts.

Wasch, S: The role of baccalaureate faculty in continuing education, Nurs Outlook 28:116, 1980.

Chapter 9

Factors influencing selection of teaching method

The teaching-learning process is an interactive process, facilitated through one or more planned learner-teacher interactions. An instructional or teaching method specifies how the teacher will interact with learners to effect the desired learning outcomes. A teaching method delineates the general features of this teacher-learner interaction by describing the technique, strategy, and kinds of learning activities used to promote learning.

Today's educator has an ever-widening array of methods available for providing continuing education to nurses. Unfortunately, no definitive data exist to support the accurate selection of the "right" teaching method, nor is there any clear-cut evidence that any one method is assuredly and consistently superior to any other. Fortunately, a variety of instructional methods may be appropriate for a given learning experience, and learning does not hinge solely on the instructional method employed. Techniques can be adapted or combined for various teaching purposes, and each method has certain identifiable caharacteristics that can direct educators in appropriately using them.

This chapter is devoted to describing factors to consider in selecting teaching methods, together with how and when to use currently available teaching methods. As you consider each of these teaching methods, remember that the most reliable indication that a teaching method is effective is whether or not the intended learning occurs.

Given that no one "right" teaching method exists and that a variety of methods may be appropriate for achieving the same instructional purposes, how does an educator decide which teaching method to use? A number of factors influence selection of the most appropriate teaching method. In a general order of their degree of influence, the following factors should govern teaching method.

SPECIFIC LEARNING OBJECTIVES

Remember that learning is evidenced and inferred from a change in the learner's behavior: a change in what the learner knows (cognitive learning), feels (affective learning), or does (psychomotor learning). The single most influential factor governing selecting a teaching method is the performance desired in the learner as an outcome of the teaching-learning experience. In general the "best" teaching method for any kind of teaching instruction is the one that best helps the learner meet the desired objectives. Consider the three following objectives:

1. The learner will be able to *define* the term *myocardial infarction*.
2. The learner will be able to *calculate* the electrical axis using a 12-lead ECG.

3. The learner will be able to *record* a 12-lead ECG.

You would intuitively know that for the learner to attain these objectives, you would need to employ different kinds of teaching strategies. A lecture or group discussion might be appropriate for learning how to *define myocardial infarction*, but would be less appropriate for learning how to *calculate* the electrical axis and even less helpful for learning how to *record* a 12-lead ECG. Conversely, practice in *recording* ECGs would not be helpful in learning how to *calculate* an axis nor in learning how to *define myocardial infarction*.

Guideline. The teaching method selected should provide the learner with practice in performing the behavior specified in the objective; the instructional technique should match as closely as possible the performance specified in the learning objective.

LEARNERS' ABILITIES, PREVIOUS BACKGROUNDS, EXPERIENCES, AND NEEDS TO PARTICIPATE IN LEARNING

Learners' familiarity and experiences with a teaching method can influence their ability to profit from that teaching method. If, for example, learners are unfamiliar with the group process technique, they are less likely to profit from a group discussion or a nursing team conference than from a more familiar method. If they have developed the habit of falling asleep during lectures, then lectures may prove to be a fruitless teaching method. Likewise, if nurses are unfamiliar with even the rudiments of physical assessment, they are not likely to profit from weekly bedside nursing rounds.

Guideline. The learning method you choose should be consistent with the capabilities and previous experiences of learners.

All learners, especially adult learners, need to participate actively in the learning process. As discussed in Chapter 8, the extent of learning is often proportional to the degree of learner participation. Thus the teaching method you select should maximally involve learners as active participants in the learning process.

SUBJECT MATTER UNDER DISCUSSION

In much the same way as desired performance governs selecting the teaching method, the subject matter discussed in relation to that performance should also govern your choice. If the subject matter consists of "principles of hemodialysis" and "techniques of arteriovenous shunt care," the principles could probably best be taught and reinforced by a lecture with illustrative demonstration, whereas techniques would likely require return demonstration with instructor feedback.

Guideline. The teaching method selected should reflect the subject matter under discussion.

RESOURCE AVAILABILITY FOR THAT TEACHING METHOD

At times the physical facilities or equipment needed to use a particular teaching method are unobtainable or not presently feasible. A lack of flexible seating arrangements may preclude selecting the group discussion method, whereas the unavailability of an auditorium may make lecturing to a large group impossible. The limited patient populations involved may diminish the value of using the clinical nursing rounds technique, and the lack of available funds to purchase manikins or models may obviate the possibility of using a laboratory experience to practice clinical skills.

Even though a particular teaching method may be judged the most appropriate vehicle for instruction, unless it is also readily available, financially feasible, and practical for the situation, it may not be very useful.

Guideline. The teaching method selected should be readily available, affordable, and realistic for the circumstances of the setting.

LEARNERS' NEEDS FOR VARIATION IN TEACHING METHODS

Remember learners' needs for novelty in the teaching-learning process. Continuous use of the same teaching method may be proportionately less effective over time, because it can become boring and monotonous. Regardless of how good the teaching method is, its effectiveness is difficult to maintain when not interrupted—at least intermittently—by a variation in teaching approaches.

Learners also need variation in teaching methods because they have different learning styles. Some learners will learn best by concrete (hands-on) learning experiences, whereas others may gain the most from group discussion, clinical rounds, or even lectures.

Guideline. Choose the teaching method from a well-developed repertoire of techniques. Varying techniques should be deliberate.

RELATIVE EFFICIENCY OF THE TEACHING METHOD

When one or more teaching methods may be equally effective in attaining the objectives, one method may be judged superior to the others because it is more economical for learners or instructors. This may be an economy of time, cost, resource support, facilities, availability, accessibility, or some other factor. If, for example, new orientees learn the principles of peritoneal dialysis as well by lecture as they did by laboratory demonstration, but learned them in half the time with the laboratory method, then the laboratory method would be the more efficient effective teaching method.

Guideline. Given a choice among equally effective teaching methods, choose the method that is the most economical of time, cost, or other significant factors.

INSTRUCTOR'S FAMILIARITY AND EXPERTISE WITH THE TEACHING METHOD

Regardless of the purported effectiveness of any teaching method, if the instructor is unfamiliar with the technique, inexperienced in its method, or unable to use it effectively, its potential value to that instructor is nullified. In an attempt to appear contemporary, educators may get swept into the premature use of whatever technique is the current fad in educational circles. Learners can sense an instructor's lack of familiarity and facility with a given instructional method and can be expected to respond with resentment and dissatisfaction if their learning needs are not met. A need for variety and novelty in teaching methods does not justify their inappropriate or unskilled use. Keep in mind that the teaching process serves the learning process. The converse does not hold true.

A tried and true maxim in education says educators tend to teach the way they were taught; because most of us were taught by lectures we tend to teach by lectures. As you learn more about instructional techniques, you must learn to strike a balance among this following trio of tendencies:

1. The tendency to teach exclusively as you were taught
2. The tendency to use methods before you are skilled at them
3. The tendency to be reluctant in experimenting with new techniques

Guideline. While being open to both experimentation and variation in established teaching methods, the teaching method selected should be one the educator is skilled in using.

INSTRUCTIONAL SETTING

For many practical and, at times, ethical reasons, certain teaching methods are typically employed in various learning settings: classroom, laboratory, and clinical. A group discussion concerning patient management problems is not appropriately located at the bedside any more than the refinement of physical assessment skills is appropriately located in a library. The very nature of the learning activity will usually dictate where it should be held.

Guideline. The teaching method selected

should be appropriate to the setting where it will be employed. At some early point before initiating the instruction, each objective should be assigned to its most appropriate setting: classroom, laboratory, or clinical.

● ● ●

The next three chapters describe a variety of teaching methods according to the setting in which they are typically employed and the degree of learner participation they require. Each chapter also provides some guidelines for using each kind of teaching method. Remember that learning is the aimed for end; the teaching methods employed can undergo nearly limitless adaptation and modification as long as they lead to the desired learning outcomes.

REFERENCES
Teaching methods in nursing

Arnold, J: Let's discuss teaching strategies, JNE **17**:15, 1978.

Clark, CC: Classroom skills for the nurse educator, New York, 1978, Springer-Verlag New York, Inc.

de Menses, M: Split brain theory: implications for nurse educators, Nurs Outlook **28**:441, 1980.

de Tornyay, R: Strategies for teaching nursing, New York, 1971, John Wiley & Sons, Inc.

Ferrell, B: Attitudes toward learning styles and self-direction of ADN students, JNE **17**:19, 1978.

Foley, R, and Smilansky, J: Teaching techniques: a handbook for health professionals, New York, 1980, McGraw-Hill Book Co.

Jernigan, DK: Testing—a learning not a grading process, Nurs Outlook **28**:120, 1980.

Mager, RF, and Beach, KM, Jr: Developing vocational instruction, Belmont, Calif., 1967, Fearon-Pitman Publishers, Inc.

Matejski, MP: Preparing nurses to teach—the charge and a response, JNE **19**:25, 1980.

Perry, SE: Teaching strategy and learner performance, JNE **18**:25, 1979.

Rees, C: Teaching for coronary care unit emergencies, J Contin Educ Nurs **11**:39, 1980.

Sanford, ND: Teaching strategies for inservice and staff development educators, J Contin Educ Nurs **10**:5, 1979.

Schweer, JE, and Gebbie, KM: Creative teaching in clinical nursing, ed 3, St. Louis, 1976, The C.V. Mosby Co.

Tapper, M: Teaching methods and techniques for staff development, J Contin Educ Nurs **8**:72, 1977.

Cognitive styles

Crancer, J, and Maury-Hess, S: Games: an alternative to pedagogical instruction, JNE **19**:45, 1980.

Rezler, AG, and French, RM: Personality types and learning preferences of students in six allied health professions, J Allied Health **4**:20, 1975.

Whitkin, HA, et al: Field–dependent and field–independent cognitive styles and their educational implications, Rev Educ Res **47**:1, 1977.

Chapter 10

Teaching methods for the classroom setting

Teaching methods for the classroom setting generally involve minimal to moderate degrees of learner participation. The range of available teaching methods for the classroom includes the lecture and various forms of group discussion such as nursing care conference, nursing team conference, case study, incident process, peer participatory conference, Conex laboratory, and brainstorming.

The classroom setting is usually the locus for cognitive or content learning. This is distinguished from both the laboratory setting, where cognitive and process learning is emphasized, and the clinical setting, where process learning is the major focus.

When the classroom is used, the educator must be certain that the principles of both the teaching-learning process and those of adult education are put into operation. Whether you are a novice or a veteran classroom educator, it is often helpful to review these principles and verify their implementation. In general you will want to be sure you are taking into account that learning:

1. Occurs as a functional unity
2. Is a social activity
3. Is influenced by the physical environment and psychological climate in which it occurs, the manner in which it is organized and communicated, the nature and timing of reinforcement, the pace and meaningfulness of instruction, and the nature and characteristics of adult learners

As you review the precepts of classroom teaching, remember that they represent the accumulated experience of much trial and error in the educational process. If you incorporate these principles into your classroom teaching, you will find that the usefulness of this setting can be dramatically improved over what it all too often is like. The setting alone does not determine the extent of learning, but how you use your setting and the principles of learning and adult education. Especially in the classroom, where these precepts are often neglected, you should double-check that they are taken into account during instruction.

LECTURE

The lecture is, by far, the most time- and tradition-honored method of teaching. Most of today's adults were taught by this method, so that many—both learners and instructors—equate teaching with lecturing.

The lecture holds the unique distinction of being not only the most widely used, but also the most frequently misused and abused form of instruction. It is a personable vehicle for orally transmitting information and, at its best, does so in a fairly organized, systematic and naturally evolving manner. At its worst, the lecture anesthetizes audiences with monotone litanies of unrelated accumulations of trivia for the learner to regurgitate later, reiterates the known and the obvious, or confuses the almost-knowns. When poorly used, the lecture can preclude learner feedback and response, transforming an audience into a sea of note-taking sponges.

If used with care, the lecture can be extremely efficient as a cost- and time-effective method of summarizing, updating, assimilating, and correlating large bodies of knowledge in a given area. When well organized in a developmental sequence, it can disseminate the expertise and insight of a single instructor to an audience limited only by seating capacity and the adequacy of acoustics.

Appropriateness for teaching. The lecture method is appropriately used for teaching when the instructional objectives center on learners' attaining such cognitive abilities as definition, recall, identification, relation, synthesis, explanation, description, understanding, interrelation, generalization, and differentiation among complex concepts. Lectures can be used to provide learners with the factual data needed to prepare for affective or psychomotor learning by supplying them with the opportunity to think abstractly and to understand theories and hypothetical applications. Lectures can be used to clarify intricate ideas, delineate important concepts, assimilate principles from a multitude of diverse disciplines, critique, motivate, and stimulate budding interests in new areas of conjecture, and entertain multiperspective approaches to issues and problems.

Guidelines for use. In preparing a lecture, planning is of the utmost importance. Some useful guides at the planning stage include the following:

1. Use the instructional objectives to formulate an outline of the key points to be covered.
2. Limit the outline to words and phrases to reduce the likelihood of "reading" the lecture.
3. Be certain that the outline introduces and develops concepts in a clear, logical sequence based on previously known learning and intentions for future learning

needs; supplement the outline with vivid examples and illustrations.

4. Plan on prefacing the lecture with objectives to be attained, key points to be discussed, the injection of thought-provoking issues, problems, and questions, and a summary of previous coverage on the topic. These measures will generate learner involvement, provide for learner orientation to the lecture, and alleviate the mental strain of needing to integrate numerous complex concepts. Lighten the mental load by alternating known and simple concepts with more complex concepts; explain the application of concepts by using clinical examples with which learners can empathize.
5. Double-check that you have allotted adequate time for considering and integrating more difficult concepts. Marking your lecture notes with the time required for covering certain sections may be helpful in judging approximate time distribution for content. Avoid the tendency of attempting to teach everything known about a given topic.
6. If unforeseen events could impinge on the amount of available instructional time, plan for this by highlighting keypoints to be covered. Then, should these circumstances arise, you will have your priorities already ordered. If segments of the lecture require significantly more or less time than you originally planned, make note of this for subsequent revision in your future time allotments for that topic.
7. Distribute the class outline before the lecture so that learners will be able to more readily follow the presentation. A distributed outline including all key points of the lecture, reduces the need for copious note-taking. If learners can be assured that all the important points are already noted in

the handout, they will be able to devote their attention to listening and integrating rather than trying to copy every word.

8. Have all support materials (supplements, handouts, audiovisual software and hardware) available and functional well in advance of the lecture time.

9. Plan for at least 10-minute breaks after every 50 minutes of instruction.

You should do the following to implement the lecture more effectively:

1. Exemplify enthusiasm for the material by using an energetic yet conversational tone of voice. Avoid being overly dramatic, affected, or listless. Vary the pitch, intensity, and rate of delivery, while maintaining the projection and modulation necessary for effective communication.

2. Use a microphone whenever necessary.

3. Vary the pace and nature of the delivery by interrupting the steady flow of the presentation with pauses. Energize learners by offering intriguing thoughts to ponder, discussions and learner reaction, clarification and reiteration of major points, and the practical application of theory to practice. Do not get so involved with teaching theory that you fail to allot adequate time to making the lecture real and useful to learners.

4. Make yourself aware of any tendencies you may have to use habitual phrases ("you know"), vague terms ("routine care"), or distracting movements and gestures (constant pacing). Focus on being natural and relaxed. Videotape your presentation or ask a peer to critique your presentation style.

5. Find a comfortable posture and location where you can be seen and heard clearly.

6. Develop your ability to recognize learners' nonverbal responses to instruction. Differentiate among facial expressions and body language that provide cues indicating understanding rather than bewilderment or confusion, agreement rather than disagreement, boredom rather than frustration, and alertness rather than fatigue. Face the learners and respond to their nonverbal reactions as readily as you would to their questions or requests for clarification. Many learners simply will not offer verbal feedback. You will have to read it by frequently scanning their faces.

7. Verify nonverbal feedback and the level of understanding by soliciting applications of concepts discussed, posing problems related to the topic, calling for questions, or interjecting discussion and critique.

8. Remember that learning always takes precedence over covering the material.

9. Keep in mind that much of what you know was learned by listening to lectures; emulate the features of lecturers you learned the most from and avoid subjecting your audience to practices you abhorred as a student.

GROUP DISCUSSION

Group discussion is another format very familiar to nurses. When used as a teaching method, group discussion consists of a purposeful meeting of two or more individuals who collectively gather to share, deliberate, exchange, and critique perspectives regarding some specific issue, situation, problem, or topic of mutual concern. The climate for exchanging ideas and information may be either formal or informal and requires some form of leadership to direct, focus, and summarize the discussion. This technique capitalizes on the aggregate knowledge, abilities, and experiences of group members who come together for the purpose of reaching some conclusion, consensus, or resolution of a problem.

Appropriateness for teaching. Group discussion is appropriately used for teaching the following:

1. How to formulate, organize, and coherently express one's perceptions and positions on issues and situations
2. The dynamics of group process and the collective management of problems
3. Problem-solving skills: how to identify, approach, reconsider, constructively critique, and weigh various elements in the problem-solving process
4. Affective behaviors; critical and analytical thinking in a cooperative atmosphere, and consciousness-raising on relevant issues and topics.
5. The skills required for effective communication and interpersonal relations
6. Effective and attentive listening to the views expressed by others
7. Areas open to multiple interpretations, when hard data and concrete facts are less available

Guidelines for use. Group discussion can be an effective teaching technique in the following situations:

1. The instructor has a thorough working knowledge of group dynamics in learning.
2. Learners have been provided with clearly defined topics and objectives. The agenda should be available enough in advance of the discussion period for participants to prepare adequately for it and to substantiate their views.
3. Seating arrangements and acoustics facilitate conversation among members of the group.
4. Group members know one another or share a similar need to accomplish the established goals.
5. The discussion leader (instructor, assigned or naturally emerging member of the group) (a) initiates the discussion by reviewing the objectives and clarifying the issue or topic to be addressed, (b) maintains and facilitates continued exchange of information by all participants, (c) discour-

ages the monopolization or misdirection of discussions, (d) identifies significant areas of discussion that have been neglected or only superficially explored, (e) ignites interaction by posing intriguing and thought-provoking questions or comments relevant to the topic, and (f) periodically and terminally summarizes conclusions that have been reached.

Various forms of group discussion are available for the classroom. Some are very commonly used by nurses and nursing students whereas others may be less familiar. Especially in adult continuing education, when both active participation in learning and the exchange of experiences and backgrounds are such valuable ingredients of learning, it is worthwhile to consider using one or a number of these group discussion methods.

Nursing care conference

When some particular aspect or problem related to individual patient care arises, a nursing care conference may be planned to manage the situation more effectively. The initiating event is usually some obstacle or problem arising in providing nursing care for a specific patient, although the need may be one expressed by either the patient, the family, or the staff nurses involved with the patient's care. The conference may be scheduled or spontaneous, and usually proceeds informally in an effort to find alternative and more effective solutions to the problems at hand.

Management and leadership of the conference are usually vested in the nurse most closely involved with that patient's care, whereas others (head nurse, clinical nurse specialist) are used as resources and consultants and may be able to broaden perspectives or suggest novel approaches or informative readings.

Whether lasting a few minutes or many hours, the nursing care conference is designed to provide direction and alternative approaches to improved nursing care of an individual patient.

In addition to its value in resolving nursing care problems, the nursing care conference may be used for assessing the overall quality and effectiveness of the care of a given patient.

Nursing team conference

When team nursing began its preeminence over functional nursing, the nursing team conference emerged as a useful vehicle for communication among members of a given team. In the nursing team conference, the nursing care provided for one, some, or all of the patients under the care of that team is appraised, modified, and later reappraised for its quality and comprehensiveness. Especially when a team may consist of multiple groups of professionals from one or more disciplines and of paraprofessionals and nonprofessional workers, clear communication among team members more readily assures the maintenance of quality and continuity of care.

Regardless of their position within the organization, team members usually empathize with one another and interrelate more effectively when they can participate collectively in resolving problems for patients under their care. As compared with the nursing care conference, the nursing team conference may be more broad in scope and less in depth for a given patient. The role of the group leader or educator is essentially the same as with the nursing care conference.

Case study

At times, the complexity, novelty, or uniqueness of a particular patient situation warrants more formal comprehensive, and detailed study and consideration. In these instances, a nursing case study may be used for presenting the findings and assessment of the patient and for reviewing and evaluating the nursing interventions taken or proposed for the patient's care. In some cases the patients themselves actively participate in the presentation by describing their clinical histories, symptoms, responses, and reactions to their health problems or therapy.

Responsibility for the presentation is usually vested in the staff members who provide the patient's nursing care. The focus is on providing a detailed and comprehensive account of one particular patient situation that, by its very nature, demands additional learning and study by those responsible for the patient's care. Especially for the self-directed adult learner, the case study provides a forum for meaningfully combining learning with nursing practice.

The educator can facilitate using the nursing case study by identifying potential patients for presentation, assisting the presenter in obtaining valid clinical assessments, and directing the presenter to relevant sources of information (books, journal articles, audiovisual programs). The educator may also provide guidance in the process of leading and managing the discussion period that follows the presentation, critiquing the learning experience, and offering suggestions for its improvement.

Staff nurses can learn from the patient, from the presentation, and from the discussion period that summarizes this information. Previously learned concepts of care can be applied and new ones can be identified and evaluated.

Incident process

The incident process is a group discussion technique that fosters the development of skills in reasoned inquiry. It is used as a basis for eliciting sound clinical decisions.

As described by the Pigors, the incident process involves selecting and presenting (written or oral) a critical incident that requires some type of decision. Either the instructor or one of the participants functions as a group leader by presenting the incident for group consideration and analysis. Once the incident has been described, group members must then investigate the incident by soliciting from the group leader further information and facts bearing on the decision about the case. The group leader is the most thoroughly familiar with all aspects of the incident. A period of time is then alloted to fact-gathering and analysis, after which the key factors influencing the incident and its related decision are delineated. The outcome of an incident process consists of a synopsis of the incident and the decision reached to resolve it. The factors or issues bearing on the incident that comprise the rationale for decision making must also be described. On the basis of these underlying factors and their interrelationships, the causes of the incident are identified, which provide the impetus and direction for making the decision. The group's outcome is then compared with the actual facts and the resulting decision to evaluate the validity of the decision.

Especially in critical care nursing, critical thinking processes, sound rationales for decision making, and direct intervention in patient welfare are requisite practitioner skills. The incident process may be a valuable adjunct for improving the efficiency and validity of individual problem-solving skills in decisions regarding patient care, may teach affective content useful in interpersonal effectiveness with families, peers, and co-workers, and may illustrate the application of analytical approaches to practice and patient care management issues.

Peer participatory conference

Krawczyk describes the peer participatory conference (PPC) as a mode of group discussion particularly attuned to adults' need to participate more dynamically in the learning process. In a PPC the instructor relinquishes the role of group leader and functions as a moderator having an equal status with the other 8 to 10 participants.

A concept related to broad areas of responsibility for patient care is selected by the instructor, usually on a weekly basis. Each group member is responsible for preparing a brief (approximately 10 minutes) description of how that concept (patient teaching, altered family roles, pain, effects of culture, effects of hospitalization) applies to her patient's situation, what interventions were taken, and what her evaluation was. Following this progress report, the member's peers and the instructor critique and evaluate the presentation, and offer additional insights and suggestions for intervention related to the concept for that week.

Krawczyk emphasizes that for this technique to be of value the nurse participants must be able to maintain their patient assignment over some predetermined and fairly long period of time. Perceived advantages of the PPC include its providing weekly feedback and constructive critique of patient care, an enhanced scope of learning with multiple applications of a given concept modified by individual circumstances, interactively using peers as resources, and building self-confidence as a contributor to the learning process.

The PPC would seem to be an especially useful vehicle for conveying applications of theory and, perhaps, research findings and affective notions to the realities of the practice setting. Transferring learning would also be enhanced as the concept of the week is applied to widely variable patient situations.

Conex laboratory (Conex lab)

A significant amount of nursing practice involves the affective realm of learning, that is, feelings, reactions, engendered emotions, controversial issues and viewpoints, and ethical and other professional concerns. These directly and indirectly affect a nurse's practice, yet are often less than optimally learned if only discussed rather than experienced. To provide for more meaningful learning in this area, Bradshaw suggests the Conex lab format.

A Conex lab is a classroom teaching method that provides for the acquisition of affective learning through group discussion of a single issue influencing nursing practice. Rather than focusing on learning content or psychomotor skills, a Conex lab emphasizes thoughts and feelings. Separate sessions are concerned with issues such as religion and nursing, sexuality, dependency, management of change, and death and dying and their effect on clinical nursing practice. Each Conex lab deals with experiences and perspectives shared in a single area of influence.

Groups are kept small (not more than 12) to promote full participation by all members. Adequate time (2 to 4 hours) is allotted for expressing and considering all viewpoints and experiences of members. The sharing of experiences and the reflections on these sharings are followed by closure activities to gain perspectives on the issue or concept and to formulate generalizations. If participants are to gain maximally from this method, the instructors must also be willing to share their personal experiences and feelings as openly as group members.

One particularly intriguing and potentially good starting session is a Conex lab centered around humor. In this lab instructors and participants share goofs and blunders that were humorous episodes while working with people, reflect on the therapeutic use of humor in nursing practice, and reinforce the notion that nursing can be fun.

As in the peer participatory conferences, the Conex lab can be helpful for conveying affective content, applying theory to practice, and making learning meaningful for adult learners.

Brainstorming

Brainstorming is a group problem-solving technique that aims at developing and stimulating creative thinking when conventional approaches to problem solving have been fruitless. Unlike many other variations of group discussion, brainstorming is most effective with larger groups of individuals (at least 25), especially those who are less constrained by rigid, analytical approaches to problem solving.

In as informal a setting as possible, participants are encouraged to generate as many novel and eclectic ideas to solve the problem as possible. Quantity, novelty, and originality are the premiums sought. As ideas are suggested, a recorder lists them so they are easily visible to the entire group. When additional ideas are no longer forthcoming, the session culminates with an evaluation of the usefulness of each suggested approach and with a decision on the most acceptable course of action. As a problem-solving technique, brainstorming is probably the least used and most enjoyable approach available.

REFERENCES
Lecture

Cooper, SS: Teaching by telephone, Nurs Educ **4:**10, 1979.

de Tornyay, R: Strategies for teaching nursing, New York, 1971, John Wiley & Sons.

Ebel, KE: The craft of teaching, San Francisco, 1976, Jossey Bass.

Hayter, J: How good is the lecture as a teaching method? Nurs Outlook **27:**274, 1979.

Postman, N, and Weingartner, C: Teaching as a subversive activity, New York, 1969, Delacorte Press.

Thompson, R: Legitimate lecturing, Improv Coll Univ Teach **22:**163, 1974

Group discussion

Anderson, NE: The use of the seminar as a teaching technique with senior undergraduate nursing students, JNE **19:**20, 1980.

Bradshaw, CE: Concentrated experiential learning laboratories, JNE **17:**32, 1978.

Cooper, SS: Methods of teaching—revisited: brainstorming, J Contin Educ Nurs **9:**16, 1978.

Cooper, SS: Methods of teaching—revisited: informal discussion, J Contin Educ Nurs **9:**14, 1978.

Cooper, SS: Methods of teaching—revisited: Nursing care conference, J Contin Educ Nurs **10:**28, 1979.

Cornwell, JB: How to stimulate—and manage—participation in the classroom, Training HRD **16:**40, 1979.

Eaton, S, Davis, G, and Benner, PE: Discussion stoppers in teaching, Nurs Outlook **25:**578, 1977.

Geis, G: Student participation in instruction, J Higher Educ **47:**249, 1976.

Kirkis, EJ: We let our students do inservice, RN **42:**91, 1979.

Krawczyk, RM: Peer participatory conferences: a dynamic method of nursing instruction, JNE **17:**5, 1978.

Pigors, P, and Pigors, F: The incident process—a method of inquiry, Nurs Outlook **14:**48, 1966.

Yeaw, EMJ: Problem solving as a method of teaching strategies in classroom and clinical teaching, JNE **18:**16, 1979.

Chapter 11

Teaching methods for the laboratory setting

The laboratory method of teaching can encompass a wide variety of teaching strategies, from the traditional biology, chemistry, or physics experimental laboratory to the research laboratory or even the audiovisual laboratory.

In nursing, the term *laboratory* can be interpreted broadly to include all forms and settings for clinical experiences or more narrowly to imply a setting for learning that is wholly or partly a mock-up of the clinical setting, located apart from the actual patient bedside area. For the present discussion, *laboratory* refers to a facility or process designed to provide learners with near real or simulated experiences using the equipment, materials, procedures, skills, or situations found in the actual clinical practice setting.

The purpose of the laboratory is to offer learners an opportunity for direct and supervised experiences in using theory for problem solving, for developing, testing, and applying previously learned principles, and for executing and practicing clinical skills, techniques, and abilities. In the laboratory, learners are given an opportunity to confront the realities encountered in applying and interrelating precepts and principles that must be put into operation in the course of daily nursing practice.

The laboratory is a conjunctive learning setting intended to serve as a bridge between the content learned in the classroom and the process (i.e., application of content) practiced at the bedside. It comprises various means for simulating psychomotor, problem-solving, affective, and interpersonal skills and for interacting with the people, equipment, events, and experiences the nurse is likely to encounter in actual clinical practice.

Like classroom teaching methods, laboratory teaching methods bring together theoretical content and scientific principles that underlie clinical practice at a location removed from patient care areas. As remote learning experiences, laboratory methods may be—but are not necessarily—somewhat less meaningful and efficient to learners. Unlike the actual clinical setting, however, the laboratory setting provides learning experiences in a more controlled, consistent, and structured environment for learning that is virtually hazard free to patients, families, other staff, and learners themselves. Because laboratory experiences are situated closer to the real world of clinical practice than are classroom methods, they expedite transfer of learning. Because they are safely removed from this real world, however, they offer some of the following advantages over teaching in the clinical area itself:

1. It is easier to supervise and guide learning when learners are concentrated in one geographical area rather than dispersed over many clinical units.
2. It is easier to assure the breadth, scope, quality, and comparability of learning experi-

ences when the innumerable variables confronted in actual patient situations are removed. Without control, these variables may preclude structuring and learning from the clinical experience.

3. The types and variety of learning experiences are more readily available than in the clinical setting where it is often impossible to obtain an adequate number of the right patients available at the right time for the right learners.

4. The congestion of learners all vying for certain types of patients at the same hours is alleviated.

5. Without the obstacles, complexities, and uncertainties inherent in using the clinical area as a learning setting, some learning experiences may be more effectively learned by being duplicated in the laboratory.

6. It is more feasible to provide the trial, practice, review, and pacing of learning because these can be duplicated innumerable times.

7. Learner errors in understanding, executing, and applying theory to practice occur more safely without potential harm to patients, families, or staff members.

8. Learner embarrassment, anxiety, feelings of inadequacy, and uncertainty in the clinical setting can be minimized to augment the likelihood of positive reinforcement of satisfactory clinical performance.

Laboratory experiences can serve as an adjunct to either classroom or clinical learning experiences. As in any other learning setting, the instructor functions as the guide and facilitator of learning, whereas the learner should be the active participant. This holds more true in the laboratory than in the classroom because the learner's direct involvement in the learning process is notably and measurably increased in the laboratory. Depending on the nature of the learning format, direct instructor involvement may be moderate (demonstrating procedures, using simulated models), minimal (feedback on return demonstration, role-playing), or nonexistent (allowing learner to learn by discovering her own mistakes).

When the laboratory is used as a learning setting, the following guidelines may be helpful:

1. Insofar as possible, schedule laboratory experiences at times when they will best complement both classroom and clinical learning experiences.

2. Be just as rigorous in defining objectives of the laboratory learning session as in defining classroom learning objectives.

3. Prepare learners by clearly stating the learning objectives, and by defining the tasks to be accomplished and the criteria of successful performance. When appropriate and necessary, provide detailed instructions with emphasis on order of execution.

4. Decide how the laboratory experience will be managed:
   a. To what extent structure and specificity will be necessary for the learning experience
   b. To what extent learners will be allowed to make mistakes and find their own ways in learning
   c. When and how you will intervene in guiding learning
   d. How you will relate this learning experience to classroom and clinical learning experiences
   e. How you will illustrate transferring the outcome of this learning experience to other comparable situations
   f. How you will evaluate learner performance
   g. How you will provide for learner integration and evaluation of the learning experience

DEMONSTRATION

In their basic training, nurses have to acquire and refine a multitude of psychomotor skills. A large majority of these clinical skills are at least initially learned by observing another's performance—the instructor, clinical preceptor, role model, or even an actor in an audiovisual program.

Especially when the technique or action is unique, new, or complex, the requisite behaviors are usually accompanied by paced explanations of appropriate underlying principles that correlate with each step or phase of the total procedure. To provide direct opportunity in performing the activity, the exhibition of model performance is followed by a period in which learners must replicate or do a return demonstration of a like performance under instructor guidance and feedback. Simultaneously using visual, auditory, and tactile sensory paths, the learner can see how to perform the activity, hear explanations of rationale and relevant concepts, and manipulate the objects and materials used in the actual procedure.

Observation (visual and auditory exposure) alone is insufficient for a learner to acquire skill; it is unrealistic to expect learners to be able to perform a given activity if the only learning experience provided is observation. Learners should not be expected to jump the knowing vs. doing chasm without instructor bridging. If you want the nurse to be able to perform the skill, you must provide for performance in the learning experience. Remember to match the learning experience with the behavior sought in the instructional objective.

Appropriateness for teaching. The demonstration method is appropriate for teaching how to operate and use biomedical equipment, perform techniques, carry out the sequential steps of a procedure, apply and illustrate principles, and test theories.

Guidelines for use. Before a demonstration, the instructor should do the following:
1. Identify the objectives and related content to be covered
2. Enumerate the key points, terms, and principles to be emphasized

3. Assemble and pretest all equipment and materials used in the demonstration; do a trial practice of all necessary steps
4. Organize the sequence of steps so that unnecessary details and steps are deleted
5. Select a location where learners can readily hear and view the demonstration
6. Attempt to secure conditions that most closely approximate those the learner will encounter in the clinical setting (for example, performing the demonstration in an unoccupied patient room using standard hospital equipment and supplies

When it is time for the demonstration, it is helpful if the instructor first:
1. Reviews the purpose and objectives for viewing the demonstration, emphasizing key points
2. Proceeds through the sequence of activities slowly enough for learners to grasp pertinent concepts and explanations, quickly enough to sustain learner attention, and frequently enough that each step in the sequence is understood and integrated with that which precedes and follows it

Immediately following the demonstration, the instructor should:
1. Offer learners the opportunity to raise questions, obtain clarifications, and review as necessary
2. Provide adequate time, preceptors, and materials for learners to do the required operations to attain mastery and to reach objectives for the session
3. Offer guidance, support, review, and feedback on learner performance
4. Allow for learner evaluation of the session
5. Modify future demonstrations based on learner feedback

SIMULATION

Simulation techniques comprise another category of teaching methods adaptable for direct transfer to the clinical setting. They can be categorized as laboratory methods because simulations attempt to replicate at least part and, at times, nearly all of the essential aspects of a clinical situation so that the situation may be more readily experienced, understood, managed, and evaluated when it later occurs. The more closely the processes and conditions of a simulation resemble the reality it is intended to represent, the greater the potential for transferring learning to that situation.

Whereas it must be borne in mind that no imitation of reality ever equals confronting the reality itself, simulations can be extremely useful in approximating reality in a more controlled environment focusing on specific learning objectives. Except for providing the actual clinical experience of the situation, simulations are very likely the next best option for providing certain types of learning experiences that are otherwise unobtainable.

Some of the values of simulations are that they:

1. More directly and actively involve learners in the learning process, while engaging learner interest and enjoyment
2. Provide for immediate feedback and reinforcement of learning
3. Approximate reality more closely than other available teaching methods
4. Simplify reality by focusing only on the aspects intended for learning, while providing a more holistic appreciation of that reality
5. Can be used without incurring the risk of adverse effects on patients or learners
6. More nearly bridge the theory-practice gap
7. Can provide for more meaningful and lasting learning experiences than can verbal or observational experiences; can allow learners to learn from mistakes and faulty problem solving
8. At times, reduce the time required to learn

9. Offer a vehicle for teaching affective and interpersonal behaviors that are otherwise difficult to provide
10. Capitalize on the adult's reservoir of experience and aptitudes
11. Can, incidentally, be both a novel and enjoyable learning medium
12. Accelerate learning by compressing into a single learning experience what might have taken days or weeks to obtain in the clinical setting

Appropriateness for teaching. Simulation techniques seem to be particularly appropriate for teaching decision-making, problem-solving, communication, and affective behaviors, as well as behaviors involving a complex interplay of social and interpersonal skills. Especially when learning requires a large measure of experience to grasp its essence, simulations of the experience may often be the only realistic way to approach teaching it.

Many simulation teaching methods are relatively new to nursing curricula, so that except for a few familiar techniques, nurses in a hospital may be largely unfamiliar with their use. Just as they are being found to be useful adjuncts to basic nursing programs, however, simulations are gradually working their way into continuing education programs in nursing.

The categories of simulation techniques considered here include physical simulations, simulated patients, simulated patient or clinical situations, written simulations, role-playing, and simulation games. Each possesses its own unique guidelines for use; these are mentioned in their respective sections.

Physical simulations

Physical simulations include a wide array of devices available for demonstrating, practicing, and refining many complex clinical skills. They include items such as Laerdal Medical Corporation's Resusci-Anne, Recording-Anne, Arrhythmia-Anne, adult and infant intubation manikins used for CPR and advanced CPR skills, training models for learning peripheral and central venipuncture, and the traditional Mrs. Chase patient models used to teach basic bedside skills such as bathing, positioning, suctioning, and ostomy care.

Physical simulations are a subcategory of audiovisual training aides, distinguished from other models by being scaled to real-life anatomical proportions. They are used for the actual practice of the specific skills, rather than only for illustration or clarification of anatomy, physiology, or scientific principles. Their value lies in the hands-on experience they provide for learners in acquiring and mastering clinical skills. In much the same way that these models are being used to teach physical diagnosis to medical students, they are proving to be worthwhile adjuncts to nursing education for both teaching and evaluating skills acquisition.

Guidelines. Using physical simulations requires that the instructor be thoroughly familiar with the models used and, preferably, be able to maintain and make minor repairs, know their idiosyncrasies and variations from real life, and make modifications for their easy use. As with other learning experiences, objectives and criteria for performance must be outlined and shared with learners.

Simulated patients

A second type of simulation involves using other individuals—peers, the instructor, or even professional actors—who pose as patients. Simulated patients are assigned predetermined sets of symptoms, problems, personalities, family, social and medical histories, or illnesses for the nurse learner to elicit, assess, or plan care for as she would in a real-life work situation. Unlike physical simulation such as using manikins, patients are real human beings—not inanimate objects transiently and mechanically imbued with life-like features.

Simulated patients are used most extensively in teaching physical assessment skills. They have proven to be a useful teaching strategy in medical schools for the last decade and are gradually appearing in nursing curricula. Using simulated patients is a valuable tool for teaching nurses how to elicit a health history, perform patient assessments, and arrive at nursing diagnoses to plan nursing care. Because most simulated patients are basically healthy individuals, the learning experience usually focuses on learning normals and normal variants rather than abnormals or the pathological conditions actually seen in clinical situations.

Guidelines. The individuals functioning as simulated patients must be adequately instructed and prepared for their assigned roles. They must be willing to maintain their roles as patients, to be poked, probed, percussed, palpated, and auscultated as determined by the learning objectives, and be capable of responding as programmed to the learner's queries. Their health histories, past and present symptoms, social and family problems may be wholly contrived or, for realism, mixed with their own personal data. Persons selected to serve as patients must be able to maintain a primary focus on meeting learner needs rather than their own, through natural, spontaneous, and credible responses.

The instructor is responsible for deciding on the necessary features of each needed patient type and for communicating this protocol to the prospective patient. Guidelines should be provided to patients on how they are to respond to certain questions or situations. As with using any other teaching medium, the instructor is responsible for evaluating the effectiveness of simulated patient performance.

Simulated situations

In much the same way as fire drills are used to teach individuals how to respond in case of a real fire, certain patient, unit, or hospital situations may also be contrived to provide learners with analagous experiences in managing them. Situations such as managing problem patients, supporting a dying patient, or handling a complex case may be constructed, depicted in real life staging, or viewed on film or transparencies for the learner to formulate the appropriate responses. Each scenario is constructed to elicit critical behaviors in the learner as determined by the learning objectives.

Videotaped simulated situations may be helpful in facilitating mastery of observational skills needed by nurses and in teaching clinical procedures and interviewing techniques.

Guidelines. For learners to gain from simulated situations, they need to recognize clearly the objectives and purposes of the session and the expected outcomes. This information will help learners focus on salient aspects of the situations as they will need to do in real life to learn the behaviors required to manage the situation effectively. Each session should be preceded by a review of its objectives and followed by a discussion of its effectiveness in meeting these objectives.

Written simulations

Rather than portraying problematic clinical situations in live or staged video formats, they may be presented as handwritten, typed, or computer-written clinical scenarios. As with other types of simulations, written simulations are valuable teaching devices that enable the instructor to circumvent having only a limited number of the necessary types of learning experiences for a large number of learners. Because they do not involve many of the costly or time-consuming features of other simulations (hiring and training simulated patients, videotaping equipment and personnel, expensive and fragile manikins or models), written simulations are especially attractive teaching vehicles for the busy and budget-conscious educator.

Written simulations can be used for instruction and evaluation of a wide variety of learner skills: in critically analyzing complex situations,

setting priorities, identifying and defining issues relevant to a problem, developing diversity in approaching a problem, efficiently using resources and ancillary personnel, directing the activities of subordinates, effectively managing administrative issues, and budgeting time and materials economically.

More than a decade ago, de Tornyay suggested that written simulations should have a place in nursing curricula, although their use is still somewhat limited today.

Guidelines. When using written simulations, the problem situation must be as plausible and close to a real-life situation as possible. Once the initial scenario is defined, learners are free to select among a number of possible options that vary in their degree of appropriateness to that situation. Each option that could potentially be selected has prepared feedback supplied for it. On making a decision, the learner is given this feedback to see the results of that decision. Once a decision has been reached, the learner may then be given a chance to rethink the consequences of the decision and select another option. Feedback provides the reinforcement necessary for affirming sound decision making and for discouraging faulty problem solving.

Sophisticated computerized programs may require the technical and programming expertise of an educational technologist, whereas less complex simulations may be formulated by the instructor.

Role-playing

Role-playing has been used extensively in nursing. Affective and psychosocial aspects of nursing have virtually cornered the exclusive use of this technique, although its use need not be so limited.

Role-playing is a spontaneous enactment of a true-to-life situation. Once the educator has defined the focus or problem of the role-play, she must construct an appropriate situational context and assign salient roles. The role-play is then executed until all relevant behaviors have been demonstrated, at which point the play is terminated and the entire group discusses it and its implications.

The actors may be volunteers from the learner group or, in some circumstances, the instructor. Although participants in the role-play are briefed, the dialogue and interpersonal exchange proceed extemporaneously without script or prompting, based on actors' perceptions of how they would behave in this situation.

As with other simulation techniques, role-playing enables participants—actors directly and observers indirectly—to develop process skills through the experience of situations representative of those they will later encounter in real life.

The purpose of role-playing is to teach processes rather than factual content. The primary educative value of the role-playing technique is its ability to teach interpersonal processes such as effective listening, communication, interviewing, patient teaching, and the behavioral aspects of providing psychosocial support to patients and families. Role-playing may be used to assist in teaching nurses to elicit a patient's health history, to work together with patients and families in designing an appropriate plan of nursing care, to provide patient education classes, and to counsel families of terminally ill patients.

A second effective use of role-playing is in fostering the development of affective skills that require learners to acknowledge and deal effectively with the delicate interplay of values, emotions, and feelings commonly found in clinical nursing situations. These include sessions dealing with ethical issues in nursing, managing conflict, facilitating planned change, and handling emergencies. Rather than merely talking about these affective areas, role-playing provides learners with a nonthreatening atmosphere in which they can actually experience and deal with the situations as they arise. In this context, role-playing serves as a dramatic and inherently involving way of illustrating and motivating required learning so that it is meaningful and readily applicable to the learners. As a simulation, it also circumvents the potentially hazardous effects on patients and nurses of saying or doing something inappropriate in a situation.

Guidelines. Unless this technique is managed effectively, role-playing may be little more than entertainment. Some guidelines for effectively using this technique include the following:

1. The capability and facility of the instructor in using role-playing as a method of instruction should heavily influence its use. Secure others skilled in using this technique rather than attempting to construct and use role-playing situations not within your range of capability.
2. Select topics appropriate for this technique (i.e., process vs. content learning).
3. Succinctly and clearly define the situational context and avoid extraneous roles.
4. Judiciously cast the roles to optimize learning potential in the experience.
5. Clearly communicate the objectives of the session to both learners and participants.
6. Insofar as possible, minimize discomfort or anxiety of the actors by encouraging their natural and uninhibited presentation.
7. Closely monitor the enactment for poignant events and developments that should be noted later in the discussion period.
8. Maintain and guide players within their assigned roles.
9. Limit the enactment period to the time required to meet the objectives—usually not more than 10 to 15 minutes.
10. Use the discussion period following the role-playing to:
    a. Reexamine and analyze the observed behaviors of depicted roles as they emerged from the situation
    b. Analyze the behaviors in roles as they were actually presented rather than what they might reveal about individual participants who portrayed them

c. Summarize and generalize learning outcomes in relation to the objectives

d. Identify direct and indirect implications of this experience for nursing practice

e. Elicit suggestions on how the role-playing process could be revised and improved for future use

Simulation games

A simulation game is a teaching technique that further optimizes the advantages of simulation by structuring the simulation within a game format. This teaching method especially facilitates learning because the simulation format encourages safe, meaningful, and relatively controlled interaction among participants in experiencing some process or aspect of reality, while the game format fosters learner interest and motivation by providing a fun way of learning. Simulation games may be used to introduce or provide an overview of some phenomenon, to offer practice in applying classroom learning, or to predict or evaluate learner performance.

As a learning tool, simulation games are designed for the learners to attain specific instructional objectives. In simulation gaming, the objectives may center around the acquisition of cognitive, affective, or psychomotor learning. Games are often used to teach the less tangible areas of instruction such as interpersonal skills, work organization, communication, consciousness raising, and management principles. When the game elements are consistent with the reality they are intended to represent, their validity facilitates transferring learning to the real world.

Games may be useful for acquiring social and affective skills and, to a lesser extent, for learning factual material. As experiential modes of learning, simulation games aim at assisting the learner in better understanding events and phenomena so they will be more capable of managing these situations when they eventually arise in the real work situation. Simulation is intend-ed to facilitate transferring learning from the contrived to the real world. In some instances, simulation games may be used for evaluation purposes—for self-evaluation, instructor evaluation of learner performance, or even in patient teaching. Pregame and postgame conferences can be used to set the stage for learning and to extract the outcomes of learning for their application to practice.

Simulation games are not only novel approaches to learning but are inherently more enjoyable experiences than listening to a lecture or preparing for group discussion. Learning derived from personal experiences of even an analogous situation is usually more meaningful and long-lasting because it is reinforced by recalling the experience. Simulation games also incorporate many principles of adult education such as active learner participation, tapping the learner's reservoir of experience, providing meaningful learning, and giving feedback on the quality of performance.

More specifically, simulation games involve interactive activities among participants whose actions are governed and restricted by specified roles, contexts, constraints, a clearly defined set of rules, methods for clearly differentiating winners from losers, and arbitrary, predetermined endpoints for the games. Chance factors such as using playing cards or dice may be incorporated when appropriate to the intended reality. Taken collectively, the elements comprise salient aspects of a situation learners need to experience to heighten their understanding of some phenomenon.

Simulation games can be as effective as more traditional forms of instruction in learners' acquisition of cognitive and affective behaviors as long as conventional approaches to instruction are not neglected. As with any other teaching method, simulation games should only be used when they are appropriate for facilitating the intended learning outcomes. Games can be as simple as providing participants with the opportunity to experience a contrived disaster, to be physically handicapped, or to play the role of a triage nurse. Games can also be highly sophisticated and technically intricate replications of complex intellectual or interpersonal processes. Using and designing simulation games constitutes an area of expertise that often requires the advanced training of the nurse educator. Whereas courses and workshops in simulation techniques are gaining in popularity and availability, some general guidelines can be offered here.

Guidelines. Before using a simulation game with learners, be sure to read the instructor's manual carefully. Gather a group of peers or learners comparable to your intended audience and pilot test the game. Note how the instructor's role varies from provider of information to facilitator and guide of learner activity. Determine how best to introduce, interact, and summarize the activity. It may even be helpful to switch roles and experience the game from the learner's perspective. Try to identify pitfalls, problems, and likely learner responses so you can deal with these more effectively during the actual learning experience. Plan for providing seating facilities, audiovisual media, or additional handouts that may enhance the experience or its transfer to the work situation.

Be certain that you can clearly communicate the object of the game, its roles, rules, and sequence so that learners know how to start, proceed, and end the game. Decide whether learning should occur spontaneously or be directed by your delineation of the game's objectives.

Determine what your role will be during the activity. Decide what you will be watching for and how you will accomplish this. Check whether more than one proctor will be needed and how and where each will function. During the pilot testing, see which rules are most often violated and why.

Allow adequate time for a thorough debriefing at the end of the game. Make a list of principles, concepts, and key points you will want to elicit and reinforce, and decide how you will provide for these. Plan for both general and specific responses to the learning experience and its validity as a learning device. Consider how the game experience relates to past and future learning and to how it transfers to the reality of the work situation. Be certain that the moral is the focus rather than the details of the game itself.

If you have not found a game suitable for your needs and are considering designing your own, it would probably be helpful to consult the references provided on this topic beforehand. Some general guidelines for designing simulation games follow.

First, isolate and clearly specify the educational need. On the basis of that need, define the instructional objectives and the characteristics of the learner group. Verify that meeting the objective merits indirect rather than direct experience. Is direct experience too uncontrollable, costly, time-consuming, unsafe, or difficult to obtain? Is experiencing the situation really necessary to learn the required lesson? If so, simulation games may be quite appropriate for your needs. If you are less than certain about this, consider alternative teaching methods. Simulations are most appropriate for highly abstract, intangible, or novel areas of learning. Games are not universally or necessarily the most effective or efficient mode of learning.

Once you have decided that a simulation game would be an appropriate learning medium, delineate the reality situation you wish to represent. From that sample of reality, decide which of all its elements are most critical for learners to experience. You will have to be selective here and avoid attempts at including so many complexities that the message gets lost in the medium. Keep the reality situation no more inclusive than it needs to be to cover all essential aspects you wish learners to experience. Needless detail will obscure the purpose of the activity.

The representation of reality you construct should be consistent with reality itself. The roles, rules, activities, consequences, and winners should be meaningful, relevant, and true to what learners will later encounter. Keep rules brief and few and time limits reasonable.

Conduct informal and formal tryouts of the game. Make changes based on this feedback as often as necessary until the final product has earned the right to be used with an actual learner group. Sometimes a well-constructed game is better than the real thing it represents.

REFERENCES

Laboratory teaching methods

Kaelin, MS, and Bliss, JB: Evaluating newly employed nurses' skills, Nurs Outlook 27:334, 1979.

Little, D, and Carnevali, D: Complexities of teaching in a clinical laboratory, JNE 11:15, 1972.

Paduano, MA: Bringing about learning in the college laboratory, JNE 17:30, 1978.

Simulations

Atkinson, FD: Designing simulation, gaming, activities: systems approach, Educ Tech 17:38, 1977.

Barrows, HS, and Tamblyn, RM: Problem-based learning in health sciences education, Atlanta, 1979, National Medical Audiovisual Center, Department of Health, Education, and Welfare.

Cooper, SS: Methods of teaching—revisited: games and simulation, J Contin Educ Nurs 10:14, 1979.

de Tornyay, R: Measuring problem-solving skills by means of the simulated clinical nursing problem test, JNE 7:3, 1968.

Greenblat, CS: Gaming—simulation and health education—an overview, Health Educ Monogr 5:5, 1977.

Horn, RE, and Cleaves, A, editors: The guide to simulations/games for education and training, ed 4, Beverly Hills, Calif., 1980, Sage Publications, Inc.

Jeffers, JM and Christensen, MG: Using simulation to facilitate the acquisition of clinical observational skills, JNE 18:29, 1979.

Kruse, LC, et al: Utilization of a media instructional support staff in the development of a simulated learning experience: medication administration, JNE 17:27, 1978.

McIntyre, HM, et al: A simulated clinical nursing test," Nurs Res 21:429, 1972.

Pearson, BD: Simulation techniques for nursing education, Int Nurs Rev 22:144, 1975.

Wolf, MS, and Duffy, ME: Simulations/games: a teaching strategy for nursing education, New York, 1979, National League for Nursing.

Zuckerman, D, and Horne, RE: The guide to simulations/games for education and training, Lexington, Massachusetts, 1973, Information Resources.

Simulated patients

Barrows, HS: Simulated patients, Springfield, Ill, 1971, Charles C Thomas, Publisher.

Frazer, NB, and Miller, RH: Training practical instructors (programmed patients) to teach basic physical examination, J Med Educ 52:149, 1977.

Lincoln, RE, Layton, J, and Holdman, H: Using simulated patients to teach assessment, Nurs Outlook 26:316, 1978.

Sherman, JE, et al: A simulated patient encounter for the family nurse practitioner, JNE 18:5, 1979.

Stillman, PL, et al: An objective method of assessing physical examination skills of nurse practitioners, JNE 18:31, 1979.

Written simulations

McGuire, CH, Solomon, LM, and Bashook, PG: Construction and use of written simulations, New York, 1976, The Psychological Corporation.

Page, GG, and Saunders, P: Written simulation in nursing, JNE 17:28, 1978.

Role-playing

Cooper, SS: "Methods of teaching—revisited: dramatic representation: skits, J Contin Educ Nurs 10:34, 1979.

Cooper, SS: Methods of teaching—revisited: role-playing, J Contin Educ Nurs 11:57, 1980.

Lewis, FM: A time to live and a time to die: an instructional drama, Nurs Outlook 25:762, 1977.

Reakes, JC: Behavior rehearsal revisited: a multifaceted tool for the instructor, JNE 18:48, 1979.

Simulation games

Abt, CC: Serious games, New York, 1970, Viking Press.

Clark, C: Simulation gaming: a new teaching strategy in nursing education, Nurs Educ 1:4, 1976.

Crancer, J, and Maury-Hess, S: Games: an alternative to pedagogical instruction, JNE 19:45, 1980.

Davidhizar, R: Use of simulation games in teaching psychiatric nursing, JNE 16:9, 1977.

Dearth, S, and McKenzie, L: Synoptics: a simulation game

for health professional students, J Contin Educ Nurs **6**:28, 1975.

Greenblat, CS, and Duke, RD, editors: Gaming-simulation: rationale, design and applications, Beverly Hills, Calif., 1975, Sage Publications.

Hayman, J: "Games—a teaching strategy, Nurs Outlook **25**:302, 1977.

Horn, RE, editor: The guide to simulations/games for education and training, ed 3, Cranford, N.J., 1977, Didactic Systems.

Lange, CM: Matching media to learning styles, Nurs Outlook **25**:18, 1977.

Lowe, J: Games and simulations in nurse education, Nurs Mirror **141**:68, 1975.

Maidmont, R, and Bronstein, RH: Simulation games—design and implementation, Columbus, Ohio, 1973, Charles E. Merrill Publishing Co.

McKenzie, L: Simulation games and adult education, Adult Leadership **22**:293, 1974.

Morris, L, et al: Student-made, student-played games, Am J Nurs **80**:1816, 1980.

Seidl, AH, and Dresen, S: Gaming: a strategy to teach conflict resolution, JNE **17**:21, 1978.

Smoyak, SA: Use of gaming simulation by health care professionals, Health Educ Monogr **5**:11, 1977.

Teaching affective skills

Conners, VL: Teaching affective behaviors, JNE **18**:33, 1979.

Davidhizar, RE: Use of simulation games in teaching psychiatric nursing, JNE **16**:9, 1977.

Davidson, ME, and McArdle, PE: Peer analysis of interpersonal responsiveness and plan for encouraging effective reshaping—pair/peer, JNE **19**:8, 1980.

Farrell, M, Haley, M, and Magnasco, J: Teaching interpersonal skills, Nurs Outlook **25**:322, 1977.

Finley B, Kim, K, and Mynatt, S: Maximizing videotaped learning of interpersonal skills, JNE **18**:33, 1979.

Friedrich, RM, Scandrett, S, and Turock, A: Innovations in continuing education: a statewide program for systematic training in interpersonal skills, J Contin Educ Nurs **10**:29, 1979.

Hazzard, ME, and Thorndal, ML: Patient anxiety: teaching students to intervene effectively, Nurse Educ **4**:19, 1979.

Krathwohl, DR, Bloom, B, and Masia, BB: Taxonomy of educational objectives: affective domain, New York, 1964, David McKay Co.

La Monica, EL, and Karshmer, JF: Empathy: educating nurses in professional practice, JNE **17**:3, 1978.

Lewis, FM: A time to live and a time to die: An instructional drama, Nurs Outlook **25**:762, 1977.

Reilly, DE: Teaching and evaluating the affective domain in nursing programs, Thorofare, N.J., 1978, Charles B. Slack.

Rynerson, BC: Using videotapes to teach therapeutic interaction, Nurs Educ **5**:10, 1980.

Wheeler, PR: Nursing the dying: suggested teaching strategies, Nurs Outlook **28**:434, 1980.

Chapter 12

Teaching methods for the clinical setting

If nursing is regarded as a clinical practice discipline, then all the teaching methods discussed thus far are effective only to the extent that they eventually become evident in nurses' clinical practice. Knowledge of facts, concepts, and principles without the attendant capability for applying these is in a very pragmatic sense useless.

A frequent criticism of new graduate nurses is that they "know" but cannot "do." "Knowing" without the ability for "doing" is often indistinguishable from not knowing at all. A recent poll of nurse administrators in Pennsylvania supports the finding that nursing administration persists in its general dissatisfaction with the immediate products of both baccalaureate and associate degree programs, and strongly prefers the diploma-prepared nurse for employment. But even the diploma program graduate frequently needs a measurable amount of assistance from the service employing her to make the full and successful transition from knowing to doing. Even in programs that provide superlative opportunities for nursing students to acquire the knowledge and skills requisite for effective clinical practice, unless these skills are recurrently practiced first in similar and then in dissimilar clinical situations, soon after they are initially learned, they often quickly evaporate from the nurse's capabilities.

If the clinical area is at the forefront in nursing, then instruction in this setting acquires paramount importance. Clinical teaching methods are intended to provide previews of the actual experience. Insofar as clinical practice is the raison d'être for all forms of basic or continuing nursing education, then the quality and extent of these previews are highly important for their eventual performance.

Unlike the classroom teaching setting, the clinical setting offers a less controllable, dependable, consistent, or structured environment. It is frequently less than the ideal that can be so clearly presented and propagandized in the classroom. Unlike the secure confines of the classroom, the clinical setting can be frightening, anxiety ridden, and anxiety producing for both instructors and learners. Unlike the laboratory setting, the clinical setting is markedly less tolerant of mistakes, omissions, or errors in judgment, and spotlights inadequacies and potential problems that never surfaced in the laboratory settings: bleeding patients, irate physicians, patients who do not speak English, itinerant support services, double shifts, intimidating colleagues, and hefty patient assignments. What the clinical setting *does* have to offer is the reality of nursing practice.

Unfortunately, even the clinical setting can be structured in such a way that it more simulates than samples the realities there. To the degree this is true, the value of that clinical learning experience is diminished. Providing nurses with only one-to-one nurse-patient ratios throughout all of their learning experiences is an example of such an artificially designed clinical experience.

Until reality is actually experienced, the learner's perceptions of what is real will always fall short of true. This leaves the learner victim to confronting the real later when performance expectations are increased and the availability of resources is likely to be diminished.

If teaching in the clinical setting is so very crucial and indeed the primary focus for the continuing education of nurses, how can the instructor best provide for learning experiences in this setting? What elements should characterize learning in this setting? If you recall the distinguishing features of the clinical setting, you can gain the insight needed into what learning here should reflect. As with the other settings available for the continuing education of nurses, the type of learning experience provided in the clinical setting should reflect the characteristics of its environment.

The critical care unit setting is more variable, anxiety producing, and threatening to newcomers than most other clinical settings. Here, where acuity of illness, weight of professional responsibility, hectic pace, and limited margin for nurse error are a way of life, there can be virtually no assurance of ever having the right patient with the right needs available at the right time to provide for the learners' educational needs. Patients' hospital stays are usually short because of the heavy demand for critical care beds. This combined with the unpredictability of a critical care patient's clinical course makes it nearly impossible to schedule particular types of learning experiences with any degree of confidence that they will actually be available at their scheduled times. So, in planning clinical learning experiences for the critical care unit staff, the instructor would do well to always plan with the idea that the original plan may often have to be forsaken in favor of serendipitous learning opportunities. In reality, unforeseen events, emergencies, unanticipated patient care situations, and unique and unusual clinical problems are often the most meaningful

occasions for teaching in the critical care setting. Instruction here must be timely, sensitive to the setting, and flexible enough to capitalize on these occurrences as they arise so as not to waste the learning opportunities they offer.

FOUR MAJOR ELEMENTS TO CONSIDER

As discussed, teaching in the clinical setting is directed at assisting the learner to apply appropriate facts, concepts, and principles together with their affective components in providing direct patient care. To attain this end, the educator's planning should include consideration of at least four major elements:

1. Instructional objectives for the clinical area
2. Focus of clinical instructor's role
3. Components of process learning in the clinical setting
4. Intradepartmental and interdepartmental collaboration

Instructional objectives for the clinical area

As you review the instructional objectives and extract those appropriate for the classroom and laboratory learning settings, the remaining objectives should be those requiring process and interaction with patients. Objectives for the clinical learning setting should refer to learner behaviors such as applying principles, concepts, theories, and facts, demonstrating understanding of the interrelations among various concepts, and refining the performance of essential skills and procedures in actual clinical practice situations. If your objectives for the clinical area are appropriate, they should not focus primarily on the knowing or feeling components of learning, but should require learner-patient interaction and the integration of learning to the complexities of direct patient care.

Focus of clinical instructor's role

As in any other learning setting, your primary focus as the instructor is to facilitate learners' meeting the instructional objectives appropriate for that setting. Once you have identified the objectives for learners to attain in the clinical setting, your subroles center around facilitating learner attainment of these clinical objectives by functioning as:

1. An actualizer by making nursing care plans useful and real
2. A guide for learning by enhancing self-directed instruction rather than intervening directly
3. A reinforcer of material previously learned in classroom and laboratory settings
4. A resource for learning through posing and responding to questions and issues as they arise from the situation
5. A validator that learning has occurred; that is, that satisfactory performance and application have been attained
6. An evaluator of the quality and degree of learning acquired
7. A trustee of learning through conveying trust and confidence in learners' abilities to think critically, to intervene accurately and creatively, and to learn from mistakes

Components of process learning in the clinical setting

As emphasized previously, the clinical setting is the optimal learning environment for process learning activities. Ultimately, all applications of learning in the clinical setting are included within one of the four phases of the nursing process: assessment, planning, implementation, or evaluation.

Putting into operation each phase of the nursing process in the critical care unit environment requires the same fundamental abilities as it would in any other clinical setting, but usually to a greater degree. In general, nurses being groomed to function effectively in the critical care setting need additional breadth and scope of instruction in the following areas:

Assessment

1. Finely attuned development of a broad range of observational skills
2. Greater facility and expertise in assessing a patient's physiological, psychosocial, and pathophysiological status by means of an in-depth multisystem approach inclusive of laboratory and diagnostic test results
3. Effective and appropriate incorporation of biomedical instrumentation as the source for deriving many parameters of the data base
4. Reaching accurate interpretations of a large, complex, and highly interrelated data base
5. Appropriate characterization of those patient problems that can be influenced by nursing practice
6. Appropriate summarization of goals or outcomes to be sought in nursing practice
7. Identification of how patient and staff values influence assessments of patient's situation

Planning

1. Appropriate correlation between identified patient problem and the nursing interventions intended to alleviate, minimize, or manage the problem
2. Planning for nursing care that is adequate in scope and breadth of nursing interventions to reach the patient outcomes set
3. Facility in organizing a full work load that reflects the priorities of care and the amount of time available for providing care for all patients
4. Effectively formulating a plan of care that is individualized, succinctly stated, reality based, feasible under existing constraints, and clearly communicated for continuity of patient care
5. Analytical and critical thinking ability to effect sound and appropriate clinical judgments consistent with scientific rationale and recognized value systems of nurse and patient

Implementation

1. Refinement of clinical procedures initially practiced in laboratory setting
2. Capability of improvising, modifying, and troubleshooting when obstacles to implementation arise

3. Ability to respond quickly and appropriately in emergency situations
4. Putting into operation effective use of interpersonal and communication skills
5. Appropriate use of available resources
6. Increasing self-direction in assuming responsibility and accountability for nursing care requirements

Evaluation

1. Ability to identify readily criteria that will be used to determine the effectiveness of interventions selected to meet care objectives
2. Ability to perform accurate self-appraisals of performance in relation to meeting the goals of patient care
3. Appropriate identification of revisions necessitated in nursing care plan based on evaluation of its effectiveness
4. Ability to summarize succinctly and clearly an evaluation of the patient's health status over time

Intradepartmental and interdepartmental collaboration

With such a large number of health care workers participating in the care of critically ill patients, the educator must work closely with each of these groups to avoid interference and foster coordination in providing care.

It is virtually impossible to program rigidly and tightly learning experiences in the critical care setting. Learning experiences must be planned in conjunction with necessary unit activities. Although this is generally the case, some guidelines for scheduling learning activities in the clinical setting can be mentioned, as follows:

1. Consult with the head nurse or charge nurse to determine when events such as medical rounds, major therapies, patient care conferences, in-service classes, and other potential learning activities will occur so that learners may avail themselves of these opportunities.
2. Consult with the head nurse or charge nurse to determine if and when other learners (nursing or medical students, house staff) will be present on the unit to avoid or synchronize with their presence. At times, it may be better to distribute learners over the course of a day or week, whereas at other times two or more groups may gain more by working together.
3. Consult with the head nurse or charge nurse to determine regular unit staffing patterns that will be in effect. Whereas learners should not be scheduled to make up for staffing shortages, their presence on the units may secondarily complement staffing and effect improved rapport between regular staff members and learner groups.
4. Determine the number and availability of instructors or preceptors so that this resource availability coincides with learners' presence in the clinical area.
5. Consult with other professional groups and departments regarding their availability and responsibilities in the clinical area.
6. Be certain that initial scheduling of clinical rotations includes orientation to physical layout and unit routines.
7. Work with the head nurse or charge nurse in determining responsibilities and methods to be used for patient assignments to learners. Reach agreements on:
   a. Who is responsible for making assignments
   b. Whether dual assignments (staff preceptor, buddy system) will be used
   c. How the responsibility and accountability for patient care will be shared and divided if coassignments are used
   d. How and when learner will be weaned from the staff preceptor or buddy
   e. Differentiation between head nurse and clinical instructor's role with respect to learning needs and validation of learning

• • •

During the past decades, critical care nurses learned to become expert practitioners primarily through on-the-job training by their more experienced counterparts. Whereas this role model approach is still evident in the initial phases of critical care education, other methods have emerged for this purpose and are considered here: the role model and preceptor method, the performance checklist, multiple assignment, and bedside nursing rounds.

ROLE MODEL AND PRECEPTOR METHOD

Most nurses new to critical care nursing acquire the necessary knowledge and skills by exposure to learning situations provided by other nurses who already possess expertise in critical care nursing practice. These other nurses may include the critical care clinical nursing specialist, in-service or staff development instructors, head nurses, or other staff nurses. Although their positions and titles vary, they all have in common an expertise in critical care nursing practice. Ideally, they also have a willingness and ability to share this expertise in developing novice critical care nurses. Their educational responsibility is to function as role models for the critical care practitioner, exemplifying the highest standards of critical care nursing practice.

At some institutions, this clinical teaching responsibility is a shared one in which one or more of these other nurses or even other professional groups (for example, inhalation therapists, pharmacists, physicians) assume responsibility for various segments of nurses' learning experiences. Although the multidisciplinary approach to clinical instruction may offer the value of multiple perspectives on patient care, subspecialty expertise, and an initiation into collaborative professional relationships for patient care, nurses usually derive their greatest amount of learning from cues offered by their future peers, their staff nurse colleagues.

Depending on the unit's policies and procedures, and how these other nurses' roles and job descriptions are variously defined and put into operation, it may be unclear who should be responsible for teaching new nurses about their role as critical care nurses. To arrive at some broad guidelines for this decision it may be helpful to remember that the role model method of teaching is based on expertise for its legitimacy and authority: whoever is most expert and capable of effectively demonstrating that expertise should function as a role model for that aspect of staff nurses' training. Some general guidelines in this respect include the following:

1. Staff nurses: patient care routines, policies, and procedures related to patient care; unit orientation (physical layout, location of equipment); taking off medical orders, patient transfer, admission, discharge, and postmortem care; functional roles if existent (medication nurse, treatments); role as primary nurse; role as nursing team member.

2. Head nurses: unit policies and procedures related to administrative areas of responsibility, personnel policies, employment policies, procedures, and unit protocols; expanded management roles such as charge nurse, team leader, assistant head nurse, and chain of command.

3. Critical care instructors: clinical and role responsibilities requiring greater expertise and more time for development than staff nurses or head nurses are able to provide; use of new equipment and introduction to new procedures; ongoing in-service programs; supervising orientation process.

4. Clinical nurse specialists for critical care: when learning requires advanced preparation that others are unable to provide; function as consultant and resource to staff nurse, head nurse and critical care instructor in areas related to clinical practice.

Because of the exceptional amount of variability and interpretation of these roles, definitive guidelines are difficult to determine. The important feature to be reemphasized is that the best qualified person be selected as the instructor for a particular aspect of learning. A clinical nursing specialist may be deemed the most appropriate person to teach theoretical and skill segments to the nurse. But if this clinical specialist has never worked as a staff nurse in the unit, or is unfamiliar with the detail of the unit and its policies and procedures, she is likely not the most appropriate person to be conveying this information. Likewise, if the staff nurse is limited in her ability to explain certain patient problems or the rationale for therapeutics employed, the head nurse, critical care instructor, or clinical nursing specialist should be sought for this instruction.

If the intricacies of a particular area of patient care cannot be adequately explained by any of these resources, an individual with expertise in the area should be solicited to provide that instruction. For example, if a unit that previously employed inhalation therapy technicians to administer all chest physiotherapy decided to change its policies so that nurses would now perform this function, and if none of the other nurses were well acquainted with this procedure, an inhalation therapy technician might be the most appropriate instructor. Insofar as possible, always match nurses' learning needs with an instructor who possesses the greatest amount of expertise for teaching in that area. Blindly vesting all of the responsibility for instruction in one person may result in new nurses failing to obtain the most relevant learning experience.

The preceptor model is a vehicle for providing one-to-one role modeling of a present staff nurse with the new staff nurse. It is rooted in the logical assumption that the best role model for the new staff nurse is an experienced colleague in the same role. Thus, experienced staff nurses serve as preceptors for new staff nurses, experienced charge nurses for new charge nurses, and experienced head nurses for new head nurses. As a general rule, this is true. Under certain circumstances, however, it may not always be valid. As long as the preceptor is truly a competent practitioner and effective teacher who recognizes the limitations of her expertise, and calls on others as resources when appropriate, she can likely provide these new staff nurses with meaningful learning experiences. If she is less than wholly competent and well versed in her practice, unable to teach, or fails to use appropriately other resources, she may prove more of a hindrance than a help in the development of the new nurse.

The preceptor or buddy is typically co-assigned with the new nurse for a specified period of time, specifically, until the novice is capable of functioning independently. The new nurse may assume the experienced nurse's schedule or vice versa to maintain continuity of instruction. Together with her preceptor, the new nurse functions in all aspects of the staff nurse's role as a practitioner in critical care nursing.

The scope of the preceptor or role model's responsibility includes the following:

1. Identifying behavioral outcomes needed by all new staff nurses on that unit
2. Assessing present capabilities of the new nurse in relation to these necessary knowledges and skills
3. Verifying abilities and knowledge allegedly possessed by the new nurse
4. Specifying learning needs not already met by previous experience
5. Setting priorities of learning needs
6. Mutually planning with the new nurse how these learning needs will be best met
7. Providing learning experiences designed to meet these learning needs
8. Mutually evaluting effectiveness of learning experiences in meeting learning needs
9. Communicating progress of the preceptorship to learner and head nurse, both verbally and in writing
10. Keeping current records on progress of the preceptorship

11. Seeking additional resources for learning when appropriate: media, other nurses, other professionals

When the new nurse is able to function more independently, she is gradually weaned from the preceptor or buddy, whom she seeks as a first-line resource.

As mentioned in Chapter 7, the preceptor model may also provide a more reality-based learning experience for the novice than might be provided by instruction from someone other than a staff nurse. For new graduates, this is an important feature of orientation to the real practice of nursing and helps in countering the tendency for reality shock and disillusionment with the profession. The preceptor method of teaching may also assist in integrating the new nurse into her peer group, acquaint her with her support systems, diminish the threat of the critical care environment, and foster professional colleagueship.

Hohman describes a similar application of the preceptor model with a group of primary care nurses. Her approach, the mentor system, is used on an ongoing rather than orientation basis with teams of primary care nurses. As a team leader, the nurse mentor functions primarily as a role model in setting and putting into operation high standards of patient care, patient teaching, family counseling, and in providing instruction in the principles underlying patient care.

Chapter 7 described a number of desirable and undesirable traits for selecting classroom and clinical instructors. In addition to possessing these traits, nurses who are to function as role models, preceptors, buddies, or mentors should be selected on the basis of the following criteria:

1. Knowledge: The preceptor should be able to provide accurate and adequate explanations of principles underlying the nurse's role with regard to patient care, and interaction with families and other health team members.

2. Skills: The preceptor must be able to perform correctly the clinical procedures required of her.

3. Experience: The preceptor should be experienced in the practice of critical care nursing to a degree sufficient to enable her to troubleshoot problems, modify procedures, and demonstrate flexibility, maturity, and sound judgment in her decisions.

4. Familiarity with the preceptor role: The preceptor should be clear on her responsibilities to the new nurse, head nurse, and others responsible for the nurse's training and should know how and when to use available resources.

5. Familiarity with principles of the teaching-learning process for adults: The clinical preceptor should possess a working knowledge of principles of adult education and the teaching-learning process as previously outlined and know how to put these into operation, how to identify problems in the educational process, and how to seek resources if necessary to resolve these problems.

6. Willingness to assume preceptor role: The preceptor should be voluntarily functioning in this role rather than being coerced, pressured, cajoled, or otherwise forced into it. Not all nurses wish to function as preceptors and not all nurses function satisfactorily even though they may be willing to assume the additional duties. The good preceptor is both willing and competent to function in this capacity; the former does not negate the need for the latter.

PERFORMANCE CHECKLISTS

McCaffrey describes a criterion-referenced checklist that may be used to teach complex clinical skills to nurses. The term *criterion-referenced* refers to there being a stated criterion or accepted standard of performance specified for each skill.

The checklist (Example 12-1) is developed by

first delineating each behavior or step required for the successful performance of a procedure. Any necessary criteria for this performance are included in the stated behavior. Some steps in the procedure are deemed as "critical" or "essential" and must be incorporated as described for "successful completion." Other behaviors may only be "desired" ones and are not absolutely necessary to achieve for satisfactory performance.

Because the checklist specifies exactly what is expected in the performance of this skill, the nurse prepares herself through self-directed pursuit of her resources (library, media, observation of peers, critical care instructors) at her own pace. When she feels fully prepared to perform the skill, she seeks out the instructor who will verify the quality and inclusiveness of her peformance by using the same checklist.

In addition to fostering principles of adult education, this method of teaching may potentially reduce learner anxiety and uncertainty

---

Example 12-1. Recording a 12-lead ECG

INSTRUCTIONS: As part of your orientation to this unit, you must learn to properly record a 12-lead ECG. The checklist that follows delineates the steps necessary to perform this clinical skill. You may use the checklist for learning how to acquire this skill; the unit in-service instructor will use the *same* form to evaluate your performance of the skill. Steps marked with an asterisk are "essential steps" that must all be included for your performance to be rated as "successfully completed."

	Done	Not done
1. *Prepares patient and equipment*		
a. Verifies patient's name	☐	☐
b. Introduces self and explains purpose and elements of procedure to patient	☐	☐
c. Plugs in grounded single channel ECG recorder	☐	☐
d. Turns power switch to "on"	☐	☐
e. Checks that there is sufficient amount of ECG paper to complete recording; replaces paper roll if necessary	☐	☐
f. Draws curtain around patient's bed	☐	☐
g. Places patient in supine position at (45-degree) semi-Fowler's angle	☐	☐
h. Exposes patient's distal limbs and chest	☐	☐
*i. Prepares skin surfaces on limbs and chest by cleansing with alcohol pad and mildly abrading friction	☐	☐
*j. Applies conductive material (alcohol pad, electrode gel) to underside of each of four electrode plates without allowing leakage of material when plate is secured	☐	☐
*k. Securely attaches each designated electrode plate to its appropriate limb without straining or kinking cable wires	☐	☐
*l. Records patient's name, date, and time on ECG paper	☐	☐
2. *Standardizes ECG for time and voltage*		
a. Turns control knob to "run"	☐	☐
b. Centers stylus on ECG paper	☐	☐
c. Verifies paper speed is 25 mm/sec	☐	☐
d. Turns lead selector switch to "STD"	☐	☐
e. Presses STD button (1 mV) and verifies presence of a 10 mm boxed deflection; adjusts to 10 mm deflection if necessary	☐	☐
f. Verifies sensitivity switch is on "1"	☐	☐
g. Verifies all waveforms are observable; if voltage inadequate, increases sensitivity to "2"; if voltage excessive, decreases sensitivity to "½"	☐	☐

Continued.

Example 12-1. Recording a 12-lead ECG—cont'd

3. *Records six frontal plane leads*
   - *a. Records at least five ECG complex cycles for each of the six frontal plane leads ☐ ☐
   - *b. Records frontal plane leads in standard order: I, II, III, AVR, AVL, AVF ☐ ☐
   - c. Identifies each frontal plane lead by its respective code marking: ☐ ☐

I -	AVR ----
II --	AVL -----
III ---	AVF ------

     If marking button does not operate properly, writes lead on ECG paper by hand ☐ ☐
4. *Records six horizontal plane leads*
   - a. Turns control knob to "on" ☐ ☐
   - b. Attaches small suction cup to chest lead cable ☐ ☐
   - c. Applies small amount of electrode gel to each of six chest lead locations: ☐ ☐
     - V_1 = Fourth ICS, RSB
     - V_2 = Fourth ICS, LSB
     - V_3 = Midway between V_2 and V_4
     - V_4 = Fifth ICS, MCL
     - V_5 = Fifth ICS, Ant AXL
     - V_6 = Fifth ICS, Mid AXL
   - d. Applies suction cup to each V position ☐ ☐
   - e. Turns lead selector to V position and power switch to "run" ☐ ☐
   - *f. Records at least five ECG complex cycles for each of the six horizontal plane leads ☐ ☐
   - g. Records chest leads in standard order: V_1 to V_6 ☐ ☐
   - h. Identifies each horizontal plane lead by its respective code marking: ☐ ☐
     - V_1 ———— -
     - V_2 ———— --
     - V_3 ———— ---
     - V_4 ———— ----
     - V_5 ———— -----
     - V_6 ———— ------
5. *Concludes ECG recording*
   - a. Turns power switch to "off" ☐ ☐
   - b. Unplugs ECG recorder ☐ ☐
   - c. Detaches electrodes from patient ☐ ☐
   - d. Removes all conductive material from patient's skin ☐ ☐

---

over others' expectations of her performance, provide for consistency in the quality and nature of requisite clinical skills, promote professional responsibility and accountability for learning, and diminish the subjectivity, cost, and time required for performance evaluation. This checklist may also assist fledgling preceptors in their evaluation of a peer's performance by clearly indicating the criteria of satisfactory performance.

Although the checklist method is less adaptable for procedures requiring a significant amount of variability tailored to the patient's situation (providing emotional support), a vast array of skills can be taught through this method of instruction.

MULTIPLE ASSIGNMENT

In 1969 Hatrock described an approach to teaching clinical skills to nurses that offered an alternative to the one-patient-to-one-nurse approach. This alternative involved assigning three learners to the care of a single patient. One learner functions as the doer and is responsible for all direct patient care. A second functions as the researcher, who collects and provides a timely and inclusive data base to the doer so that it may be reflected in the care provided. The third member functions as an observer and is responsible for monitoring the effectiveness of care administered and the interactions between doer and researcher and doer and patient.

The postulated advantages of the multiple assignment method of clinical instruction include the following:

1. Peer participation in planning and evaluation of patient care
2. More economical in numbers of patients that must be available for learning experiences
3. Reduction in learner anxiety
4. Group identification and resolution of patient care problems

A 1976 study reported by Van Den Berg found the multiple assignment method superior to the traditional assignment of one learner to one or more patients. In measures of nursing knowledge (multiple choice items), concept usage (open-ended question items) and learner self-esteem index (Barksdale's building self-esteem items), learners assigned to the multiple assignment method showed greater amounts of improvement than did those who received the traditional patient assignment. Van Den Berg concluded that this teaching approach appears to be more effective than traditional approaches in the acquisition and application of concepts related to nursing practice.

The notion of grouping learners for coresponsibility in a learning situation is at times very useful. In the critical care environment, this method of teaching may not only diminish a sense of wariness in a learning situation, but may also foster professional collaboration in

obtaining a complete and accurate patient assessment, a more realistic and inclusive plan of care, more effective and expert implementation of that care plan, and a more objective and valid evaluation of care. Especially for critically ill patients, who have so many parameters and facets of care to be attended to, two or more perspectives on care may be able to improve significantly the quality of the care.

BEDSIDE NURSING ROUNDS

Before the advent of primary nursing, the head nurse, charge nurse, or team leader obtained pertinent data concerning the status and treatment of patients on a nursing unit by extracting a summary of this information from the nurse assigned to that patient. Although this information may have been garnered primarily for reporting it to superiors and to the oncoming charge personnel, the sharing of information certainly contributed to the reporter's experience learned about patients and their course of illness and response to therapy. If this information is no longer shared among the nursing staff, not only is the information sharing process lost, but so is a viable learning opportunity and vehicle for improving the quality, inclusiveness, and continuity of patient care.

The notion of bedside nursing rounds is very likely an offshoot of the traditional medical rounds that transpire in all teaching hospitals. Although both types of rounds involve a bedside discussion and evaluation of a patient's status and current therapies by those involved as care givers, nursing rounds are generally more holistic in scope, extending from the patient's health-related problems to incorporate psychological, social, cultural, and educational problems. Nursing rounds may also incorporate the patient as a more active participant in providing for the ongoing data base and evaluation of the plan of care.

Some of the other advantages that bedside nursing rounds offer include the following:

1. Providing a more meaningful learning experience than methods in either laboratory or classroom settings could provide
2. Locating the educational setting where the ultimate outcomes of learning are evidenced
3. Promoting a wider array of approaches to patient management
4. Fostering greater commitment to and continuity in selected plans of care arrived at by group consensus
5. Providing a mechanism to monitor and improve quality and continuity of patient care
6. Enabling learners to individualize and to set priorities for care from validated data base assessments
7. Demonstrating a wide range of normal variants and presentations of abnormal findings as they actually exist to afford relevant and meaningful learning experiences
8. Illustrating how to modify techniques, procedures, and other nursing interventions based on patient situations and real-life constraints

Bedside nursing rounds can be used to do the following:

1. Develop and finely tune patient assessment skills through direct observation, palpation, percussion, and auscultation of the real patient
2. Integrate laboratory and diagnostic data bases with the nurse's ongoing clinical assessment of patients
3. Stimulate peer review and critique of care plans
4. Incorporate patient participation in the plan of care
5. Teach and reinforce principles of normal and pathological physiology and assessment of response to interventions
6. Enrich the data base by providing multiple and variable perspectives

7. Expose a larger number of learners to learning experiences available on the unit
8. Provide a vehicle for patient and family education and for resolution of problems related to the impact of illnesses on patients and families
9. Provide a forum for self-evaluation and instructor's evaluation of learning
10. Foster self-directed learning activity that is immediately applicable
11. Enhance all phases of the nursing process
12. Develop ability to synthesize, organize, and cogently present the totality of a patient's situation to peers for their consideration
13. Foster enhanced self-confidence in assuming accountability for patient care

Nursing rounds can be conducted in a number of ways. At first, the instructor will likely take a more active role in structuring and managing the rounds. Once participants have decided on the most useful format for rounds, the instructor role may recede to that of a consultant resource, supplementing learners' efforts by offering additional instruction, suggesting role modeling, or setting standards of care.

The essential phases of planning for rounds include the following:

1. Determine the maximum number of learners who will participate in rounds. Most critical care units are short of space and overcrowding readily occurs; probably not more than three to four learners should be used; if nursing is one of many groups who perform bedside rounds, reduce the number of participants.
2. Select patients who will be presented during rounds, provide for a mechanism to prevent overuse of patients, and accommodate for such events as family visits, diagnostic tests, treatments, medications, and meals. When at all possible, patients'

willingness and ability to participate should be elicited.

3. Decide how patient presentations will be conducted.
   a. Learner may be given freedom to decide this with instructor functioning as resource or source of guidelines and suggestions.
   b. Content and duration of presentation should be agreed on. Presentation usually incorporates a summary of patient history, significant current clinical problems and clinical findings (laboratory, diagnostic, physical), verification of clinical findings, and synopsis of patient problems.
   c. Decide how patient will be asked to participate and how patient will be prepared.
   d. Decide criteria for terminating presentation: criteria of patient fatigue, deterioration in patient status, and meeting objectives of bedside rounds.
   e. Determine how concluding conference will be conducted for discussion of abnormal and problematic findings, identification of appropriate nursing interventions, specification of criteria that will be used to determine effectiveness of care, and planning or revising plan of care.

Like any other teaching method, bedside nursing rounds are intended to supplement and reinforce other learning experiences. Because they deliver the instruction to the forefront of nursing, however, they are potentially a most viable, meaningful, and reality-based vehicle for clinical instruction. When planned for the bedside critical care practitioner, nursing rounds provide an enriching learning experience complemented by elements of quality assurance and a truly professional colleagueship in nursing practice.

In summary, many teaching methods are available to the critical care nurse educator that may be considered in making the final decision about which method to use for meeting a specific instructional objective. Tailor your decision on the basis of the appropriateness of the method for facilitating learners attaining the objective. Remember to incorporate principles of adult education and those of the teaching-learning process. An illustration of how to match instructional objectives with teaching methods is provided in Appendix B. Evaluating how well objectives and learning experiences are matched is the subject of Chapter 13.

REFERENCES
Clinical teaching methods

Blake, KJ: Introducing new techniques and equipment, Superv Nurs **9**:21, 1978.

Gudmundsen, A: Teaching psychomotor skills, JNE **14**:23, 1975.

Hardy, LK: Keeping up with 'Mrs. Chase': an analysis of nursing skill-learning, J Adv Nurs **5**:321, 1980.

Harrell, JRS: Orienting the experienced critical care nurse, Superv Nurs **11**:32, 1980.

Hogan, R: Making clinical assignments, Nurs Outlook **24**:496, 1976.

Infante, MS: Toward effective and efficient use of the clinical laboratory, Nurs Educ **6**:16, 1981.

Jeffers, JM, and Christensen, MG: Using simulation to facilitate the acquisition of clinical observational skills, JNE **18**:29, 1979.

Knopke, HJ, and Diekelmann, NL: Approaches to teaching in the health sciences, Reading, Mass., 1978, Addison-Wesley Publishing Co.

Leonard, A: Client assesment, JNE **18**:41, 1979.

O'Shea, H: Reinforcing clinical study, Nurs Outlook **18**:59, 1970.

Pearson, BD: Considerations for student clinical assignments, JNE **16**:3, 1977.

Rauen, KC: The clinical instructor as role model, JNE **8**:33, 1974.

Schweer, JE, and Gebbie, M: Creative teaching in clinical nursing, ed 3, St. Louis, 1976, The C.V. Mosby Co.

Shortridge, L, et al: Opportunity to learn physical assessment in a continuing education course, J Contin Educ Nurs **8**:6, 1977.

Stritter, FT, and Flair, MD: Effective clinical teaching, Bethesda, MD., 1980, National Medical Audiovisual Center, Department of Health and Human Services.

Sullivan, K, et al: From learning modules to clinical practice, Nurs Outlook 25:319, 1977.

Wiedenbach, E: Meeting the realities in clinical teaching, New York, 1971, Springer-Verlag New York, Inc.

Yeaw, EMJ: Problem solving as a method of teaching strategies in classroom and clinical teaching, JNE 18:16, 1979.

Role model and preceptor method

Burke, W, Lukes, JJ, and Mansell, E: The preceptorship, an integral unit of the curriculum in community and family medicine, J Comm Health 3:271, 1978.

Cason, CL, Cason, GJ, and Bartnik, DA: Peer instruction in professional nurse education: a qualitative case study, JNE 16:10, 1977.

DePaolis, M: The need for teaching competencies in clinical instructors, AANA J 48:50, 1980.

Dell, MS, and Griffith, E: A preceptor program for nurses' clinical orientation, J Nurs Admin 7:37, 1977.

Goldsberry, JE: From student to professional, J Nurs Admin 7:191, 1977.

Haller, JA: Preceptorship—a vital ingredient in medical evaluation, Pharos 4:27, 1978.

Hohman, J: Nurse mentor system cuts costs, boosts quality of patient care, Hospitals 53:93, 1979.

Knauss, PJ: Staff nurse preceptorship: an experiment for graduate nurse orientation, J Contin Educ Nurs 11:44, 1980.

Levenstein, A: The nurse's role as teacher, Superv Nurs 9:20, 1978.

Maraldo, PJ: Better nursing care through preceptorships, RN 40:69, 1977.

May, L: Clinical preceptors for new nurses, Am J Nurs 80:1824, 1980.

McGrath, BJ, and Koewing, JR: A clinical preceptorship for new graduate nurses, J Nurs Admin 8:12, 1978.

Moyer, MG, and Mann, JK: A preceptorship program of orientation within the critical care unit, Heart Lung 8:530, 1979.

Personett, JD: The primary educator, JNE 16:38, 1977.

Pilette, PC: The mentor relationship, Nurs Outlook 26:329, 1978.

Rauen, KC: The clinical instructor as role model, JNE 8:33, 1974.

Rosenbaum, BL, and Bake, B: Do as I do: the trainer as a behavior model, Training HRD 16:90, 1979.

Williamson, JA, and Therrien, BA: The nurse preceptor. In Williamson JA, editor: Current perspectives in nursing education, vol 2, St. Louis, 1978, The C.V. Mosby Co.

Performance checklist

del Bueno, DJ: Performance evaluation: when all is said and done, more is said than done, J Nurs Admin 7:21, 1977.

Kelly, K: CPR—to certify or not to certify, Superv Nurs 11:34, 1980.

McBride, H: Flexible process—an alternative curriculum option: part 3. Clinical evaluation, JNE 18:20, 1979.

McCaffrey, C: Performance checklists: an effective method of teaching, learning and evaluating, Nurs Educ 3:11, 1978.

O'Leary, MM, and Holzemer, WL: Evaluation of an inservice program, J Nurs Admin 10:21, 1980.

Wyman, J, and Ferneau, K: Developing a criterion-referenced tool, Nurs Outlook 25:584, 1977.

Multiple assignment

Delorey, PE: Multiple assignments: rehearsal for practice, Am J Nurs 72:292, 1972.

Gustafson, DD: Student peer evaluation: a successful adaptation for observed home visits, JNE 19:4, 1980.

Hatrock, B: Multiple student assignments, Nurs Outlook 17:40, 1969.

Jackson, BS: An experience in participant observation, Nurs Outlook 23:552, 1975.

Saxon, J: Multiple asignments—try them, Am J Nurs 75:2183, 1975.

Van Den Berg, EL: The multiple assignment: an effective alternative for laboratory experiences, JNE 15:3, 1976.

Bedside nursing rounds

Bauer, CU: The clinician's use of nursing rounds. In Popiel, ES, editor: Nursing and the process of continuing education, ed 2, St. Louis, 1977, The C.V. Mosby Co.

Holm, K, et al: A teaching-learning experience: nursing rounds, JNE 17:33, 1978.

Jackson, BS, and Mantle, DD: Teaching patient assessment: the pros and cons of clinical rounds, JNE 16:24, 1977.

Malasanos, L, and Tichy, AM: The bedside clinic—nursing rounds as a teaching strategy, JNE 16:10, 1977.

Unit IV

EVALUATION

Chapter 13

The purposes and functions of educational evaluation

COMPONENTS OF EVALUATION

Planning, designing, and implementing educational programs do not guarantee a good program. The only way to verify the outcome of any learning experience is through a process of planned and systematic evaluation.

Evaluation is the process by which a judgment is made concerning the relative value of something. It is a largely subjective process that considers the various outcomes and effectiveness of an endeavor and then ascribes some qualitative assessment to those outcomes. The ultimate aim of evaluation is not merely arriving at the value judgment, but rather using such appraisals as a basis for subsequent decision making about the endeavor.

For evaluation to improve an educational program, its decision-making structure must be fortified by an efficient appraisal mechanism. An efficient evaluation process is useful in its form and content, virtually continuous in its occurrence, systematically ordered in its planning, inclusive in its coverage, and synchronous in its timing to the events and outcomes it seeks to monitor. Unless this process provides valid, timely, coherent, and useful appraisals, evaluation becomes an academic exercise.

Educational evaluation provides value judgments about both the educational process and its outcomes, and decisions can then be made for improving both.

In the education of critical care nurses, the educational process is directed at nurses attaining the cognitive, affective, and psychomotor capabilities that constitute competent critical care nursing. To the extent that evaluations verify that nurses attain these capabilities, the educational process is judged valid and effective. When evaluation reveals that they have not attained these capabilities, it may suggest the process variables that need to be modified to produce the desired ends. Evaluation, then, has a reciprocal relationship to both instructional objectives and the learning experiences provided to meet these objectives.

Measurement

An evaluation is the product of a measurement and some standard or criterion against which the measurement is compared. *Measurement* is a more objective process than evaluation. Measurement determines the amount, extent, magnitude, capacity, or degree to which some characteristic or attribute is present in some object or person. Measurement is the core of evaluation because it provides the raw data necessary to make an informed evaluation. Like evaluation, measurement incorporates the accumulation of observations with respect to some standard unit of measurement (such as 60 inches, 50 kilograms, 30 milliliters). Unlike evaluation, measurement is purely a quantitative assessment that passes no judgments (such as short or tall, emaciated or obese, adequate or inadequate) on the data.

Standard or criterion

The *standard* or *criterion* against which measurements are compared is a common reference point for making such comparisons. The standard may be held to a personal (value system), collective (standards of patient care), or universal (kilogram) degree, be real (ruler) or imagined (expectations), or be constant (time) or variable (attitudes). Regardless of its nature, the criterion functions as the standard of measurement for a given phenomenon to be compared with to render an evaluation of that phenomenon.

In educational evaluations, measurements are taken for various reasons by many different individuals and groups who seek information about a multitude of pertinent aspects of the educational process and its outcomes. These groups derive their observations at different times and in different places. Because the parties seek measurements of different aspects of the overall educational process, the tools and techniques used to derive measurements, the criteria against which the measurements are compared, and the nature and form of the resulting appraisal all differ.

A desire for sound decision making necessitates that one approach an investigation of the evaluation process with the same or greater degree of scrutiny than that applied to all preceding aspects of the educational process. The remainder of this unit will examine each aspect of the necessary investigation: the why, who, what, when, where, and how of the evaluation process.

EDUCATIONAL PROGRAM EVALUATION (THE WHY)

The evaluation process may be undertaken for any one of a number of reasons. As mentioned previously, educational evaluation is typically conducted to examine both the process and the product of the educational program.

Product versus process evaluation

Product evaluation is performed to determine whether instructional and program objectives have been attained or the degree to which these have been attained. *Process evaluation*, by contrast, examines the operational or procedural design and its implementation to appraise its effectiveness in meeting program and instructional objectives. Taken together, the findings of process and product evaluation provide the collective information necessary for *program evaluation*, the value judgment assigned to an entire educational program.

Functions of educational evaluation

The various functions of educational evaluation may be conveniently grouped according to whether they contribute more toward product or toward process evaluation. The potential functions provided by product evaluation include the ability to:

1. Determine whether the instructional objectives have been attained
2. Clarify, reinforce, and redefine instructional objectives
3. Appraise, certify, or differentiate attained learning
4. Motivate and positively reinforce learning through self-appraisal
5. Determine the nature and degree of behavioral change associated with learning
6. Differentiate present from previous level of competence

7. Diagnose the nature and extent of learning problems
8. Provide constructive feedback to learners
9. Predict future performance (aptitude tests)
10. Estimate present performance capability (achievement tests)
11. Determine present level of performance (power tests)
12. Determine speed of performance (speed tests)
13. Identify areas in need of remedial instruction (diagnostic tests)
14. Determine whether agreed on standards of performance have been met (mastery tests)
15. Differentiate degree of learning based on levels of performance
16. Positively reinforce learning by boosting morale and edifying learning attainment
17. Provide a focal point for learning by focusing attention on the important aspects to be learned
18. Promote learner's personal and professional growth

The potential functions served by process evaluation include the ability to:

1. Make decisions regarding subsequent planning, development, and implementation
2. Improve the effectiveness and efficiency of instruction
3. Adapt instruction to individual needs and abilities
4. Justify programming continuation or expansion
5. Provide feedback that promotes improvement in the teaching-learning process
6. Determine the effectiveness of various teaching methods and formats
7. Provide a mechanism for quality control in educational programming
8. Provide answers to questions that will arise regarding the educational process
9. Provide for accreditation and certification of educational programs

COMPARISON OF EVALUATION IN FORMAL VERSUS CONTINUING EDUCATION

The evaluation process used for continuing education programs is substantively the same process used in formal, academic education. Evaluation in a hospital-based program of continuing education for nursing differs from that in a formal educational setting primarily in its focus. Evaluation in formal academic settings is primarily aimed at verifying learning acquisition, whereas evaluation in a service setting is primarily aimed at verifying the application of learning to the practice or work setting.

Formal and hospital-based continuing education differ in the following variables that may influence both the outcome and the process of educational evaluation.

Focus. Participants in formal educational programs in nursing focus on obtaining a degree or diploma. Peer performance is used to evaluate the achievement of primarily theoretical competencies and the acquisition of learning. The credit system perpetuates a grade-oriented approach to learning. Participants in a program of continuing education in nursing, by contrast, focus on obtaining currency, clinical proficiency, and career mobility within the profession. Individual performance and achievement are the primary concerns, and emphasis is placed on extending theoretical to practical competence in the work setting. Continuing education is performance oriented and is primarily concerned with applying learning to the practice setting. There is no inherent reason why service-based programs of continuing education could not concurrently be degree-granting courses. Such programs are gaining popularity, but remain today more the exception than the rule.

Participant attendance. In academic settings, participants may be more easily scheduled and assembled for classes; participation may be mandated; and participants have common reasons for attending. In continuing education, participant attendance is a function of the participant's interest in and evaluation of the learning experience. Attendance typically cannot and should not be mandated, and participants may have widely varying reasons for attending.

Resources. In formal academic settings, organizational resources are all directed toward meeting educational goals. In the hospital setting, however, resources devoted to educational endeavors are often extremely limited in number and kind.

Nature and amount of evaluative data. In formal academic settings, a moderate array of data is readily available for a number of learning variables. The data necessary for evaluating continuing education programs consist of a wide array of many similar and dissimilar variables and are usually more difficult to obtain.

Instructors. Formal academic settings usually have a more homogeneous group of instructors in their expertise in the instructional and evaluation processes. In clinical settings, the instructor-to-learner ratio is usually low and the total number of evaluators is fairly circumscribed. In continuing education settings, the instructor-to-learner ratio may be exceedingly high, with a significant variability in the instructional and evaluative expertise of instructors. The wider variety of individuals who participate in the evaluative process in a hospital-based program of continuing education reflects the large number of individual evaluators.

Nature of learning experiences. In continuing education programs, learning experiences are usually much shorter and more limited in scope and depth than their academic counterparts. Likewise, the learning environment and the number of variables in the learning experience are much less structured and controllable. The content areas of academic learning experiences are well defined, whereas the content areas of continuing education programs may be unlimited in their extension.

Learners' standards of evaluation. In academic settings, learners usually estimate their performance based on the outcome of teacher-made tests and performance on standardized tests. Continuing education learners, on the other hand, use the realities of the practice setting as their primary standard for evaluation.

• • •

In summary, evaluation in continuing education differs from evaluation in formal programs of education more in its focus and scope than in its nature. Evaluation in continuing education extends well beyond acquiring learning to applying learning in the practice setting. In addition to its pragmatic focus, the service setting houses a greater number of groups and individuals who may influence and participate in evaluating educational programs offered there.

The ability to alter the scope and focus of evaluation suggests that the evaluation process is somewhat pliant, capable of adjusting its dimensions and components to the decisions it must direct. Depending on the number and type of decisions it must guide, the evaluation process may operate at varying levels and encompass a variable number of steps.

LEVELS OF EDUCATIONAL EVALUATION

The evaluation process may potentially extend through five progressively higher levels of evaluation. The level to which the evaluation process proceeds is dependent on three factors: the purposes for performing the evaluation, the nature and amount of resources available for the evaluation process, and the proficiency of evaluators at each progressive level.

The five levels of educational evaluation are as follows.

1. Satisfaction-reaction ("happiness index").

The satisfaction-reaction level of evaluation attempts to determine the participants' satisfaction or reaction to the material and to the learning experience. It bears no necessary relationship to learning anything. In general it determines the participants' initial and superficial responses to the learning experience, frequently supplied as participants hastily depart from the offering. Responses are usually categorical, summary statements, and nearly reflexive. At times the format of the response form may discourage negative responses by requiring additional time to complete them. Although this is usually the least time-consuming and costly vehicle for evaluating educational programs, it is also the least valuable and most subject to potential sources of bias less prevalent at other levels of evaluation.

2. Attainment of learning (instructional objectives). The attainment of learning level of evaluation is usually tied to program and instructional objectives with variable degrees of cohesion. The attempt here is to verify that learners have some degree of behavioral change (cognitive, affective, or psychomotor) as a result of participating in the learning experience. This level of educational evaluation is typically the culmination of most evaluation efforts in formal educational programs and may represent the logistical limits that outside (extramural) continuing education services may be able to provide. Most traditional classroom, teacher-made tests function at this level. They are reasonably easy to provide and do not necessitate any inordinate expense.

3. Transfer of learning to practice. Transfer of learning to practice is a continuation of the evaluation effort that provides follow-up of one or more behavioral changes (learning) that have been transferred into practice. Assuming the evaluation process is sound, this may be the most meaningful and valid level of evaluation for a practice-oriented profession. Unlike their outside counterparts, hospital-based continuing education programs have the potential for this type

of extended evaluation. Even at this limited extension, however, the complexity and sophistication of the evaluation process become increasingly greater and require delineating competency standards of critical care nursing practice. Precedents and expertise in evaluation at this level usually diminish, whereas the evaluation process becomes more difficult to design and implement. This level of evaluation is therefore performed less frequently and less adeptly.

4. Effect on patients. Effect on patients comprises a further extension of the evaluation process to determine if the transferred learning actually results in improved patient care. Patient outcomes are the measuring device at this level. Evaluating improved service to patients requires that one delineates patient care standards and makes sure that additional expertise in the evaluation process is available. Accordingly, the number of variables that may influence the evaluation outcomes expands.

5. Effect on the organization, system, and profession of nursing. Effect on the organization, system, and profession of nursing, the highest potential level of educational evaluation, is rarely afforded. At this level, norms and criteria for comparison of outcomes may be extremely limited and frequently unavailable. The monetary and expert personnel resources required for a truly comprehensive evaluation at this level are frequently unobtainable. In reality, representative segments of this level of evaluation may be available to the educator for sampling, but are frequently not pursued.

PROCESS OF EDUCATIONAL EVALUATION

In evaluating the educational process and its outcomes, you will reach a valid appraisal only if you approach the investigation systematically. This section has addressed the first step in this process by describing the many possible reasons for performing an educational evaluation. Knowing the general purpose and potential functions of evaluation, you must then determine which of these reasons constitute a rationale in the circumstances of your particular setting. If the primary purpose of evaluation is to provide a basis for subsequent decision making concerning the educational process and its outcomes, then the next logical series of steps includes the following:

1. Identifying *what* needs to be evaluated:
   a. What questions will need to be answered in the decision-making process
   b. What decisions will need to be made
   c. What criteria will be used in the evaluation
   d. What form data should be in to answer these questions
2. Specifying *who* should be involved in the evaluation process:
   a. Who desires evaluation information
   b. Who will need to be contacted to obtain evaluation data
   c. Who is in the best position to evaluate which aspects of the educational process and its outcomes
3. Determining *when* the evaluation information should be obtained:
   a. When is the optimal time to collect each type or category of evaluative data
   b. When is a reasonable time to schedule collecting evaluative information
4. Determining *where* evaluations should occur:
   a. Where settings are available to evaluate learning
   b. Where various types of learning are most likely to be evidenced
   c. Where other locations are for evaluating.
5. Determining *how* the evaluation process will proceed:
   a. How to select or design an adequate number of representative types of instruments for measuring or collecting each type of data necessary
6. Executing the evaluation process
7. Organizing and summarizing the information obtained
8. Analyzing and interpreting the information obtained to arrive at an evaluation of each pertinent area for decision making
9. Reporting the information and evaluations reached to individuals and groups needing these for decision making
10. Following through and participating in decision-making processes regarding the educational process and its outcomes
11. Modifying subsequent planning for the evaluation process based on decisions made from the evaluation

REFERENCES

The measurement and evaluation of learning

Chase, CI: Measurement for educational evaluation, ed 2, Reading, Mass., 1978, Addison-Wesley Publishing Co.

Ebel, RL: Essentials of educational measurement, ed 3, Englewood Cliffs, NJ, 1979, Prentice-Hall, Inc.

Gronlund, NE: Constructing achievement tests, ed 2, Englewood Cliffs, NJ, 1977, Prentice-Hall, Inc.

Gronlund, NE: Measurement and evaluation in teaching, ed 3, New York, 1976, Macmillan Publishing Co.

Nunnally, JC: Educational measurement and evaluation, New York, 1972, McGraw-Hill Book Co.

Thorndike, RL, and Hagen, E: Measurement and evaluation in psychology and education, ed 4, New York, 1977, John Wiley and Sons, Inc.

The evaluation of education in nursing

Abruzzese, R: Evaluation—what does it mean? Nurs Educ **5**:30, 1980.

Cowart, ME, and Burge, JM: Evaluation by jury, Nurs Outlook **28**:329, 1979.

Hitchens, EW: Evaluation: the graffiti technique, JNE **18**:46, 1979.

Jackson, MO: Instructor and course evaluation based on student-identified criteria, JNE **16**:8, 1977.

Kelly, RL: Evaluation is more than measurement, Am J Nurs **73**:114, 1973.

Lange, C: Using media in evaluation, Nurs Outlook **25**:241, 1977.

Marriner, A, Langford, T, and Goodwin, LD: Curriculum

evaluation: wordfact, ritual, or reality, Nurs Outlook **28**:228, 1980.

Meleis, AI, and Benner, P: Process or product evaluation? Nurs Outlook **23**:303, 1975.

Miller, M: Designing practical continuing education program evaluation forms, J Contin Educ Nurs **12**:6, 1981.

National League for Nursing: Generating effective teaching, New York, 1978, National League for Nursing.

Evaluation of formal versus continuing nursing education

Carroll, M: Evaluation of programs and individual courses. In National League for Nursing: The community college and continuing education for health personnel, New York, 1978, National League for Nursing.

Cornwell, JB: Quality assurance and control in training, Training HRD **17**:33, 1980.

Mitsunaga, B, and Shores, L: Evaluation in continuing education: is it practical? J Contin Educ Nurs **8**:7, 1977.

Smith, CE: Planning, implementing and evaluating learning experiences for adults, Nurs Educ **3**:31, 1978.

Wolanin, MO: Continuing educational approval committee works toward evaluation of nurse outcomes, J Contin Educ Nurs **10**:31, 1979.

Zemke, R: You can evaluate bottom-line results, Training HRD **17**:6, 1980.

Chapter 14

Evaluation of educational programs: preliminary determinations

WHAT NEEDS TO BE EVALUATED: AN OVERVIEW OF HOSPITAL-BASED EDUCATIONAL EVALUATION

Evaluation is performed for a number of groups and for a wide variety of purposes. The most immediately relevant segment of evaluation is in relation to attaining cognitive, affective, and psychomotor competencies as specified in the instructional objectives. Because of its importance to the entire evaluation process, the measurement and evaluation of learning will be the focus of Chapters 15 and 16. The balance of this chapter will address the *what, who, when, where,* and *how* of service-based educational evaluation. The first section describes what types of evaluative information are pertinent for various groups within the hospital setting. The form in which this evaluative data should be provided to arrive at answers necessary for that group's future decision making, when the data form is not obvious, is given in parentheses. Many program evaluations are less inclusive than this. Consider these as potential areas for evaluation, and select those most relevant to your particular needs and decisions.

In relation to learners

1. Attaining learning and transferring learning to work setting (observable performance behaviors)

2. Degree to which individual expectations and objectives were met (opinion surveys, questionnaires)
   a. Overall level of satisfaction with program
   b. Perceived attainment of instructional objectives and program goals (rating scale or checklist marks)
3. Perceived omissions or unnecessary inclusions in content and learning experiences:
   a. Areas in need of lesser or greater emphasis
   b. Perception of most and least useful or meaningful segments of program
   c. Suggestions for improvement (narrative data)
4. Learning difficulties (diagnostic data)
5. Learner appraisal of curriculum, instruction, faculty, facilities, learning setting, evaluation, and instructional methods and materials (rating scale or checklist marks)

In relation to curriculum (see also Chapter 7)

1. Need for refining or revising program and instructional objectives
   a. Content selection, coverage, and emphasis
   b. Program format
2. Flexibility of curriculum
3. Degree of consistency between instructional or program objectives and content selection (observable learner competencies for different content areas in the form of scores, marks, ratings; participant reaction data in narrative or rating form)

In relation to instruction (see also Chapters 7 to 12)

1. Level of instruction
2. Allotment of hours
3. Organizing, sequencing, and scheduling learning activities
4. Effectiveness of various teaching methods and instructional strategies
5. Degree of consistency between actual learning experiences and instructional objectives
6. Effectiveness of various instructional media in meeting learning objectives
7. Effectiveness and availability of learning resources: audiovisual hardware, software, books, models (observable learner competencies in relation to instructional and program objectives in the form of scores, marks, or ratings)

In relation to faculty (see also Chapter 7)

1. Self-appraisal of performance (rating data)
2. Knowledge of subject matter (student and program director rating data)
3. Preparation, organization, delivery, enthusiasm, expertise, ability to role model, use of appropriate teaching methods and materials (observable learner competencies, learner and program director ratings)

In relation to learning environment (see also Chapter 8)

1. Perceived degree to which it helped learning (learner, instructor, and program director ratings)
2. Adequacy and availability of physical facilities: size, seating, acoustics, comfort, number (anecdotal notes, subjective data)

In relation to hospital and nursing administration (see also Chapter 6)

1. Cost-effectiveness of program (statistical data)
2. Recruitment and marketing costs (dollars per participant)
3. Turnover, attrition, retention (relative percentages, ratios)
4. Number of lost patient care hours (hours per participant)
5. Need for adjusting budgetary allocation
6. Whether to continue, discontinue, or expand program funding (cost-benefit ratio)

7. Appropriateness of program dates, number and type of participants for agency goals (cost-benefit ratio in relation to subjective data)
8. Degree to which program met JCAH requirements for in-service or continuing education (comparative data on compliance with JCAH standards)
9. Whether program met hospital and departmental goals (compare estimated data with stated objectives of department and hospital)

In relation to critical care unit administration and staff (see also Chapters 1 and 6)

1. Effect of program on the need for staff nurses, staffing patterns, mix or staff scheduling (staffing data: full-time equivalents, nurse to patient ratio, comparative data on hours of care and staffing budget)
2. Effect of program on efficiency, attitude, and morale of nurses (subjective data)
3. Transferring learning to work setting, fulfilling role expectations, and effect on position change or career advancement (ratings and narrative data on performance evaluations)
4. Effect on fostering continuing education (number of nurses pursuing formal and informal continuing education activities)

In relation to patients

1. Effect of program on patient outcomes and quality of patient care provided (patient outcomes, audit criteria in relation to standards of care)

In relation to other hospital departments (see also Chapters 1 and 6)

1. Personnel
   a. Need for revising entry requirements for participants
   b. Need for revising contractual agreements
   c. Need for revising policies and procedures related to participation
   d. Efficiency of selection process (number of participants who successfully complete the program each year)
2. Public relations
   a. Full evaluation of program marketing, advertising, and promotion

b. Whether target population was reached, by which forms and at what cost of advertising (demographic data of participants, number of inquiries about the program, cost for each participant)

3. Audiovisual

a. Need for developing or purchasing other media hardware or software (participant, instructor, and program director reaction data, narrative data, results of summary from audiovisual review process, subjective data)

In relation to professional credentialing and accrediting agencies

1. Whether criteria for accreditation, certification, continuing education unit (CEU) approval, or credit- and degree-granting were met

In relation to program operation and administration (data from all preceding areas are collectively evaluated to make decisions regarding the following)

1. Efficiency of whole program
2. Appropriateness of program policies and practices
3. Adequacy of resources and staff personnel in support of program
4. Appropriateness of program goals
5. Approaches to revisions in outcomes or process
6. Whether roles and responsibilities are clearly defined
7. Need to replace, remove, or augment faculty
8. Comparative cost-effectiveness of various teaching methods
9. Efficiency and effectiveness of application processing, interviewing, and selecting participants
10. Relationship and currency of needs assessment to program objectives, content, learning experiences, and evaluation process
11. Whether the organizational structure facilitates meeting program goals
12. Whether the principles of adult education and the teaching-learning process are being put into operation
13. Adequacy of faculty selection and review processes

14. Adequacy of financial and support resources
15. Adequacy of administrative support

In relation to the evaluation process

1. Whether all necessary evaluative information has been obtained
2. Whether results of evaluation have been incorporated into program planning and operations
3. Whether all significant parties have been represented in the evaluation process
4. Whether the measuring instruments are valid and reliable
5. Whether a sufficient number of evaluation tools were used for the evaluation

Focus on evaluating learning

The preceding section delineated an extraordinarily comprehensive evaluation of hospital-based educational programming. As the person responsible for critical care nursing education, however, your most immediate concern is with evaluating learning as it influences critical care nursing practice. Before discussing further details of the evaluation process, it is best to examine more closely just what aspect of learning you actually intend to evaluate.

Critical care nursing practice and organizational and educational needs are all dynamic phenomena that vary with time and local circumstances. As they are altered, your program and instructional objectives must be synchronously modified to remain relevant and meaningful. Some educational programming may be aimed at the continued development of a virtually limitless variety of clinical proficiencies of staff nurses: advanced programs for staff development, general continuing education, programs for position change, career development, or improving weak areas in performance evaluations.

At other times, educational programming is aimed at learners attaining very specific proficiencies and capabilities for clinical practice: the essential elements contained in unit orientation, unit in-service programs on using new equipment or procedures, attaining hospital certification for basic cardiac life support, defibrillation, drawing arterial blood gases, or interpreting ECG strips. Staff development programs are likely situated somewhere in the gray area between these two categories.

Not only do the instructional objectives and learning experiences vary in each case, but what you need to evaluate also varies. In the first, more general category, evaluation typically focuses on the degree to which different learners met the instructional objectives: of all the learners who learned the most? In the second, more specific category, you would care less about how much one learner learned in relation to others and more about whether each individual learner met highly specific and prescribed instructional objectives. The first aims at evaluating *achievement,* whereas the second aims at evaluating *mastery* or *competency.* The major difference between the two is whether the evaluation process terminates with verifying that the instructional objective was attained (mastery or competency) or continues above or below the objective to determine the relative degree to which it was attained (achievement).

Approaches to educational evaluation

Evaluation of achievement: the traditional approach. The measurements used for educational evaluation in most schools, including schools of nursing, evaluate relative achievement. Conventional approaches to evaluation measure the degree to which learners attain the instructional objectives. In its most traditional form, evaluating achievement attempts to differentiate among the performance levels of learners. It assumes that given a large enough group, a few learners will attain high degrees of learning, a few low degrees of learning, and most will be somewhere in the middle. The resulting form of evaluation data is comparative: percentiles or letter or numerical grades are assigned in relation to other learners' performance.

In formal education, evaluation has largely focused on teaching rather than learning, on attaining cognitive learning (knowing) rather than transferring or applying knowledge (doing). Learners with relatively similar entry abilities and experiences (or lack of these) are subject to a relatively fixed set of learning experiences distributed over a prescribed period of time, and leave programs with dissimilar capabilities and achievement levels. Instructional objectives originate more often with the teacher than with the practitioner. Competition between learners is keen, and grades are the most concrete measures of success. Regardless of how much any learner learned, the costs of the educational and evaluative processes are fixed. There is no guarantee that any two learners derive the same learning from the experience.

Evaluation of mastery or competency: an alternative approach. A difficulty inherent in traditional forms of education and evaluation is that whereas *knowing* is usually a prerequisite condition for competent *doing,* knowing alone is not a sufficient condition for doing. In a practice discipline such as nursing, that knowing and doing are two different things is all too frequently heard in the hue and cry of nursing service personnel with respect to newly graduated nurses: "It is not that they do not know their job; the problem is that they are not able to do it!"

Competency is a more inclusive phenomenon than simply an additive mixture of unrelated bits of the right behaviors. Isolated bits of knowledge or having the right feelings is not an adequate index of competency, and the abilities to perform isolated skills are not a full definition of competency. Nurse educators have been wrestling for some time with the problem of producing graduates who have a more realistic balance of knowing and doing rather than one at the expense of the other.

This dichotomy between what a nurse knows

and what she is able to do has been assisted by the following two merging forces:

1. A resurgence of the role of service- or agency-based nursing educators whose responsibility is to bridge this gap for the benefit of the agency and the patient.
2. A recognition from other spheres of education and training that a "knowledgeable practitioner" is not an inherent contradiction in terms, nor is it impossible to produce one.

Both of these forces emphasize that instructional objectives have to be closely tied to what the practice setting requires of the practitioner: that in practice, the bottom line is doing, not merely knowing. Regardless of the nurse's educational preparation, if she cannot demonstrate a certain level of competency in her assigned role, she is of little value to the patient or to the agency. In the work setting, practitioners use competency as the evaluation standard: how one practitioner performs in comparison with her peers is less relevant than how she performs in relation to existing performance standards.

Clinical educators and trainers in other related practice settings emphasize that teaching is less important than learning, that applying and transferring knowledge is of greater value than merely possessing it. These educators are impressed that given adequate time and appropriate learning activities suited to their learning style and background, virtually all learners can attain the desired competencies by many different means. They note the time, money, and other resources wasted on reteaching things learners already know, that many learners can achieve learning objectives in a shorter than usual time, and that instructors can be relieved of monotonous and inefficient use of their time to be free to work with learners with learning problems. Trainers recognize that the demands of the work setting require evaluating an individual's overall competency rather than merely what a worker knows, feels, or can accomplish as

an isolated skill. The job of in-service educators and other professional trainers is not only to develop employees to their fullest potential, but to do so only after assuring that each employee in a given position obtains a certain essential, required level of performance. Competition among learners and the allocation of letter grades are not pertinent when the learner's only competition is with herself.

This alternative approach to educational evaluation is referred to as competency-based (or mastery) evaluation. Its emphasis on attaining required, critical competencies in practice seems to merit some consideration by critical care educators. Competency-based evaluation is only one facet of competency-based education (CBE), which emphasizes the ultimate, long-range outcomes of education and clarifies the relationship between a learner's meeting isolated instructional objectives and attaining overall competency in a field. CBE does not deemphasize the degree to which learning objectives are met, but calls attention to the pragmatic realities that (1) the entirety of the educational process is subservient to the ultimate outcomes of learning and (2) some of the ultimate outcomes of learning are critical or essential for competent performance in the work setting, whereas others are of lesser importance.

Standards of reference in educational evaluation

As discussed previously, evaluations are derived from considering measurements in relation to some agreed reference point or standard of measurement. Just as one may compare the length of an object to a yardstick that indicates inches or to a meter that indicates centimeters, so one may also measure learning using different standards of measurement. Just as one would derive different numerical values (measurements) depending on the standard or criterion of measurement, so too the nature of the resulting evaluation will differ when different standards of reference are used to evaluate learning.

Norm-referenced evaluation. When achievement is evaluated, the traditional standard of reference used called *norm-referenced evaluation,* is the individual learner's performance in comparison to that of others in the peer or norm group (class, age, or sex group). Norm-referenced evaluation is a *relative* basis for evaluation because it emphasizes how well one performs in relation to how others performed. Anyone who has ever taken a standardized achievement test (SAT, GRE) or IQ test, or has benefitted or lost from the use of grading curves has been subjected to norm-referenced evaluation. With norm-referenced evaluation, you can perform very poorly in an absolute sense based on your score alone (getting 40 of 120 items correct), but do exceedingly well based on the relative performance of others taking the same or comparable test (if most of the others only got 30 of 120 items correct).

When competition, relative achievement, and differentiation among performance levels is needed, norm-referenced evaluation is the appropriate form to use.

Criterion-referenced evaluation. At other times it may be more useful to assure, through *criterion-referenced evaluation*, that each learner can perform at a clearly specified level. Suppose, for example, you were responsible for having all the staff nurses trained in Basic Cardiac Life Support (BCLS) according to the American Heart Association standards for CPR. Even if nurse A's level of performance far surpassed that of nurses B, C, and D, this is no guarantee that anyone's performance met the Heart Association standards. The relative performance levels of any of these nurses are meaningless; each individual's performance is judged as satisfactory or not in relation to whether it meets the Heart Association's prescribed performance standards. This is called criterion-referenced evaluation because the evaluation is based on performance in relation to some prescribed performance level. Criterion-referenced evaluation is generally an *absolute* evaluation method: either the performance meets the prescribed standard or it does not; degrees of achievement greater or lesser than the established standard are largely irrelevant for evaluation purposes.

As you might expect, competency- or mastery-based evaluation, with its emphasis on the mastery of specified competencies, typically incorporates criterion-referenced evaluation. In considering the remaining elements of the evaluation process, it will be necessary to return to other aspects of evaluation where the differences between various types of reference standards and approaches to evaluation exist.

SPECIFYING WHO SHOULD BE INVOLVED IN THE EVALUATION PROCESS
Some general considerations

The responsibility for assessing, planning, and implementing various phases of an educational program has been emphasized as a shared responsibility. If the appraisal of this collective effort is to be as efficient as the preceding phases of the educational process, evaluation must likewise be a shared process. The more inclusive and encompassing the evaluative information, moreover, the more likely the resulting judgment will be accurate.

Obtaining an accurate picture of how effective and efficient the educational process and its outcomes are entails identifying groups or individuals who:

1. Are in the best position to supply certain categories of evaluative information
2. Participate as learners in the program
3. Participate as providers or support personnel in the program
4. Participate as planners or designers of the program
5. Use the evaluative data for making decisions about the program
6. Will be directly or indirectly affected by the evaluations

How many individuals and groups participate in program evaluation and the composition of this group will depend on the scope and purposes established for the program. Remember that learning is not the only variable that requires evaluation; logistics, operations, and processes cannot afford to be neglected.

Some suggested participants

A comprehensive program evaluation may enlist some or all of the following groups:

1. Program participants: learners and their peers
2. Program faculty: instructors, preceptors, and peers in the nursing in-service department
3. Clients of participants: patients, families, and other consumers
4. Staff nurses of the critical care units
5. Administrators: hospital, nursing, and unit
6. Resource and support personnel: clerical and professional (audiovisual, personnel, public relations, and budgetary support)
7. Program director and staff members
8. Advisory committee members, if appropriate
9. Professional groups: JCAH, state nursing associations, professional organizations such as the American Association of Critical-Care Nurses, local colleges and universities

DETERMINING WHEN TO EVALUATE

The optimal number, frequency, and timing of evaluations are determined primarily by the purpose for performing the assessment and by the type of decisions and information sought. In general, evaluations should be performed as follows:

1. In sufficient number to provide an adequate sampling of the outcomes and behavioral performances to be evaluated
2. With a sufficient variety of different methods to overcome the inherently limited validity and scope of any one assessment tool
3. Frequently enough to detect significant changes over time in the variables assessed
4. At the times most likely to provide the data sought

Formative evaluation

In relation to the time over which evaluative data are collected are two main categories of evaluation: formative and summative. *Formative evaluation* is conducted throughout the implementation phase of the educational process. Its purpose is to monitor the ongoing operational processes of teaching, learning, and related support activities to enhance the efficiency and effectiveness of these operations. Formative evaluations are usually dynamic and informal, spontaneous and immediate in effect, sensitive to discrete incidents, and limited in the sphere of decisions they influence. The primary value of formative evaluation is its ability to detect areas needing modification, revision, or improvement and to make necessary corrective adjustments to resolve problems expeditiously before the program has been completed. It should combine systematically scheduled evaluations together with an informal openness to serendipitous findings. The majority of formative data should be searched for, not found by accident.

Examples of formative evaluations include the following:

1. Preentrance or screening tests administered before enrollment in an educational program to determine if individuals have the requisite capabilities necessary to enter the program
2. Pretests administered on entry to assess levels of performance in relation to the program objectives before the learning experience

3. Diagnostic tests administered during a course of study to identify the areas or reasons for learning difficulties
4. Quizzes administered at the end of fairly discrete subdivisions of the program (lesson, unit, course, midprogram) to assess learning in certain content areas or to assess cumulative learning
5. Self-assessment guides (study guides) to enable the learner to assess developing competencies

Summative evaluation

In contrast to the continual focus of formative evaluations, *summative evaluations* have a terminal focus. Rather than concentrating on the unfolding educational process, summative evaluations examine the ultimate outcomes and final products of the program to provide a synopsis of its overall or net value. Summative evaluations are directed at effecting improvements and necessary revisions in subsequent rather than current programming activities. The conclusions reached in these final judgments are usually more static and formal, more anticipated or planned, and less timely in immediate effects but more far-reaching in the decisions they influence. Because they incorporate data from numerous sources, summative evaluations' primary purpose is to provide the information needed for making major decisions regarding the program: whether or not to fund the program, to continue with the original design, or to modify substantially designs or procedures.

Some examples of summative evaluation include the following:

1. Posttests aimed at determining whether a learner has successfully completed a program or not (in mastery or competency-based evaluation), and what the learner's final score or grade will be (achievement evaluation)
2. Certification examinations that determine whether an individual meets all of the requirements for certification
3. Questionnaires, checklists, or rating scales devised to obtain overall impressions of program design, instruction, and outcomes from both learners and instructors
4. Balance sheets that tabulate the cost-benefit ratios of an entire program

To direct effectively the educational and administrative decision-making processes, evaluation should be incorporated into an organized schedule of assessments that coincide with the availability of the information and the sequencing of events it monitors. Neither formative nor summative evaluation alone is sufficient; each must be planned to complement the other if all phases of the program are to benefit maximally.

Foresight and experience will assist you in learning when and how often to evaluate various facets of the educational process. If you miscalculated anywhere, the lack of availability or access to data when you need it for a decision will indicate your omission.

WHERE TO EVALUATE

Evaluation is best done wherever the information sought is most likely to be available. Deciding where to evaluate is therefore primarily a function of what needs to be evaluated.

Settings for evaluating learning

In evaluating learning, the cognitive behavior of knowing, the affective behavior of feeling or valuing, and the psychomotor behavior of doing can be observed best in one or more of three different locales. Many cognitive behaviors (definition, recall, identification, recognition, specification, explanation, description) are most often evident in the classroom, whereas higher intellectual functions (synthesis, integration, analysis, application) may be more readily observed in the laboratory or clinical setting.

Affective behaviors pose particular difficulties

in evaluation because they lack standardized definition and their appraisal criteria are often imprecise. A learner's true dispositions, inclinations, attitudes, and beliefs often remain hidden behind a façade of "how the instructor expects me to say I feel." Attempting to locate evidence of affective learning is a reminder that affective behaviors require some object, context, or situation for the learner to experience and respond to. In a classroom, written simulations, simulated situations, media vignettes, or case presentations may elicit evidence of affective behaviors. In general, however, the closer the context is to actual practice, the more likely valid evidence of affective behaviors will be demonstrated. Laboratory sessions, with simulated situations involving patients culturally and socioeconomically different from learners, or role-playing sessions are useful places to seek affective evaluation. The clinical unit may be the best of all locations because it provides learners with true samples of life to experience, to reflect on, to analyze the values in, and to select the most appropriate course of action, based on a commitment to a value position.

Psychomotor behaviors require an opportunity for at least simulated performance of skills in a laboratory. Assuming patient safety and learner anxiety are monitored, the ideal setting for the evaluation of psychomotor behavior would be at the bedside. The laboratory may be more appropriately used to evaluate minimum and safe competencies, whereas the clinical area is used to evaluate continued learning transfer and the refinement of minimum skill competency.

Other settings for program evaluation

Program evaluation entails more than merely evaluating learning. Your evaluation itinerary should include making frequent visits back to all three learning settings to evaluate the instructional processes there. Evaluate the administrative and logistical aspects of the program by visiting the critical care administrative, the hospital administrators' and nursing administrators' offices. Plan on stops at the personnel, public relations, audiovisual, in-service, and nurse recruiter's offices. Schedule a block of time for compilation, review, and analysis in your own office and, perhaps, a few on-site visits to speak with representatives of local universities and professional certifying and accrediting agencies. Finally, find comfortable nooks in the hallway and cafeteria of your agency to derive some informal feedback only available in these settings.

HOW THE EVALUATION PROCESS WILL PROCEED
Planning for measurement and evaluation

Putting into operation and coordinating the evaluation of an educational program demands as substantial an investment of time and energy as in any of the preceding stages of the educational process. To reap the best returns on your investment, a systematic approach is again advisable.

As an educator, your most immediate concern is with evaluating learning. The various cognitive, affective, and psychomotor capabilities that collectively determine competency in critical care nursing practice may be appraised by using various evaluation instruments and methods. This section first considers some precepts and benchmarks that apply to all types of devices used for evaluating learning and then focuses on the procedural elements of test construction, use, and scoring procedures appropriate for evaluating different types of instructional objectives. Then, the transition from measurement to evaluation is marked by describing various grading systems and the statistical analysis of evaluation data. How to obtain evaluative data to answer decisions regarding related aspects of the educational process such as curriculum and instruction, use of resources, administrative matters, and the concerns of participating groups is discussed. The cumulative result of these interrelated assessments will comprise the basis for evaluating the entire educational program.

Preliminary considerations. As you approach the definitive tasks of evaluating learning, you should bear some helpful guiding precepts in mind. Strictly interpreted, these principles apply most directly to written forms of evaluation, but their spirit should also pervade performance evaluations.

The nature and form of evaluation should be directly related to its intended purpose and function. It is axiomatic that the basis of program evaluation be rooted in the objectives established at the outset for the program. Evaluation of learning, in turn, must emanate from and return to answer the set instructional objectives.

Individual test items, the functional units of evaluation, should symmetrically balance with their corresponding objectives: the behavior, content, and conditions contained in evaluation items should be those set forth in the instructional objectives. If the objective requires that the learner demonstrate the *application* of principles, whereas the evaluation device only requires *recall* from rote memory, the inconsistency between specified and evaluated behaviors results in the evaluator not knowing if the objective was attained or not.

Evaluating higher mental processes (understanding, application, differentiation, discrimination, synthesis, description) is often neglected in favor of evaluating those easier to test (recall, recognition, identification). Unless the specific makeup of the evaluation device is monitored, it is easy to aim short in evaluating the cognitive levels you are really interested in learners attaining. A judicious amount of attention should therefore be paid to assuring that the evaluation items are directly related to the learning objectives.

An adequate number and variety of measurements are required for reaching true appraisals. The more limited the range, scope, number, and types of measurements, the less confidence you can place in the validity of the evaluation. Conversely, the more encompassing the range, scope, number, and types of measurements, the more secure you can then be that the evaluation is accurate and true. Especially when the ultimate outcome is as broad a category as clinical competency in critical care nursing, the range of objectives necessary to adequately sample measurements of competency is inherently large; successful performance of an inadequate number of activities cannot validly generate the designation "competent."

The evaluation process should reflect the priorities already assigned to various outcomes of the program. Just as the amount of instructional time allotted to certain objectives corresponds to their relative importance in the curriculum, the weight or emphasis of evaluation should be distributed according to this same set of educational priorities. If you spent one fourth of the instructional time teaching anatomy and physiology, one fourth teaching pathophysiology, and one half on applying principles of care, then the same proportions should be allotted to evaluating learning in these areas.

If your intention is to evaluate gullibility, trick and catch items can be very effective. If you need to identify trivia addicts, evaluating minutiae can be very helpful. If you do not need to evaluate these behaviors, then these test items are inappropriate.

Identify what the important outcomes of learning are and evaluate these in proportion to their importance. Besides finding out the answers for the questions you need to answer, you will also find that you sleep better at night. Emphasizing one thing while instructing and testing for another while evaluating not only violates the precepts of sound evaluation, but is also less than fair to learners.

Learners, by and large, are not mind readers. When you intend to measure certain aspects of a learner's peformance, it is always most helpful to tell the learner this. In constructing test items, check to be sure that what you are measuring is what you intend to measure. Shaking heads, staring blankly into space, and an open palms-up gesture are all indications from the learners that you have not clearly communicated the task to be accomplished and evaluated. Test situations or items need clear, precise, unambiguous definitions of the performances required if learners are to be treated humanely. Avoid concealing your intentions in a high-powered vocabulary only exceptional learners can decipher or in such complexity that learners lose track of what the problem was. Be as clear, direct, and brief as possible in posing the evaluation situation.

Measurements should not be mistaken for evaluations. Remember that measurements are only raw data; their meaning, significance, and interpretation are determined by evaluation. Measurements therefore should not be taken as prima facie evidence of performance; their face value depends on the exchange rate that evaluation sets. Depending on the evaluation criteria, a score of 75 could be interpreted as satisfactory, marginal, or failing. Measurement data are only data, not evaluations.

Benchmarks of measurement. Sound decision making for educational programming relies on a sound evaluation process to guide it. A sound evaluation process in turn depends on the integrity of the measurement process that underlies it. The legitimacy of decisions, is therefore directly related to the legitimacy of measurement.

How can you determine the degree of confidence you can rightfully ascribe to measurements? How can you tell if the data, scores, or marks are meaningful and useful for making those important decisions? Although a number of factors may influence how useful any given set of evaluation measurements is, the primary determinants are the validity, reliability, and usefulness of the test or measuring instrument.

Before you can rightfully formulate evaluations you should have some rational basis for believing the test instruments used for measurement are capable of producing the intended information consistently and repeatedly and that they are feasible and practical to use in your setting.

Validity, reliability, and usefulness are the benchmarks of all evaluation measurement. Of this trio, validity is the most important attribute of an evaluation tool; without it, reliability and usefulness are virtually meaningless commodities and the decision-making processes build on a groundless base.

These benchmarks provide an indication of the degree of confidence placed in the measurement data. Ideally, all three characteristics are maximally present in each evaluation tool. In reality, each is present to a greater or lesser degree, rather than to an absolute degree of "there" or "not there."

Because you will need to depend on these benchmarks for determining the quality of the measurements obtained, you should examine each more closely to better understand the attribute and to be able to determine the degree to which it is present.

Validity. Validity may be defined as the degree to which an evaluation device (test) measures what it was intended to measure. The validity of any test is always judged in reference to a specific purpose. If, for example, a comprehensive multiple-choice test is used to evaluate learning at the end of a 3-week ICU course and is also the test used to screen applicants for entry into this program, the validity of the test for measuring learning must be determined apart from its validity as a screening device; the same test may be highly valid as a posttest and virtually invalid as a screening device. Multiple test devices may all be used for a single purpose (for example, measuring learning), or a single test may be used for multiple purposes. In each instance, validity must be determined for each discrete instrument and evaluation purpose.

In its most basic form, validity refers to the degree to which the test situations or items elicit the behaviors, content, and conditions called for in the instructional objectives. If test situations or items are appropriate correlates of the instructional objectives, the measurement outcomes should be valid indexes of whether or not that objective was attained. Conversely, if the intended purpose of the evaluation is to determine if a nurse can "apply principles of crisis intervention" and the test item only requires that she "list the steps of crisis intervention," "listing" is not a valid measure of the nurse's ability to "apply" principles.

Validity estimates may report any one or more of three different types of validity: content validity, criterion-related validity, and construct validity.

CONTENT VALIDITY. Content validity refers to the degree to which the behaviors and content areas in the evaluation items are representative of the ones called for in the instructional objectives. In assessing content validity, the educator is determining both the inclusiveness and the precision of the evaluation tool, that is, if all of the behaviors (cognitive, affective, psychomotor) called for are in fact present somewhere in the tool and if they are present in their appropriate proportion.

To appraise a measurement tool for content validity, first identify the behaviors and corresponding subject matter called for in the objectives. From the relative amount of instructional time allotted for each objective, determine the weight the objective was given in the course. Then check that the evaluation tool requires a demonstration of the same behaviors and content areas specified in the objective. Finally, verify that the weight allotted in the evaluation device is the equivalent of that allotted for instructional time. For example, a 12-hour CCU course has three course objectives:

1. The orientee will be able to attach a patient to a cardiac monitor as described in the CCU procedure book.
2. The orientee will be able to accurately identify all 15 ECG strips contained in module I.
3. The orientee will meet the requirements for certification in Basic Cardiac Life Support (BCLS).

Objective 1 was deemed least important and therefore was allotted only 2 hours (17%) of the instructional time; objective 2 was deemed important and therefore was allotted 4 hours (33%) of the instructional time; objective 3 was deemed most important and therefore was allotted 6 hours (50%) of the instructional time. When the evaluation tool is examined for content validity, not only would the same behaviors and subject matter have to be present, but if the total number of evaluation items were 60, 17% of these (10 items) would have to be related to the content areas and behaviors of objective 1, 33% (20 items) would have to be related to the content areas and behaviors of objective 2, and 50% (30 items) would have to be related to the content areas and behaviors of objective 3.

For most classroom tests, the appraisal of content validity is provided by a consensus of experts in the subject area. To the extent that evaluation items apportionately represent the instructional objectives, content validity is ascribed. Hospital-based nursing educators are likely to use content validity as their primary method for determining the overall validity of classroom tests, especially those for cognitive learning objectives.

You may also hear of the term *face validity*. Face validity refers to whether a measuring instrument seems—from its superficial appearance—to represent the content areas and behaviors it is intended to represent. It differs from content validity in that the appraisal of face validity is largely superficial and random rather than comprehensive and systematic. The evaluator is also typically not a true expert in the relevant field. Because this type of appraisal does not provide any validity for the evaluation process, it should not be seriously entertained as a form of validity.

CRITERION-RELATED VALIDITY. Criterion-related validity refers to the degree to which an individual's performance on one measuring instrument correlates with present or future performance on another related instrument. As its name implies, criterion-related validity requires that the initial test results be compared with results on some valid criterion measure or standard related to the initial performance. If the second performance is a suitable criterion measure of the first, then performance on the initial measure could be used to predict performance on the second measure.

Because criterion-related validity may involve the prediction of either another present performance or a future performance, the types of validity it provides are appropriately designated as *concurrent* or *predictive validity*.

Concurrent validity refers to the degree to which performance levels on one test correlate with performance levels on a second test taken at essentially the same time. Because a nurse's ability to correctly draw an ABG sample is partly a function of her knowledge about the technique, the critical care educator might be interested in comparing the relationship between a nurse's score on a written test (cognitive performance) related to arterial puncture with her score from a rating scale appraisal of clinical performance of arterial puncture.

Predictive validity refers to the degree to which performance levels on one test correlates with performance levels on a second test taken in the future. As the critical care educator, you might be interested in determining the relationship between a nurse's posttest scores for the nurse orientation program and her clinical performance evaluation 6 months later. You might also be interested in determining how well posttest scores in a CCRN preparation course can predict a nurse's subsequent scores on the actual CCRN examination. If the scores correlate closely, you have a reasonably valid basis for then predicting the latter from the former.

One difficulty encountered with criterion-related validity is reaching consensus on what constitutes a valid criterion measure. For many areas of measurement, locating suitable and practical criteria is a major obstacle.

The term *correlation* has been used here a number of times in describing criterion-related validity. A correlation expresses the degree of relationship between two things. As a statistical index of relationship, correlations are determined by computing this relationship as a correlation coefficient abbreviated as "r."

The numerical value of a correlation coefficient (r) may range from -1.0 to $+1.0$. If two sets of scores are directly related to one another so that as one increases (or decreases), the other set likewise increases (or decreases), the sets of scores are said to have a high positive correlation. High positive correlations have correlation coefficients (r values) that approach $+1.0$. If the two sets of scores had a perfect positive correlation, then as one set of scores increases (or decreases) by a certain amount, the other would likewise increase (or decrease) by the same amount. Lesser degrees of positive correlation (between 0.0 and $+1.0$) indicate that the direct relationship is proportionately less than the maximum. Fig. 2 illustrates how a perfect positive correlation would appear, and Fig. 3 illustrates how a less than perfect positive correlation would appear, plotted on a graphic design called a scattergram. If no relationship existed between two sets of scores, the value of r would be 0.0 (Fig. 4), implying that no association can be determined between the two entities. Negative correlations are equally important to determine. When values are inversely related to one another, the rise of one is associated with a fall in the other. Figs. 5 and 6 illustrate how two variables may possess comparably high degrees of negative correlation.

Calculating a correlation coefficient is beyond

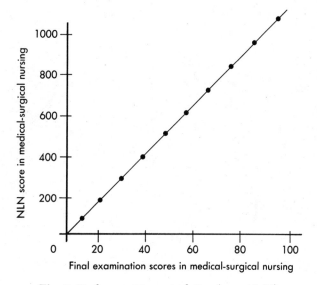

Fig. 2. Perfect positive correlation (r = +1.00).

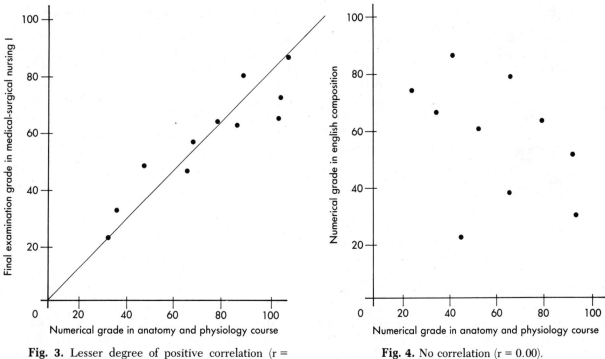

Fig. 3. Lesser degree of positive correlation (r = +0.70).

Fig. 4. No correlation (r = 0.00).

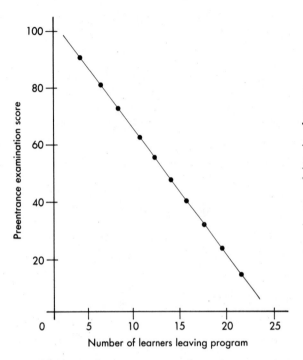

Fig. 5. Perfect negative correlation (r = −1.00).

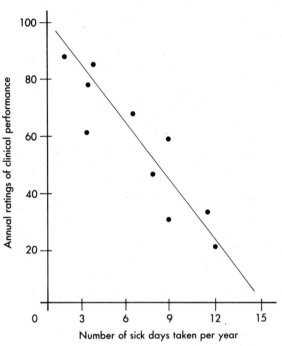

Fig. 6. Lesser degree of negative correlation (r = −0.70).

the scope of this book, but may be found in any reference on descriptive statistics.

CONSTRUCT VALIDITY. Construct validity is the third and least often used type of validity. Constructs are abstract, theoretical, or intangible qualities (such as anxiety, critical-thinking ability, or insight) assumed to be the basis for certain kinds of behavior. Construct validity refers to the degree to which specific constructs are represented in the measurement device. To the degree that these items appropriately and comprehensively measure the constructs, the results of the measurement are explainable by the constructs contained there.

Construct validity is most often employed with measures of affective behavior. If, for example, you were interested in assessing a nurse's "empathy" for the families of ICU patients, you would need to determine what the constituents of "empathy" are and design an evaluation device to measure these.

A problem with assessing construct validity immediately arises because of the limited number of available and valid tools with which to measure these qualities. Construct validity generally requires a substantial review of the literature and research findings related to the construct or its subcomponents, and typically is used more in personality and intelligence testing. Construct validity may require that numerous correlations be made and demonstrated repeatedly among subcomponents to substantiate the final correlation.

Reliability. Reliability refers to the stability of measurements over time, the comparability of results between different measuring instruments or between different raters, the ability to generalize results from one situation to another, or the degree of consistency within a single test. If, for example, you had reason to doubt that a cardiovascular pressure monitoring system was working properly, you might attempt to evaluate its integrity by taking multiple readings over a specified period of time to see if the trends remained essentially similar. You might change your measuring device and cross-check the comparability of readings between the transducer monitoring system and a water manometer system, or you could ask a colleague to see what readings she obtains. You could also check to determine if the same transducer system and monitoring unit had been recently used on other patients and whether any questionable readings had been obtained. Finally, you could double-check your equipment by calibrating it again.

Next to validity, reliability is the most important attribute of a measuring device. Reliability is an essential prerequisite for validity, so that the low reliability of a measuring device necessarily limits its validity; the converse is not true. If you took blood pressures with both an arterial monitoring system and a sphygmomanometer cuff and the cuff measurements consistently gave you readings of 10 mm Hg below that of the transducer system, the cuff measurements, although highly consistent in their margin of error, would nevertheless be invalid readings of true arterial pressure. Even high degrees of reliability do not then assure validity.

Reliability, like validity, is always in reference to the purpose for which measurements are obtained; a certain bed scale may be highly reliable for weighing adult patients, moderately reliable for weighing children, and not at all reliable for weighing infants and neonates.

As mentioned earlier, a number of methods can be used to determine reliability. One category focuses on administrating or constructing an objectively scored measuring device, whereas another category focuses on subjectively scored measurements. Each method for determining reliability provides the educator with somewhat different information and implications regarding reliability. When reporting or evaluating how reliable a measuring instrument is, therefore, it is important to know which type of reliability is referred to fully to understand its

impact on the value of the instrument.

Methods for determining reliability that focus on test administration or construction include measures of stability, equivalence, and internal consistency.

One way of determining an instrument's reliability is to determine its temporal stability (consistency of measurements over time). *Stability reliability* refers to how repeatable the results of measurement are when the same test is administered to the same persons under the same conditions at two different times (T1 and T2). Because the same test is given on both occasions, stability may also be called *test-retest reliability*. It is determined by calculating a correlation coefficient called a reliability coefficient.

The intervening time period between tests, the waiting period between T1 and T2, can vary from days to months or even years, depending on the purpose for the retesting. For example, a critical care educator may be interested in determining the reliability of an evaluation tool for measuring staff nurses' understanding of the principles involved with using the intraaortic balloon pump. To determine how reliable the evaluation tool is, the educator could retest the same nurses 2 weeks apart. If the educator needed to provide long-term follow-up of nurses who had completed a lengthy ICU course, the second testing could be scheduled for 6 months or 1 year following completion of the course.

As the intervening period between test and retest varies, some potential problems arise that may influence the confidence with which reliability coefficience can be interpreted. Short intervening periods between T1 and T2 may elicit falsely high reliability coefficients because the examinees can easily recall the test items and how they responded to them in T1, or their familiarity with the test (T2) may reduce the anxiety they felt in T1. Long intervening periods on the other hand, allow many other variables to enter the test situation: the nurses may acquire a significant amount of learning, their ease or skill in test-taking may improve, their lives or work situations may drastically alter, or it may become increasingly more difficult to replicate closely the situation and conditions present at the initial testing. In general, test-retest reliability coefficients in the order of at least 0.4 are desirable for classroom tests.

A second method in this category attempts to verify reliability by computing the correlation between scores from two different tests that supposedly measure the same thing. Assuming the two test instruments measure the same things (behaviors and content areas) under the same conditions, they should produce virtually the same results. This is termed *parallel, equivalent,* or *alternate form reliability*.

When employed to measure only equivalence, a single test occasion is used to administer both tests to the same individuals. A reliability coefficient is then derived from a comparison of the results of each. The statistical device used to determine this coefficient is called the Pearson Product Moment Correlation Coefficient. If T2 is truly an equivalent (parallel, alternate) form of T1, the results should be highly consistent with each other. Euivalent forms of the same test may also be administered with a specific intervening time period. Assuming this intervening period is significant (i.e., more than just the time it requires to complete either test), the correlations derived would indicate two types of reliability: equivalence and stability.

The problem with the equivalence reliability method is that frequently T2 is not really equivalent to T1. Equivalence implies that each individual test item and the overall test has precisely the same range and scope of behaviors, content, difficulty, and discrimination as the other. Constructing a test instrument with this degree of precision is a formidable task, even for experienced and knowledgeable educators. In reality, then, many alternate or parallel forms of the same test really are not interchangeable; they simply are not the same test.

A second problem encountered with using this reliability method is that it assumes the examinees and test conditions remain unchanged. Even if T2 were administered directly after T1, the influence of test-taking skill, fatigue, and review of the content from the initial testing may be significant in determining the scores and the correlation between scores. Because these factors may influence reliability, they need to be borne in mind when making interpretations. They do not necessarily obviate the results, but must be considered during evaluation.

Internal consistency reliability, the last method in this category, considers the consistency of performance on items within the same test. Instead of administering the same test on two different occasions or constructing two comparable tests to be given in a single test period, this method involves constructing a single test administered on a single occasion. Because it is economical of both instructor and examinee time, internal consistency reliability is the most common procedure used to determine test reliability.

Constructing an instrument for estimating reliability by this method usually proceeds in one of two ways. The *split-half method* involves dividing the total test into two equivalent halves that measure the same thing. This can be accomplished by matching the items so that the second half of the test is an alternate form of the first half or so all evenly numbered items are matched with their odd numbered equivalents. Two separate scores are thus derived from this one test and compared with one another to estimate the degree of reliability between the scores. The split-half method computes reliability by using a statistical device called the Spearman-Brown Prophecy Formula.

An alternate way to compute reliability is to compare the two scores from each test in terms of how many high versus low scorers get the item correct and how much spread versus homogeneity of scores was produced. This method uses a statistical device called the Kuder-Richardson Formula (KR20 or KR21).

The second category of methods for determining reliability is useful when scores or measurements must be derived from the subjective judgments of raters who use some form of checklist or rating scale as the measuring instrument. To determine how reliable these instruments are, two different approaches may be used. The first calls for two or more raters to use the same rating device in rating the exact same performance. Videotape or good vantage points must be provided so that the performance being rated is in reality the same. The simultaneous ratings of the same performance are then compared with one another, providing for *inter-rater reliability*.

A second way to determine the reliability of subjectively scored measurements is to have the same rater observe the same performance (usually on some permanent record such as film) at two different times. Because the rater is the same in both instances and the performance being rated is held constant, this is referred to as *intra-rater reliability*. Inter-rater reliability considers agreement between raters, whereas intra-rater reliability considers agreement by the same rater over time. In general, the greater the number of raters involved with estimating reliability, the more accurate will be the results of that estimate.

From the preceding section, it is clear that many factors may influence reliability and the overall implications of any given estimate of reliability. When establishing acceptable reliability levels is a problem (if values consistently are less than 0.3), you may be able to attribute the problem to one or more of the following:

1. Too few items in the test (restricts the number of behaviors and content areas represented)
2. Some variation or error in test construction or administration
3. Lack of objectivity in scoring
4. Too many test items that are too difficult
5. Too few persons taking the test (an inadequate sample size)
6. Errors in calculating reliability
7. Testing for an inherently unstable variable

VALIDITY AND RELIABILITY IN COMPETENCY-BASED, CRITERION-REFERENCED EVALUATION. The standard methods employed for determining reliability and some types of validity are largely inappropriate to use in criterion-referenced evaluation because they depend on the spread or variation in scores. Criterion-referenced evaluation is only concerned with whether the criteria were achieved or not; it has no attendant interest in other degrees of achievement. The typical variation or spread of scores desired in norm-referenced evaluation of achievement is, therefore, of no use in criterion-referenced evaluation of competency. In criterion-referenced evaluation, these attributes are satisfied only to the extent that the nature and number of criteria identified are, in reality, true and reliable indicators of the specified competency.

Usefulness. Usefulness is the third major attribute any measuring device needs to have. Regardless of an instrument's validity and reliability, if it is unwieldy or requires excessive resources to construct, administer, complete, score, or interpret, it is not likely ever to be put to use. Like validity and reliability, usefulness is also a matter of degree and an attribute considered in light of the other benchmarks of evaluation. Unlike the other benchmarks, however, an instrument's usefulness is a more or less independent attribute, assessed with different criteria and on very different grounds. In determining the usefulness of an evaluation device you may wish to consider some or all of the following areas:

Test construction

1. Are the resources required to construct the device already available in the immediate vicinity or will they have to be secured externally?
2. Is it reasonable and justified to expend the time, budget, and support services toward constructing this device?

3. How much time will test construction require?

Test administration

1. Will available personnel be able to administer the device or will outside experts need to be secured?
2. Are the directions for taking the test already included in the device or must they be given in advance?
3. How long will it take to administer the test?
4. How many and what type of individuals are necessary for administering the test?
5. Are verbal, written, or both types of directions needed for administering the test?
6. Are directions self-explanatory or will detailed verbal directions need to be provided?

Test completion

1. What is the average amount of time required for taking the test?
2. What are likely to be the shortest and longest times required for completing the test?
3. Does the test format facilitate ease of test completion? Is the test copy legible, free of errors, and visually satisfactory? Are the parts of the same item located on the same page? Are all related sections grouped together?
4. Do answer sheets (if used) correspond correctly with each item? Are they easy to use?

Test scoring and interpretation

1. How long will it take to score and interpret results?
2. Are responses to be scored by hand, stencil overlay, computer, or by some other device?
3. Is interpretation of test results a relatively easy, straightforward, and clearly-defined matter?
4. Will experts be needed for interpreting the results? At what cost?
5. How many people will be required for scoring and interpreting the test results?

Test cost

1. How much will each of the preceding cost?
2. What is the total cost for using this evaluation device?
3. Can cost-effectiveness be increased?

• • •

Now that some precepts and essential attributes of all evaluation devices have been reviewed, it is time to address the procedural elements of constructing and implementing various evaluation devices and methods.

REFERENCES
Evaluating continuing education in nursing

Arney, WR: Evaluation of a continuing nursing education program and its implications, J Contin Educ Nurs 9:45, 1978.

Bille, DA: An experience with formative evaluation, J Contin Educ Nurs 7:25, 1976.

Bille, DA, and Fitzgibbons, M: Evaluating CE: quantification or involvement? Nurs Admin Q 2:1, 1978.

Clark, CC: The nurse as continuing educator, New York, 1979, Springer-Verlag New York, Inc.

Collart, ME: An overview in planning, implementing, and evaluating continuing nursing education, J Contin Educ Nurs 7:9, 1976.

del Bueno, DJ: The cost of competency, J Nurs Admin 5:16, 1975.

del Bueno, DJ: Evaluation of a continuing education workshop for inservice educators, J Contin Educ Nurs 8:13, 1977.

Goodykoontz, L: Evaluating a continuing education program, J Contin Educ Nurs 11:25, 1980.

Keeler, JD: The process of program evaluation, Nurs Outlook 20:316, 1972.

Kibbee, P: Developing a model for implementation of an evaluation component in an orientation program, J Contin Educ Nurs 11:25, 1980.

Magner, MM: Developing and evaluating inservice programs, Superv Nurs 9:10, 1978.

Mitsunaga, B, and Shores, L: Evaluation in continuing education: is it practical? J Contin Educ Nurs 8:7, 1977.

O'Leary, MM, and Holzemer, WL: Evaluation of an inservice program, J Nurs Admin 10:21, 1980.

Popiel, ES: Course evaluations. In Popiel, ES, editor: Nursing and the process of continuing education, ed 2, St. Louis, 1977, The C.V. Mosby Co.

Staropoli, CJ, and Waltz, CF: Developing and evaluating eductional programs for health care providers, Philadelphia, 1978, J.A. Davis Co.

Wolanin, MO: Continuing educational approval committee works toward evaluation of nurse outcomes, J Contin Educ Nurs 10:31, 1979.

Mastery- or competency-based evaluation

Barrentine, MM: A contract for mastery learning. In National League for Nursing: Generating effective teaching, New York, 1978, National League for Nursing.

Block, JH, editor: Mastery learning, New York, 1971, Holt, Rinehart and Winston.

Crehan, KD: Item analysis for teacher-made mastery tests, J Educ Measure **11**:255, 1974.

Davis, JH, and Williams, DD: Learning for mastery: individualized testing through computer-managed evaluation, Nurs Educ **5**:9, 1980.

del Bueno, DJ: Competency based education, Nurs Educ **3**:10, 1978.

del Bueno, DJ: The cost of competency, J Nurs Admin **5**:16, 1975.

del Bueno, DJ, Barker, F, and Christmyer, C: Implementing a competency-based orientation program, Nurs Educ **5**:16, 1980.

Hart, E, and Marsico, T: Creative approaches to nurse-midwifery education. I. Mastery learning: an approach to individualizing learning, J Nurs Midwif **20**:17, 1975.

Jones, P, and Zemke, R: Talking with Malcolm Knowles: the adult learner is a "less neglected species," Training HRD **14**:16, 1977.

Litwack, LL: A system for evaluation, Nurs Outlook **24**:45, 1976.

Litwack, LL: Meeting the challenge of clinical evaluation. In National League for Nursing: The challenge of clinical evaluation, New York, 1979, National League for Nursing.

Mueller, DJ: Mastery learning: Partly boon, partly boondoggle, Teach Coll Rec **78**:41, 1976.

Perry, SE: Teaching strategy and learner performance, JNE **18**:25, 1979.

Peterson, CJ: Development of competencies in associate degree nursing, New York, 1978, National League for Nursing.

Pinkney-Atkinson, VJ: Mastery learning model for an inservice nurse training program for the care of hypertensive patients, J Contin Educ Nurs **11**:27, 1980.

Sonnen, BE: Bloom's theory of school learning, J Contin Educ Nurs **12**:38, 1981.

Voight, JW: Assessing clinical performance: a model for competency, JNE **18**:30, 1979.

Norm- versus criterion-referenced evaluation

Bower, FL: Normative- or criterion-referenced evaluation? Nurs Outlook **22**:499, 1974.

Deets, CA: Evaluating CE programs, AORN J **26**:152, 1977.

Gronlund, NE: Measurement and evaluation in teaching, ed 3, New York, 1976, Macmillan Publishing Co.

Gronlund, NE: Preparing criterion-referenced tests for classroom instruction, New York, 1973, Macmillan Publishing Co.

Kneedler, J: Criterion referenced measurement for one continuing education offering: pre- and postoperative visits by operating room nurses, J Contin Educ Nurs **7**:26, 1976.

Krumme, US: The case for criterion-referenced measurement, Nurs Outlook **23**:764, 1975.

Martuza, VR: Applying norm-referenced and criterion-referenced measurement in education, Boston, 1977, Allyn and Bacon.

Popham, WJ, editor: Criterion-referenced measurement: an introduction, Englewood Cliffs, N.J., 1971, Educational Technology Publications.

Pounds, E, and Askins, BE: Criterion-referenced teaching and testing, AORN J **21**:862, 1975.

Wyman, J, and Fernau, K: Developing a criterion-referenced tool, Nurs Outlook **25**:584, 1977.

Test validity, reliability, and usefulness (see also Meaurement and evaluation of learning)

King, EC: Determining and interpreting test validity, reliability and practicality, Nurs Educ **4**:6, 1979.

Loustau, A, et al: Evaluating students' clinical performance: using videotape to establish rater reliability, JNE **19**:10, 1980.

Talmadge, H: Statistics as a tool for educational practitioners, Berkeley, Calif., 1976, McCuthan Publishing Corp.

Thorndike, RL, and Hagen, E: Measurement and evaluation in psychology and education, ed 4, New York, 1977, John Wiley and Sons, Inc.

Chapter 15

Measurement of learning

TERMS USED IN EDUCATIONAL MEASUREMENT

The measurement of learning involves designing and constructing measuring devices that enable the educator to determine the attainment of learning. The measurement of achievement requires that the degree of learning be evidenced, whereas the measurement of mastery requires only that a specified level of learning be evidenced. In either case, a measuring device and an adequate number of opportunities for demonstrating learning that collectively verify the degree of learning attainment are necessary.

A measurement *method* is an overall approach, technique, or strategy for measuring learning such as classroom or clinical methods of evaluation or subjective or objective methods of measurement. A measuring *instrument* refers to any means, tool, or device used to measure the degree of learning attainment. The most commonly employed measuring instrument is a test. A *test* is a written or situational occurrence that provides one or more instances for the learner to demonstrate learning. These individual instances or samples of demonstrated learning that collectively comprise a test are called test *items*.

A wide array of methods, instruments, tests, and items are available to the educator for measuring learning. They vary in their appropriateness for measuring different types of learning, in their ease of construction, administration, and scoring, in their usefulness and appropriateness for various settings, and in the types of evidence they provide for evaluation. Selection from this array is, unfortunately, often limited to only the few methods with which the educator is most familiar.

The following section describes a systematic process for educators to use in designing a plan to measure learning. Just as architects design a blueprint for a building to be properly constructed, educators should design a blueprint for evaluation to be properly provided.

DESIGNING A BLUEPRINT TO MEASURE LEARNING

A well-designed plan to measure learning should contain the following five major steps:
1. Identify the instructional objectives the test must measure.
2. Design a test blueprint that orders the collective behaviors and content areas included in the test.
3. Assign a relative importance to each behavior and content area.
4. Allocate a corresponding amount of emphasis to measuring learning of these behaviors and content areas.
5. Construct a table of test specifications that reflects the proportionate emphasis given to the behaviors and content areas contained within the test blueprint.

Step 1: Identify instructional objectives the test must measure

Just as the instructional objectives are the focal point for all preceding phases of the educational process, they also guide the educator in measuring and evaluating learning. As mentioned in Chapter 5, the clear delineation of behaviors and content areas described in the instructional objectives suggests not only the most appropriate teaching method but also the most appropriate evaluative method. Because the measurement of learning aims at determining if these behaviors and their related content areas have been learned, they are the logical starting place for evaluation. Example 15-1 lists the instructional objectives that could be used for a unit on the nursing care of a patient with a myocardial infarction (MI). This set of instructional objectives can also illustrate the other steps in designing a plan to measure learning.

Example 15-1. Instructional objectives for unit on MI patient

---

1.1 Describes the functional anatomy of the cardiovascular system *(cognitive)*
Instructional objectives: (all cognitive)
  1.11 Defines terms pertaining to the cardiovascular system with respect to their anatomical features.
  1.12 Identifies the macroscopic structures of the cardiovascular system.
  1.13 Identifies the microscopic structures (ultrastructures) of the cardiovascular system.
  1.14 Identifies the anatomical features of cardiac muscle cells that differentiate them from skeletal and smooth muscle cells.
  1.15 Identifies the anatomical sequence of electrical depolarization.
  1.16 Specifies the direction and circuit of systemic, pulmonary, and coronary blood flows.
  1.17 Compares and contrasts differences in musculature of the four heart chambers.
  1.18 Compares and contrasts differences in morphology of systemic arteries and veins and pulmonary artery and aorta.
  1.19 Differentiates between morphological structure of sinuses of Valsalva and that of venous and heart valves.
1.2 Describes cardiovascular physiology and electrophysiology *(all cognitive)*
Instructional objectives: (all cognitive)
  1.21 Defines the major anatomical components of the cardiovascular system according to their primary functions.
  1.22 Defines the meaning of terms related to generation and dissipation of an action potential.
  1.23 Defines terms related to venous capacitance and basic electrical properties.
  1.24 Identifies Starling's law of the heart.
  1.25 Identifies hydrostatic and osmotic pressures contributing to capillary fluid exchange.
  1.26 Identifies terms related to electrical properties of cardiac muscle.
  1.27 Identifies classic ECG changes associated with an MI.
  1.28 Specifies the hemodynamic events associated with electrochemical stages of myocardial muscle contraction.
  1.29 Specifies physiological responses to stimulation of major nervous system receptors in the heart.
  1.211 Specifies the electrocardiographic representation of electrochemical events associated with one cardiac cycle.
  1.212 Specifies and computes correct values of cardiac output and mean arterial pressure without aid of given formulas.
  1.213 Compares and contrasts general functions of the four heart chambers in relation to their morphological features.
  1.214 Compares and contrasts the primary functions of systemic arteries with systemic veins and pulmonary artery with the aorta in relation to their morphological features.

Continued.

Example 15-1. Instructional objectives for unit on MI patient—cont'd

    1.215 Compares and contrasts the features of impulse conduction during the absolute refractory period with those of the relative refractory period.

    1.216 Compares and contrasts the physiological outcomes of aerobic versus anaerobic cardiac metabolism.

    1.217 Compares and contrasts the electrocardiographic changes associated with myocardial ischemia, injury, and infarction.

    1.218 Differentiates between the direction of blood flow through the sinuses of Valsalva with that of blood flow through the venous and cardiac valves.

    1.219 Differentiates between the mechanical phase of myocardial contraction during which coronary perfusion occurs and that during which systemic perfusion occurs.

1.3 **Describes the psychosocial dynamics of adjusting to an acute, life-threatening illness** *(affective and cognitive)*

Instructional objectives:

    1.31 Defines terms related to adjustment to any stressful situation. *(cognitive)*

    1.32 Defines affective connotations of "the heart". *(cognitive)*

    1.33 Defines and identifies stages of psychosocial recovery from an MI as described by Cassem and Hackett. *(cognitive)*

    1.34 Defines and identifies defense mechanisms commonly used by MI patients. *(cognitive)*

    1.35 Identifies factors influencing body image and self-concept. *(cognitive)*

    1.36 Identifies influence of family on patient's adjustment to an MI. *(cognitive, affective)*

    1.37 Identifies environmental and social factors contributing to stress of CCU patient. *(cognitive, affective)*

    1.38 Identifies sources of chest pain from causes other than MI or angina. *(cognitive)*

    1.39 Specifies protective use of denial. *(cognitive, affective)*

    1.311 Specifies therapeutic value of work in relation to one's self-concept. *(cognitive, affective)*

    1.312 Specifies purpose of including family in patient's recovery process. *(cognitive, affective)*

    1.313 Specifies effects of residual symptoms on body image. *(cognitive)*

    1.314 Compares and contrasts stages of psychosocial recovery from an MI to Kübler Ross's stages in grief reaction. *(cognitive)*

    1.315 Compares and contrasts anxiety with fear; resignation with resolution. *(cognitive)*

    1.316 Compares and contrasts perceptions and objective reality. *(cognitive)*

    1.317 Differentiates and discriminates between patient situations requiring supportive interventions with those requiring reality orientation. *(cognitive, affective)*

    1.318 Differentiates and discriminates between therapeutic and pathological use of denial. *(cognitive, affective)*

    1.319 Differentiates and discriminates between potential supportive and nonsupportive family interactions with patient. *(cognitive, affective)*

1.4 **Develops a systematic plan of nursing care for the MI patient, based on appropriate anatomical, physiological, and psychosocial principles, pathophysiological features of MI, and nursing care objectives** *(cognitive and affective)*

Instructional objectives:

    1.41 Defines terms related to epidemiological features of MI: precipitating factors, etiologic factors, and type A personality. *(cognitive)*

    1.42 Defines terms related to nursing interventions for MI patients. *(cognitive)*

    1.43 Identifies purpose and rationale of nursing interventions based on prevention of physiological and psychosocial complications of an MI. *(cognitive, affective)*

    1.44 Identifies classic signs and symptoms of an MI. *(cognitive)*

    1.45 Identifies cardinal signs of respiratory or cardiac arrest. *(cognitive)*

    1.46 Identifies adventitious pulmonary sounds from their description. *(cognitive)*

    1.47 Identifies more common cardiac dysrhythmias from a description of the P, QRS, and T wave. *(cognitive)*

    1.48 Specifies the objectives of nursing intervention for the physical and psychosocial recovery of an MI patient. *(cognitive, affective)*

Example 15-1. Instructional objectives for unit on MI patient—cont'd

1.49 Specifies the steps in the nursing process. *(cognitive)*

1.411 Specifies precipitating events and risk factors in the etiology of an MI: physical and psychosocial. *(cognitive)*

1.412 Specifies appropriate nursing interventions in supporting the patient's physical and psychosocial adjustment to an MI.

1.413 Specifies appropriate nursing interventions in supporting the family's adjustment to the patient's MI. *(cognitive, affective)*

1.414 Specifies the criteria for evaluating outcomes of nursing interventions. *(cognitive)*

1.415 Specifies the potential consequences of physical and psychosocial complications of an MI: dysrhythmias, congestive heart failure, cardiogenic shock, venous thrombosis, pericarditis, ventricular aneurysm, ventricular rupture, denial, depression. *(cognitive, affective)*

1.416 Specifies the rationale for using various cardiac drugs: digitalis, lidocaine, atropine, potassium chloride, dopamine, heparin, morphine, colace. *(cognitive)*

1.417 Compares and contrasts signs and symptoms of angina and costochondritis with those of MI. *(cognitive)*

1.418 Compares and contrasts prognostic significance of S_3 with that of S_4. *(cognitive)*

1.419 Compares and contrasts etiological and precipitating factors in an MI. *(cognitive, affective)*

1.420 Compares and contrasts one- and two-person CPR technique.

1.421 Compares and contrasts principle underlying cardioversion and principle underlying defibrillation. *(cognitive)*

1.422 Differentiates and discriminates between nursing approach priorities in care of a young man with an MI and an elderly woman with an MI. *(cognitive, affective)*

1.423 Differentiates and discriminates between planning nursing interventions for rest and quiet with patient's need for social contact in the CCU. *(cognitive, affective)*

1.5 Applies knowledge of anatomical, physiological, and psychosocial principles in administering nursing care to a specific patient with MI *(cognitive, psychomotor, and affective)*

Instructional objectives:

1.51 Demonstrates ability to focus nursing care objectives on patient's perceptions of reality and to objective reality. *(affective, cognitive)*

1.52 Demonstrates ability to set priorities of nursing care according to patient's perceptions of the immediacy of needs. *(affective, cognitive)*

1.53 Demonstrates flexibility of approach to patient problems. *(affective)*

1.54 Demonstrates awareness of interrelatedness of patient's biopsychosocial needs. *(cognitive, affective)*

1.55 Discriminates and differentiates between patient's problems and nursing problems in patient situations. *(cognitive)*

1.56 Demonstrates awareness of need for patient feedback in confirming perceptions of patient problems. *(affective)*

1.57 Coordinates nursing interventions according to their priority in meeting patient's needs. *(cognitive, affective, and psychomotor)*

1.58 Demonstrates correct techniques in using equipment in the CCU: monitor leads, oxygen mask, elastic stockings, footboard, stethoscope. *(psychomotor)*

1.59 Demonstrates ability to synthesize data to arrive at decisions for planning nursing interventions. *(cognitive)*

1.511 Demonstrates awareness of physiological hemodynamics in positioning and exercising the MI patient. *(cognitive, psychomotor)*

1.512 Initiates appropriate patient and family teaching when opportunity arises. *(cognitive, affective, and psychomotor)*

1.513 Demonstrates readiness to revise nursing interventions in light of patient perceptions and outcomes. *(cognitive, affective)*

1.514 Demonstrates individualization of nursing interventions based on confirmed patient and family needs, rather than based on rigid adherence to theoretical protocols. *(affective)*

Step 2: Design a test blueprint

To assure that a measuring instrument covers the instructional objectives with the degree of specificity intended, it is helpful to group differentially the behavioral categories with their corresponding content areas. Because learning is defined as a change in behavior and because these behaviors must occur with respect to a specific subject matter, then behavioral categories and content areas constitute the two dimensions of a test blueprint. Table 15-1 illustrates a test blueprint derived from the instructional objectives listed in Example 15-1.

As you can see, a test blueprint merely provides a two-dimensional regrouping of all behaviors and content areas found in the instructional objectives. It more clearly orders the behaviors and content areas the test should or could potentially include.

Step 3: Assign a relative importance to each behavior and content area

In Chapter 7 the procedure for allotting instructional hours was described. At that time, a value judgment had to be made regarding the priority and relative importance of each behavior in its related content area with respect to the total amount of instructional time available. To be meaningful in its emphasis, the evaluation process must correspond to the instructional process in apportioning comparable amounts of measurement according to the emphasis allotted in instructional time. In this way, the appropriate amount of emphasis in evaluation remains consistent with both the apportioned instructional time and with the relative priority of each instructional objective for the course or program. Table 15-2 illustrates how the priority of learning behaviors may be used to first assign relative percentages of instructional time that translate into relative amounts of instructional time.

Step 4: Allocate a corresponding amount of emphasis to measuring learning

Allocating a corresponding amount of emphasis to measuring learning entails making decisions on how many items to include in the test and how many to allot to each behavior and content area. The first decision is discussed in greater detail later in this section. The second decision is made on the same basis as the allocations for relative amounts of instructional time: that is, the same emphasis (percentage) given to the behavior in instructional time is similarly reserved for that behavior in the evaluation process. As illustrated in Table 15-2, once the total number of test items is determined (in this case a total of 60 items), decremental proportions of the total number of items are assigned based on the same percentages given to that behavior in instructional time.

Step 5: Construct a table of test specifications

Once the total number of test items and a breakdown of items for each behavior category have been determined, you need to subdivide the number of items assigned to each behavior category among the content areas contained within the objectives. If you refer back to the objectives listed in Example 15-1, you can see that the behavior categories are differentially applied across four major content areas.

Table 15-3 illustrates how a test specification table is constructed. Like the test blueprint, a test specification table is a two-dimensional synopsis of behaviors and content areas to be evaluated. Unlike the qualitative blueprint, however, the test specification provides a detailed and quantitative summary of all test items, cross-referenced by behavior category and related content area. It reflects the proportionate emphasis that should appear in a test and is based on the test blueprint.

Table 15-1. Test blueprint

Behavior	Functional anatomy of cardiovascular system	Cardiovascular physiology and electrophysiology	Psychosocial dynamics	Principles underlying care
Defines	Anatomical features of: Sarcomere Endocardium Myocardium Pericardium Skeleton 4 chambers 4 valves Conduction system Systemic arteries Systemic veins Systemic capillaries Coronary arterial system Coronary venous system Sinus of Valsalva	Anatomical features by their functions: Heart Heart valves Systemic arteries Systemic veins Systemic capillaries Baroreceptors Chemoreceptors Nervous system connections Meanings of terms: Threshold potential Transmembrane potential Depolarization Repolarization Refractoriness Preload and afterload Vectors Vulnerable period Central venous pressure Pulmonary arterial wedge pressure	Affective connotations of the heart: Stages of psychosocial recovery from MI "Cardiac cripple" "Ego infarction" Body image Self-concept Anxiety, denial, and depression Reality testing Adjustment, coping, and resolution Rapport Communications	Terms: Precipitating factors Etiological factors Sedentary Type A personality Cardioversion S_3, S_4 Adventitious pulmonary sounds Learning readiness
Identifies	Macroscopic structure of cardiovascular system Microscopic structure of cardiovascular system Anatomical features of cardiac cells that differentiate them from skeletal and smooth muscle cells Sequence of electric depolarization	Starling's law of the heart Hydrostatic and osmotic pressures at capillary level Terms related to electrical actions: automaticity, conductivity, contractility, irritability ECG changes with MI	Stages of psychosocial recovery Factors influencing body image and self-concept Defense mechanisms Family's influence on patient recovery Environmental factors contributing to stress of CCU patient	Purpose and rationale of nursing actions based on physical and psychological complications of MI Classic signs and symptoms of MI Cardinal signs of cardiorespiratory arrest Lung sounds Dysrhythmias Sources of chest pain other than MI

Continued.

Table 15-1. Test blueprint—cont'd

Behavior	Functional anatomy of cardiovascular system	Cardiovascular physiology and electrophysiology	Psychosocial dynamics	Principles underlying care
Specifies	Direction and circuit of systemic, pulmonary, and coronary blood flows	Hemodynamic events associated with the electrochemical stages of myocardial muscle contractions Physiological effects of stimulation of various receptors ECG representation of electrochemical events in cardiac cycle Correct values for cardiac output and mean arterial pressure without formulas given	Protective use of denial Therapeutic value of work in relation to self-concept Purpose of including family in recovery process of patient Effects of residual symptoms on body image of patient	Nursing care objectives for patient with MI 4 steps in nursing process Risk factors and precipitating events in etiology of MI Appropriate nursing interventions in supporting recovery of MI patient Criteria for evaluating outcomes of nursing interventions Psychosocial complications of MI Rationale for use of cardiac drugs
Compares and contrasts	Differences in muscular structure and functions of right atria and ventricles and those of left atria and ventricles Differences in morphology and primary function of systemic arteries and systemic veins and pulmonary artery and the aorta	Impulse conduction during absolute refractory period and during relative refractory period Outcomes of aerobic and anaerobic metabolism	Cassem and Hackett's stages and Kübler-Ross' stages Anxiety and fear Perceptions and actual reality Resignation and resolution	Precipitating and etiological factors in MI One- and two-person CPR technique Principle of cardioversion and defibrillation Symptoms of angina, costochondritis and symptoms of MI Significance of S_3 and S_4 ECG changes in ischemia, injury, and infarction
Differentiates and discriminates	Structure of sinuses of Valsalva and structure of venous and cardiac valves	Direction of blood flow past sinuses of Valsalva and past venous or cardiac valves Mechanical phase of coronary perfusion and systemic perfusion	Situations requiring supportive intervention and reality orientation Therapeutic and pathological use of denial Supportive and nonsupportive family interactions with MI patient	Nursing approach priorities to young male and elderly female MI patients Patient's need for rest and quiet environment and need for social contact in CCU

Table 15-2. Relative allotments of instructional time and relative allotments of test items

Assigned priority	Behavior category	Percent of total instructional time	Number of instructional hours	Percent of total test items	Number of test items
1	Applies	40	3.2	40	24
2	Specifies	20	1.6	20	12
3	Discriminates and differentiates	15	1.2	15	9
4	Compares and contrasts	10	0.8	10	6
5	Defines	10	0.8	10	6
6	Identifies	5	0.4	5	3
	TOTAL	100	8.0	100	60

Table 15-3. Test specification*

Behavior	Anatomy	Physiology	Psychosocial	Principles	Scoring unit totals	Percent of totals
Defines	0	1	3	2	6	10%
Identifies	2	1	0	0	3	5%
Specifies	2	1	4	5	12	20%
Compares and contrasts	1	3	1	1	6	10%
Discriminates and differentiates	1	3	2	3	9	15%
Applies and uses	3	6	5	10	24	40%
Item totals and percent of totals	9	15	15	21	60	100%
	15%	25%	25%	35%		

*Total number of objective test items: 60. Total number of scoring units: 60. Total time: 2 hours (120 min). Time per item: 2 min/item.

DETERMINING THE TYPE OF TEST ITEMS TO USE

Test items may be categorized in many different ways to determine the item they represent. Educators may classify items according to any of the following systems:

1. How responses to the items are provided
   a. Entirely learner provided (essay item)
   b. Learner selects among responses instructor supplies (multiple-choice item)
2. How items are constructed
   a. Free response by learner (short essay item)
   b. Restricted response (fill-in-the-blank item)
   c. Structured response (true-false item)
3. How items are scored
   a. Subjectively scored items requiring expert to score (essay item)
   b. Intermediate items at times requiring expert to score (short answer item)
   c. Objectively scored item anyone or a machine could score (matching or multiple-choice item)
4. Location where measurement occurs
   a. Classroom (paper and pencil tests)
   b. Laboratory (simulations)

c. Clinical setting (rating scale, film)
5. Type of learning measured
   a. Cognitive learning (traditional written test)
   b. Affective learning (videotape, simulation experiences)
   c. Psychomotor and integrated learning (checklists, rating scale, film)
6. Any combination of these

Any of these approaches can conceivably achieve the same purpose; there is no right or wrong way to classify test items. For consistency, however, the last approach to categorize test items into various types will be used here because the emphasis is to assure that the evaluation process fulfills its rightful responsibility in measuring the types of learning specified in the instructional objectives. Following a discussion of how to determine how many items to include in a test will be a discussion of each type of test item in detail according to the type of learning it seeks to measure.

DETERMINING THE NUMBER OF TEST ITEMS TO USE

No easy formulas exist to use in calculating the total number of items a test can or should include. Many factors influence this decision. Probably the most direct way to estimate the number of items you can include is to consider the specific types of items in the test and how long each item usually takes to complete. As a very rough rule of thumb, true-false or simple multiple-choice test items may require 30 to 60 seconds to complete each item, complex multiple-choice and short answer and completion items may require 1 to 2 minutes each, long matching items or short essays may require 3 to 5 minutes each, and broad essay items and other complex items may be best judged only by pilot testing or through experience.

Other factors related to this decision include the following:
1. Time available for constructing test items

2. Time available for scoring test items
3. Time available for testing
4. Number and nature (complexity, level) of behaviors and content areas that must be covered
5. Skill the instructor presently has in constructing various types of test items
6. Past experience in using tests
7. Need for attendant skills such as reading, comprehending, and assimilating long passages, computing problems and formulas, complex problem solving, constructing figures or diagrams, and care plans
8. Influence of fatigue on the examinee

Now that plans for measuring learning have been specified, it is time to consider each type of learning and the test items available for measuring each.

TRADITIONAL METHODS OF TESTING

Two pragmatic reasons exist for describing traditional methods of testing learning. First, whereas nursing is admittedly a practice discipline, competent doing is in substantial part a function of what a nurse knows. Second, continuing and academic nurse educators persistently use these methods. The suggestions delineated here may improve these methods' validity, reliability, and usefulness as instruments to measure learning.

Essay items

An essay item presents a problem or problem situation to which the examinee must formulate and organize a response. The response may be limited to a few sentences or extend over many pages, depending on the nature and focus of the postulated problem.

Uses. Well-constructed essay items are most appropriately used for measuring complex cognitive behavior such as the ability to organize, integrate, synthesize, differentiate, describe, and summarize. They offer a learner the opportunity to draw on past experience and a full breadth of knowledge in demonstrating the ability to set priorities, to think critically and logically, and to solve practical problems the work situation presents. The essay item seems to have its greatest usefulness in situations where originality, creativity, and organization are necessary to solve problems for which more than one plausible approach is available.

Some educators also see essay items as useful vehicles for measuring affective learning. The validity of using essay items for eliciting affective performance is open to question, however, inasmuch as learners quickly become adept at delivering what they know is expected and acceptable in their response. A mammoth discrepancy may exist between what a learner says she feels or would do and what she actually feels and does in the work situation.

Two supposed advantages of essay items are that they may reduce the amount of time necessary to write test items and that they give learners a larger measure of freedom in responding. These advantages, however, are gained at problematic costs that often offset them.

Limitations. Essay items have some real or potential problems of validity and reliability that often restrict their usefulness as measuring devices. Because the time available for any testing period is more or less finite, there is an associated limit to how many essay items may be included in a given test. Depending on the length and complexity of the expected response, this time restriction may severely limit the number of objectives that can be measured. As the number of content areas and performance behaviors covered is reduced, the validity of the test is proportionately diminished. The more limited the sampling of objectives is, the fewer instances of behavior are available to make inferences from for evaluating learner performance.

An attendant problem with the validity of essay items is the open-ended, ambiguous nature of some of the behaviors they request of the examinee. Directions to "discuss," "give

your opinion," or "describe" may leave both learners and instructors at a loss to be able to isolate the behaviors and content areas called for in the objective. Finally, at times options are given to learners about which items must be answered. If all learners are not responding to the same items, they may not all be tested on the same objectives.

The validity problems associated with essay items may be compounded by a difficulty in establishing reliability for them. Not only are most forms (tests-retests, equivalence, internal consistency) of reliability testing difficult to achieve with essay items, but inter-rater and intra-rater reliability are also notoriously low. The scores assigned to essay items may vary among equally expert judges, vary with the same expert at different times, vary by the individual learner (facility and quality of verbal expression, writing ability, spelling, composition, grammar, punctuation, and handwriting), vary with the learner's response to the previous item, or vary even according to the order in which the test items appear. At times it is difficult to discern whether what was written was any more important than how it was expressed.

In addition to its propensity for inconsistencies, scoring essay items is usually a slow, methodical, time-consuming, and somewhat laborious task. This devours much instructor time in scoring and much learner time in receiving feedback.

Past grievances against the essay item may have not always endeared it as a measuring device, but abuses should not be blamed for all of its shortcomings. The essay item can be a helpful vehicle to measure learning if greater attention is paid to how it is written, used, and scored.

Writing essay items. The validity of the essay item may be improved in two ways. The first way is by writing a greater number of items that call for shortened, more focused responses rath-

Example 15-2. Examples of essay items: poor and improved

Item 1	*Poor:*	Discuss the physiology of cerebrospinal fluid.
	Improved:	Outline the major structures involved in the synthesis, circulation, and reabsorption of cerebrospinal fluid.
Item 2	*Poor:*	Describe what is meant by the term *surface tension*.
	Improved:	Specify how surfactant affects surface tension in the alveoli.
Item 3	*Poor:*	Describe the various types of heart block.
	Improved:	Differentiate between atrioventricular and intraventricular forms of heart block.

er than using only a few items that require lengthy, complex answers. If each essay item is carefully focused on a limited number of behaviors and content areas, the total number of items that can be included within a given time should be increased. If more objectives are represented, the adequacy of sampled content areas and behaviors increases the potential validity of the essay examination.

The second way is by replacing unrestricted and indefinite verbs with verbs that restrict, clarify, and unambiguously delineate the performance required of the examinee. Verbs such as "contrast," "specify," "illustrate," "outline," and "list" give clearer directions to learners and facilitate greater consistency between the instructional objectives and the essay test items. Rather than requesting that a nurse "Describe the ECG features of atrioventricular conduction defects," a more focused essay item might be stated, "Differentiate between a Mobitz type I second-degree AV block and a Mobitz type II second-degree AV block." Example 15-2 illustrates how restrictive verbs can assist in improving the specificity and validity of essay items.

Once the behaviors and content areas derived from the instructional objectives are identified, check that the behaviors and content areas tested in the essay item are congruent with those in the objectives. Predetermining these mental processes and affirming their presence in the essay item will add immeasurably to the item's validity.

Administering essay tests. A final check of the essay test should affirm that all items can be answered in the time allotted, all learners are required to answer the same items, and a point value is assigned to each item so examinees may distribute their response time accordingly.

Directions provided for learners should include how much time is available for taking the test and any restrictions or expectations regarding responses such as length of response or use of specific formats (outline, SOAP).

Scoring. To counteract some of the reliability problems that beset essay items, the instructor should prepare a scoring guide for each item that defines the essential elements of the ideal response and the number of points allocated to each of these elements in determining the total point value of the item. The examinee's name may be concealed or changed to an examination number so that the biasing influence of knowing who the examinee is has been reduced.

Consistency and uniformity in scoring items may be aided by scoring all responses to the same item before moving on to the next item and by having more than one expert involved in scoring. After each item is scored, papers can be rearranged before the next item is reviewed so that the papers on the bottom of the pile are not always subject to the scorer's fatigue and variable patience levels.

Short answer or completion items

Short answer or completion items may appear in one of two forms: as a direct question or as a sentence having one or more important words deleted. The direct question requires the examinee to supply a word, a phrase, or a few sentences. The incomplete sentence usually requires the learner to supply only a word, a phrase, or a number that completes the statement.

Uses. Short answer or completion items are useful for assessing a learner's ability to recall facts, symbols, dates, or abbreviations; to define terms, processes, or principles; or to work computational problems that have few potentially correct answers. This item may also be used with numbered anatomical illustrations or diagrams of equipment for which the learner must identify the names or functions.

Some advantages of the short answer or completion item include its economy and ease of construction and scoring in comparison with essays and other items. Because each item usually takes only a brief time to answer, a greater number of items can be included in a test period, allowing for a more representative sampling of the behaviors and content areas cotained in the objectives. Guessing is reduced because the learner is not supplied with answers to select from. In addition to the enhanced validity provided by more fully sampling instructional objectives, reliability is also enhanced as long as the required responses truly represent only one potentially correct answer.

Limitations. The major limitations of short answer or completion items concern their restricted levels of cognitive assessment and problems in scoring responses. The inherent form of these items restricts their use to situations in which learners can supply the necessary few words or phrases. As a result, these items are limited to assessing more rudimentary cognitive functions such as recall and recognition of factual information. This limited focus precipitates instructors lifting statements verbatim from textbooks and lectures, and encourages learners to memorize facts and isolated bits of trivia.

In reality, few questions have only a single correct response. Ambiguously or imprecisely worded items leave themselves open to multiple interpretations, differing by shades or spectra from the instructor's original intention. This may leave instructors having to defend their key and its rationale, and leave learners openly hostile. Even when a variety of plausible responses are deemed acceptable, a content area expert is needed to differentiate among these and determine what effects, if any, shades of difference in response or misspellings will have. Although scoring should be rather straightforward with this item, the preceding limitations can make it a laborious chore.

If blanks are scattered all over the page, visual searching can become exasperating for the scorer. Some examinees will attempt to write short essays in the 2-inch blank, causing visual stress among scorers.

Writing short answer or completion items. When writing short answer or completion items, focus only on important content area elements. Be careful to pose the question or statement as clearly and precisely as possible so that it leads to only one possible brief answer. As an illustration, in Item 1 of Example 15-3, multiple interpretations are plausible for the response because the problem does not differentiate between receptive or motor speech functions and does not specify what divisional level of the central nervous system the instructor intends the learner to use. As a result, examinees could respond with any of the following and be plausibly correct: dominant cerebral, left hemispherical, Broca's, Wernicke's, tempoparietal, fronto-

Example 15-3. Examples of completion items: poor and improved

---

Item 1   *Poor:*   Speech is controlled in the _____ area of the brain.

           Improved: A patient who demonstrates motor aphasia has sustained damage to a frontoparietal section of the dominant hemisphere called _____ area.

Item 2   *Poor:*   An elevated arterial Pco_2 level is always associated with _____ .

           Improved: When arterial Pco_2 levels rise, arterial pH levels would be expected to _____ .

Item 3   *Poor:*   The _____ represents conduction time through the AV junction.

           Improved: In the ECG cycle, conduction time through the AV junction is represented by the _____ .

---

temporal, frontoparietal, motor, or association. The improved version of this item has only one correct response.

Include enough information in the question or statement so that the examinee can respond to an adequate stimulus. Avoid omitting so many words that the learner has no basis for knowing where to direct her thought processes (Item 2, Example 15-3).

Whenever numerical or symbolic responses (dosages, volumes, weights) are requested, provide the units of measurement for the response. Although you need to give an adequate amount of stimuli for the examinee to respond to, avoid dispensing unwarranted cues. These grammatical or typographical cues constitute undue advantages given to the learner. Use the "a (an)" forms of indefinite articles and keep the length of blanks uniform.

To facilitate the learner's ability to respond to the item, it is better to situate the blank at the end rather than at the beginning of the item (Item 3, Example 15-3).

Administering short answer or completion tests. Group similar forms of short answer or completion items and provide explicit directions to learners for each separate form. Specify the scoring value of each and any special instructions related to spelling variations or the need to show all computations. The scoring process may be simplified by numbering each blank and then providing a separate numbered answer sheet or by using the right- or left-hand margins for listing the responses corresponding to that item number. This will reduce the scoring time, obviate the hide-and-seek approach to locating answers, and diminish the likelihood that examinees will need to use inordinately small or illegible handwriting within a sentence.

Scoring. For scoring, you will need to devise a key of all acceptable responses. In reality, it is usually helpful to scan the answers given to items to determine if more than one interpretation was made and, if so, whether it seems plausible and acceptable. If alternate responses are deemed acceptable, they will need to be incorporated into the key. In general, one scoring unit of equal weight is assigned to each blank within a group of item forms. Alloting partial credit for answers is problematic for both instructors and learners and is best avoided by well-written and narrowly circumscribed wording.

True-false items

True-false items are declarative statements that examinees must judge as either "true" or "false." Because responses to the item are limited to these two options, this item is also referred to as an alternate or fixed response item.

Uses. True-false items are ideally suited to assessing a learner's knowledge of facts that are categorically true or false. Because most every content area possesses some undeniable constants, this item can be widely applicable over a broad range of factual subject matter. True-false items may also be useful in assessing a learner's preconceptions, misconceptions, and fallacious or mistaken beliefs.

True-false items are relatively easy to construct and respond to, are good for assessing an extensive amount of subject matter in a relatively brief time, and can result in a more representative sampling of the instructional objectives. When written to require only an indication of truth or falsity, these items can be rapidly and efficiently scored by nonexperts in the content area, by clerks, or even by computers.

Limitations. By their very nature, true-false items are restricted in the number and types of instructional objectives they can appraise. Their use is generally limited only to those content areas that can be categorized as true or false without qualification. This restricted range of applicability precipitates two undesirable results: a focus on circumscribed bits of information and a tendency to encourage rote memorization of trivia.

The alternate either-or format of these items encourages guessing; even if a learner knows virtually nothing about the content area addressed in the item, she has a 50% chance of guessing correctly.

Writing unambiguous true-false items can be an onerous task because the truth or falsity of a statement is usually contingent on a specific context, set of circumstances, or even the interpretation of the reader. These items are only designed for dealing with absolute truth or falsity; relative degrees of these attributes present problems when item writers attempt to qualify relative truths or falsehoods, forcing them into a mold they do not fit.

Writing true-false items. When writing true-false items, keep the item brief, direct, and lim-

ited to a single idea. Long, complex verbiage only adds confusion and extraneous sources of error. Reread the item as written to be certain it represents a statement that can be unequivocally and demonstrably classified as true or false without further qualification. Avoid using determiners that cue the item as true (qualifiers such as *usually, often, sometimes, typically, in most cases*) and those that cue the item as false (overly inclusive determiners such as *only, all, never, no, always*). Avoid the converse problems of hiding the focus of truth or falsity in some inconspicuous part of a word or phrase of the item and using single or double negatives that alter or reverse the focus of the item. Form can also influence a learner's response if the qualifying phrases of true items are consistently made longer and more complex than false ones.

Some of these logistical problems with writing true-false items can be diminished by employing forms other than the declarative sentence. Ambiguity in item wording may be reduced by underlining or capitalizing the focus of truth or falsity of the item so that learners know where to direct their attention in responding to the item. A fuller evaluation of the learner's knowledge and a reduced likelihood of guessing may be enhanced by combining this underlining with requiring the examinee to correct or cross out any false segments of the sentence. Providing a brief vignette as a context for a series of true-false items may also give clearer directions to learners for determining the veracity of the statements (Example 15-4).

Administering true-false tests. Be sure to select a response format that enables the scorer to decipher true from false responses; when examinees are asked to write "T" or "F," it is often uncanny how many pseudo letters are revealed that share characteristics common to both Ts and Fs. A checkmark next to the appropriate response or circling the intended response will help keep scoring dilemmas under control.

If more than one version of the true-false for-

Example 15-4. Examples of true-false items: poor and improved

---

Item 1	*Poor:*	Sleep and wakefulness are controlled by the brainstem.
	Improved:	Sleep and wakefulness are controlled by the *reticular formation*.
Item 2	*Poor:*	The mitral and tricuspid valves are *not* examples of semilunar valves.
	Improved:	The mitral and tricuspid valves are examples of atrioventricular valves.
Item 3	*Poor:*	Normal intracranial pressures range from 0 to 15.
	Improved:	Normal intracranial pressures range from 0 to 15 mm Hg.

---

mat is used, provide separate sets of instructions for each. Indicate how and where responses are to be marked and whether false segments or statements need to be corrected. Points allocated differently for each format should be described for the examinee. Because learners are quick to detect patterns in the list of responses, randomize the order of true and false statements and provide approximately a 50% distribution of each.

Scoring. If only one true-false format is used, the scoring unit or number of points for each item remains constant. When variant or multiple true-false formats are used, you will need to determine whether different point allocations will need to be used. Because some variants require more than one behavior of the examinee, decisions and problems related to assigning partial credit again arise.

Matching items

A matching item consists of a series of problem items (stems, premises) that are in some way associated with an accompanying series of possible responses or options. The separate series are arranged in a two-column format. The learner's task is to indicate which response or option corresponds to the item presented on the basis of some predetermined characteristic. The problem items are typically numbered consecutively and arranged in the left-hand column; they may occur in the form of incomplete sentences, phrases, or words. All answers must be drawn from the same set of options.

Uses. Matching items are best suited to measuring knowledge of facts and associations among these such as associating anatomical structures with their function or location, terms or concepts with their definition or symbol, principles with their application, or poisons with their antidotes. These items are limited to assessing the lower orders of cognitive functioning such as identification, recall, recognition, differentiation, and association. They can be used for appraising verbal associations or may be cast into a numbered diagram for matching the function or name of numbered parts. As with other item types that test factual knowledge, matching items can incorporate the assessment of multiple content areas in a brief time.

Limitations. Matching items share the limited focus of applicability and tendency for trivia found in true-false items. Their usefulness is limited by their inability to appraise higher cognitive levels. If each of the alternative responses can be used only once and their number is equivalent to the number of problem items, guessing and crediting through the process of elimination can reduce their validity as measuring devices. Unless lists of each column are kept rather short, many options are not reasonable alternatives for each problem item and the validity of the exercise again falters.

Writing matching items. Within each series of

Example 15-5. Examples of matching items: poor and improved

Poor matching items

A

_____ 1. Gradual deterioration in level of consciousness
_____ 2. Papilledema and respiratory alkalosis
_____ 3. Xanthochromia and elevated lumbar pressures
_____ 4. Unconscious
_____ 5. "Clear interval"

B

a. Spinothalamic tracts
b. Epidural hematoma
c. Subdural hematoma
d. C_1-C_5 lesions
e. Autonomic hyperreflexia
f. Subarachnoid hemorrhage
g. Cerebral edema
h. Cerebral concussion
i. Pyramidal tracts

Improved matching items

Nursing assessment

_____ 1. "Following admission for acute head injury, neuro status satisfactory; over the past 12 hours, however, level of consciousness has gradually deteriorated."
_____ 2. "Funduscopic exam reveals papilledema; ABG's reveal respiratory alkalosis."
_____ 3. "LP demonstrated xanthochromia and pressure of 30 mm Hg."
_____ 4. "Immediately following trauma incident, patient had transient loss of consciousness."
_____ 5. "Patient admitted to ICU following acute head trauma. Was unconscious on arrival at emergency department, then awake and alert, pupils equal and reactive to light for past 2 hours. Patient now unresponsive to all stimuli and left pupil is dilated and nonreactive to light."

Associated clinical condition

a. Brainstem herniation
b. Epidural hematoma
c. Cerebral concussion
d. Cerebral contusion
e. Subdural hematoma
f. Subarachnoid hemorrhage
g. Cerebral edema

---

a column, the set should be homogeneous so that the basis for matching remains clear. Headings over each column should specify the commonality among the included elements. This will assist examinees in understanding how the two columns relate to one another. Problems with guessing can be diminished by providing more responses than items to be matched. To facilitate test taking, state the options as briefly as possible and keep both lists relatively short. If either series has some inherent ordering, arrange that series accordingly (numerical, chronological, alphabetical) (Example 15-5).

Administering matching tests. The two-column series should be clearly differentiated by consecutively numbering one and alphabetically listing the other. Directions should include the basis for matching the items, whether options can be used more than once, whether any problems require more than one option and how and where answers are to be recorded. It is most humane to have all elements of each column located on the same page.

Scoring. No special scoring considerations are necessary for matching items.

Multiple-choice items

A multiple-choice item consists of a *stem* that formulates a problem or asks a question, a *key* that constitutes the correct or best response to the problem or question posed, and a series of alternative options called *distractors* that provide plausible but incorrect or less desirable responses to the stem.

Similar to true-false or matching items, multiple-choice items are classified as objective test items because they do not require a subject matter expert for scoring and may even be scored by a machine or a computer. They also share a common general form in that each item presents a specific problem together with a specific and limited set of choices from which the examinee must select a response.

Multiple-choice items may be cast into a number of different response formats, depending on the performance behaviors and content areas to be measured, as follows.

Correct response format is used when the key is unequivocally and demonstrably correct, whereas the distractors are absolutely incorrect. Its primary use is in measuring factual truisms and items of certainty.

Best response format is used when the key is clearly and defensibly the most desirable or appropriate response among the alternatives offered, whereas the distractors are less than optimal but also correct. Its primary use is in measuring areas having varying degrees of appropriateness or veracity, controversial issues and topics, areas where certainty and fact are relative to circumstances, or a complex, interrelated set of variables.

Multiple response format is used when the key includes more than a single option (multiple keys) or when multiple options are combined within a single key. Its primary use is in measuring more complex cognitive functions such as data interpretation and analysis, inferential and deductive reasoning, problem solving, and the determination of multiple causation or effect.

Negative response format is used when the key designates an option that is an exception, error, exclusion, anomaly, or other aberration that singles it out from the other options. Its primary use is for detecting errors or exceptions to general rules or procedures, or for emphasizing contraindications and inappropriate ministrations.

Context-dependent response format is used when the key to a number of items is in part based on information provided in a picture, graphic, illustration, or narrative preceding the item series. It is primarily used for obtaining a more holistic and meaningful frame of reference for fuller consideration of more complex phenomena as they occur in a realistic situation.

Example 15-6 illustrates examples of each of the multiple-choice response formats. Other variations of these formats, such as combining two or more aspects of the response in a single option, are also possible.

Uses. The widespread popularity of the multiple-choice item is rooted in its superior versatility, flexibility, economy, and validity in comparison to other forms of written measurement items. The multiple-choice item can appraise cognitive learning as well or better than virtually any other written test item and frequently does so more effectively and efficiently. It can measure the full range of cognitive abilities and, depending on the cognitive function and proximity between options, offer measurement at virtually any degree of difficulty level. Even among the best and brightest learners, it can require fine discriminatory powers to select appropriately among the offered alternatives.

In addition to the flexibility in design and response formats, multiple-choice items are efficient and economical to write, answer, score, and analyze. Item writing time is usually counterbalanced by improved clarity and reduced ambiguity, as well as the lessened response, feedback, and scoring times effected.

Reliability and validity are similarly enhanced by the greater breadth and scope of the coverage of objectives various forms of this item afford. Scores can be subjected to a wide array of descriptive and statistical methods of analysis and guessing can be controlled by clearly positing the problem and constructing an adequate number of homogeneous distractors. Logistical scoring problems that plague other item types (legibility of handwriting, skill in written expression, spelling, punctuation, variable degrees of

Example 15-6. Multiple-choice response formats

1. *Correct response:* When key is unequivocally correct.

    The percussion note normally heard over peripheral lung fields is _____ .
    a. Dullness
    b. Tympany
    c. Resonance
    d. Hyperresonance

2. *Best response:* When key is defensibly the most appropriate or desirable response.

    Patients should be suctioned for

    _____ .
    a. Up to 30 seconds every hour
    b. Up to 15 seconds every 30 minutes
    c. As long as necessary to clear the airway
    d. No more than 30 seconds when scheduled
    e. No more than 15 seconds when clinically indicated

3. *Multiple response:* Multiple key type.

    The chief advantages of intermittent mandatory ventilation (IMV) over traditional methods of weaning are that IMV is _____ .
    1. Safer
    2. Less physiologically demanding to patients
    3. Faster
    4. Less burdensome for staff nurses
    5. More readily accepted by patients
    Choices:
        a. 1, 2 4
        b. 1, 2, 5
        c. 2, 3, 5
        d. 2 and 3 only

Multiple response: Multiple options within single key.

Weaning from mechanical ventilation should be discontinued immediately whenever there is any evidence of _____ .
a. Hypertension, tachycardia, or anxiety
b. Hypertension, bradycardia, or diaphoresis
c. Hypotension, tachycardia, or agitation
d. Hypotension, bradycardia, or ventricular dysrhythmias

4. *Negative response*

    When administering CPR, the victim's head would *not* be hyperextended if there were any possibility of _____ .
    a. A fractured mandible
    b. An occipital fracture
    c. Cervical spinal cord injury
    d. Thoracic spinal cord injury

5. *Context-dependent response*

    On his fourth day of hospitalization for an acute MI, Mr. Rockville experiences a sudden recurrence of chest pain that is positional and radiates to his left shoulder, a fever of 102.6° F, and S-T segment elevation in nearly all ECG leads. The most likely cause of this clinical picture is _____ .
    a. Extension of the original MI
    b. Pericardial tamponade
    c. Acute pericarditis
    d. Hypostatic pneumonia

response accuracy, subjective scoring biases) that render them less reliable are virtually nullified by using the multiple-choice item.

Limitations. The limitations of the multiple-choice item are few and largely outweighed by its advantages and usefulness. In the main, the multiple-choice item is limited to written assessments of cognitive learning. Its validity and usefulness in assessing affective and psychomotor learning are less universally accepted.

Because providing attractive and functional distractors accounts for much of their effective-ness, it maybe difficult to find suitable and adequate numbers of these alternative options. As with any test item that predetermines the learner's potential array of responses, multiple-choice items inherently limit the ability to measure how well a learner can select among options that are self-determined. Guessing is likely to be a problem only when distractors are ineffective or inappropriate, if the item is unduly difficult, or if it has an insufficient number of option choices.

Writing multiple choice items. In writing multiple-choice items, an equal amount of attention must be paid to the stem and the distractors; the effective construction of each is a bit of an art.

The stem of the item may be written as an incomplete sentence or as a direct question. In either case, it should incorporate three components: (1) a clear, concise formulation of a single problem that has a single correct or best response, (2) all information and qualifications pertinent for responding to the problem, and (3) any words or phrases that would otherwise have to be repeated in each option.

The stem must postulate a problem clearly so that the appropriate solution or response to it is evident to the examinee. Ambiguity or lack of focus leaves the learner at a loss in deciding how to respond to the item. If well-informed learners and competent practitioners can anticipate the correct or best response before considering the options offered, you can be reasonably confident that the problem is clearly posed.

In delineating the problem, brevity is a virtue related to clarity. Avoid loading the stem with complex sentence structure, nonfunctional verbiage, and elaborate jargon. These elements not only precipitate unnecessary mental calisthenics, but clutter and convert the item into a measure of reading comprehension. Too much information in the stem may also increase the likelihood that more than one closely related option is correct.

As with other item types, the stem should formulate a single problem for measurement. Even if the performance required in the item consists of multiple component abilities, the overall task as described in the stem should be clearly discernible as an identifiable composite.

It seems self-evident that the stem should be written so that it has a correct or best answer, but at times it is only after a test has been reviewed by colleagues or taken by learners that you discover this is not the case. A related finding may be that the stem as written has more

than one equally correct or best option; in this case, either the stem or the proximity of options to one another must be revised.

In constructing the item, it is generally advised that all necessary information, qualifications, and repeated sections be located within the stem so that the problem is completely evident after reading only the stem and so that options may be kept as brief as possible. Following this maxim will make the multiple-choice item more straightforward and efficient and reduce the reading burden for the examinee. The information contained within the stem should be limited to information that is pertinent and directly related to formulating an accurate response.

Negative stems should be used sparingly and only as warranted. When they are employed, the negative segment should be emphasized by highlighting it with capital letters, italics, or underlining.

A final check on the stems should verify that the stem of one item does not reveal the appropriate response to other items within the test.

A perfectly written stem cannot compensate adequately for poorly constructed distractors. Unless these alternative responses are composed at least as well as the stem, all measurement value of the item can be lost. The best way to determine if the options offered are functioning well is if examinees knowledgeable in the area addressed by the item can readily identify what the clearly correct or best option (key) is, and can easily reject all other distractors, while examinees deficient in this requisite knowledge hesitate and select from among the distractors rather than choose the key.

All options to an item must be plausible, logical, and grammatically consistent with the stem. Alternatives should be internally homogeneous in their content, terminology, part of speech, units of measurement (for computational problems), frame of reference, and length. If some inherent sequence is present among the options (order of magnitude, numerical, alphabetical, or chronological order), they should be so sequenced. When the length of the option is variable, shortest to longest length can also be used for determining the ordering sequence. This can assist in discouraging guessing based solely on the length of the option. In general, the more homogeneous the options are, the better they will discriminate between the knowing and the unknowing learner.

As mentioned with true-false items, be careful that you have not used sophisticated technical terms, complex and excessive qualifications, and option lengths that are proportional to the likelihood that that option is the key. Giveaways of this sort diminish the value of the subsequent measurement data.

You must use at least three effective options to avoid reversion to an alternate (either-or) response item. For the most part, more than six options constitute a memory exercise and waste much reading time. The number of options offered is usually three to five. Use fewer when only two or three options are plausible rather than including obviously wrong or ridiculous options that surely will not be plausible in even the poorest achiever's consideration. An example of this might be:

The architecture of the mainstem pulmonary bronchi leaves the _____ lung more vulnerable to inadvertent bronchial intubation and resultant pneumonia.
    A. Right
    B. Left

If an alternate response item is not desired, the item writer must rewrite the stem to correct the problem rather than add implausible options. Usually, the optimal number of reasonable alternatives is determined by the nature of the variables being measured balanced with a need to better control guessing by increasing the number of options to four or five.

"None of the above" or "all of the above" as options are typically employed as filler options when the item writer cannot readily think of other plausible alternatives. If "none of the above" is used, it should be in computational or other factual items where the key is exactly correct. If "all of the above" is used, it should not be the key any more often than it is not.

Options that deal with numerical ranges (range of normal, dosages) should be exclusive of one another so that the correct or best response does not overlap two or more potential choices.

Administering multiple-choice tests. Multiple-choice items are typically numbered and options are lettered. Whatever method is selected should remain the same for all items and responses.

Lay out the test so that various content areas, response formats, or alternative forms of the multiple-choice item (or other item types) are grouped together. Items and their related options, especially context-dependent forms, should appear on the same page so that time is not wasted flipping pages back and forth. Make each page appear visually satisfying by not crowding or varying the location of options with respect to the stem.

Directions to the examinee should include the basis for responding to the item (correct instead of best response) and how responses should be recorded (separate answer sheet, circled, underlined).

As you review the full key, double-check that you have not introduced a recognizable pattern of correct or best responses; if necessary, randomize the key sequence so that an option's position has no relation to its tendency to be the key.

Strictly speaking, if the stem is an incomplete sentence, all options should begin with lower case letters and receive any terminal punctuation necessary. If the stem is a direct question, each option should begin with a capital letter and end with the appropriate punctuation.

Scoring. The score obtained with multiple-choice items is based on the number of items answered correctly when compared with the key.

NONTRADITIONAL METHODS OF TESTING

In Chapter 7 we discussed using instructional media in curriculum planning and implementation. A number of these media forms (slide-tapes, audio tapes, film, overhead projector, filmstrip-tapes, television) may also be used for evaluating content areas. Some provide this by means of pretests and posttests, whereas others use self-assessments or study guides. Many are rather informal and are aimed at providing immediate feedback to the adult learners who use them.

In place of written problem situations or stems, visual or auditory stimuli may be used to elicit learners' responses. Filmed or taped scenarios may serve as the basis for learners' responses to a number of test items. In addition to being very effective vehicles for evaluation, media are also a pleasant alternative to the printed word.

Computer-assisted instruction (CAI) is as valuable for evaluation as it is for instruction. Some centers combine the more traditional methods of evaluation, especially multiple-choice type items, and with the aid of computers design, administer, measure, and analyze evaluation data. The computer may assist in scoring, grading, and analyzing test scores, may be employed to generate test items, design test formats, or may identify learning problems or areas needing further clarification or remediation. Computers may also provide both rapid and detailed forms of feedback to learners. The analysis of measurement data frequently neglected by instructors can be provided quickly and efficiently by computer assistance, making test analysis a rather painless procedure and increasing the likelihood it will be performed.

Chapter 16 describes the evaluation of affective and psychomotor learning. As you review these sections, you will find that many of the teaching methods mentioned in Chapter 9 are also useful evaluation devices.

Before considering the evaluation of affective and psychomotor types of learning, however, the evaluation process for cognitive learning needs to be completed by making the transition from measurement to evaluation of learning.

REFERENCES
Traditional achievement tests

Ebel, R: Can teachers write good true-false test items? J Educ Measure **12**:31, 1975.

Gronlund, NE: Constructing achievement tests, ed 2, Englewood Cliffs, N.J., 1977, Prentice-Hall.

King, EC: Constructing classroom achievement tests, Nurs Educ **3**:30, 1978.

Lange, CM: Using media in evaluation, Nurs Outlook **25**:241, 1977.

Mehrens, WA, editor: Readings in measurement and evaluation in education and psychology, New York, 1976, Holt, Rinehart and Winston.

Miller, HG, and Williams, G: Construction of higher level multiple-choice questions covering factual content, Educ Technol **13**:39, 1973.

Murphy, SA: Improving teacher-made tests in an integrated curriculum, JNE **18**:41, 1979.

Rezler, AG, and Liu, RW: Hope for that hopeless essay test, JNE **16**:5, 1977.

Ross, GR, and Ross, MC: Using the computer to prepare multiple-choice examinations: a simplified system, JNE **16**:32, 1977.

Staropoli, CJ, and Waltz, CF: Developing and evaluating educational programs for health care providers, Philadelphia, 1978, F.A. Davis Co.

Wood, DA, and Adkins, DD: Test construction: development and interpretation of achievement tests, ed 2, Columbus, Ohio, 1974, Charles E. Merrill Books, Inc.

Chapter 16

Evaluation of learning

EVALUATION OF COGNITIVE LEARNING

The measuring items described in Chapter 15 are useful in providing valid and reliable indicators of learning. Their usefulness, however, is limited to their ability to adequately quantify learning performances. Test items provide educational measurements. They do not provide for evaluating learning performance.

To derive evaluations from these measurements, the educator must now compare an individual's performance to some criterion that functions as a reference point for evaluating that performance. As discussed earlier, the reference point against which an individual's performance is compared may be either group performance or some specified criterion level of performance; that is, evaluating learning may be either norm referenced or criterion referenced.

When the educator is interested in describing a group's overall performance or in describing an individual learner's performance in relation to that of others, norm-referenced evaluation techniques are appropriate. When the educator is interested only in describing the performance of the individual learner without relating it to the performance of others, criterion-referenced evaluation procedures are more appropriate. Hospital-based educators may find that both types of evaluations are necessary or that one or the other is needed at different times or for different purposes. For these reasons, the present section briefly describes the major concepts and

components entailed in each type of educational evaluation.

The discussion is limited to an overview of each because their definitive aspects constitute discrete and advanced studies in and of themselves that are well beyond the scope of this book. The purpose of acquainting you as hospital-based educators with the general features of educational evaluation is to acquaint you with their features and availability and to stimulate you to pursue them in greater detail as your needs for evaluation warrant.

Norm-referenced evaluation: analysis of group performance

The concepts and techniques used in norm-referenced evaluation of cognitive learning are borrowed from the field of descriptive statistics. Its parent field, *statistics*, comprises all data analysis techniques applied to quantitative information derived from groups. The mathematical study of statistics is divided into two branches, descriptive and inferential. *Descriptive statistics* comprises techniques that enable one to summarize and to characterize measurement data meaningfully and concisely. *Inferential statistics* includes analysis that enables one to validly generalize or to extend measurement findings to other comparable groups or test situations. Because norm-referenced evaluation attempts to describe an individual's performance in relation to that of others, it requires that the

Table 16-1. Scores obtained by 20 nurses in critical care pretest

Nurse	Score	Nurse	Score
A	34	K	52
B	59	L	46
C	39	M	52
D	58	N	47
E	42	O	52
F	41	P	47
G	57	Q	51
H	45	R	49
I	54	S	51
J	45	T	49

Table 16-2. Frequency distribution of critical care pretest scores

x	f	x	f
60		45	||
59	|	44	
58	|	43	
57	|	42	|
56		41	|
55		40	
54	|	39	|
53		38	
52	|||	37	
51	||	36	
50		35	
49	||	34	|
48		33	
47	||	32	
46	|	31	
			N = 20

x = score obtained
f = frequency of occurrence of that score
N = total number of scores

educator first be able to describe group performance and then to consider how the individual learner performed in relation to the group.

Suppose you just administered a 60-item multiple-choice pretest to 20 nurse orientees (n = 20) of the critical care units. After scoring all 20 tests, alloting one point (scoring unit) for each correct item out of 60 possible correct items, you reviewed the scores these nurses obtained and listed them as seen in Table 16-1. When the data appear in this form, you can see how difficult it is to derive any meaningful evaluation of overall group performance.

Some questions you would likely be asking yourself at this juncture include the following:

1. How could the data be organized so that it would be easier to recognize and to describe how the group performed?
2. Rather than considering all of these separate scores, how could I best summarize overall performance?
3. Did everyone in the group do about the same or was there a lot of variation among individual performances?

Frequency distributions. Consecutively listing these scores does not offer much meaningful information to the educator who needs to evaluate a set of test scores. Because the obtained scores are numerical values, you might logically conclude that one way to bring order to these separate scores is to arrange the scores in numerical order from the highest to the lowest attained score. The resulting tabulation (Table 16-2) is called a *frequency distribution.*

A frequency distribution is helpful as an initial device for counting (tallying, tabulating) the frequency of occurrences of any given score. Because no nurses received scores below 32, these do not need to be included in enumerating how often a specific score was obtained. Even deleting these lower scores does not seem to summarize the others adequately enough.

Grouped frequency distribution. A further refinement that presents the data in an even more summarized format is achieved by retabulating the scores according to exclusive groups called *class intervals.* This provides an even more visually convenient and economical form

Table 16-3. Grouped and cumulative frequency distribution and cumulative percentage of critical care pretest scores

Class interval	f	Cumulative f	Cumulative percentage
56 to 60	3	20	100
51 to 55	6	17	85
46 to 50	5	11	55
41 to 45	4	6	30
36 to 40	1	2	15
31 to 35	1	1	5
	N = 20		

of frequency distribution referred to as a *grouped frequency distribution*. As Table 16-3 illustrates, a grouped frequency distribution simply gathers groups of scores and determines the frequency of scores on the basis of these groups of scores rather than on the basis of individual scores. Each group or class interval should be of equal size and should not overlap with adjacent groups.

Cumulative frequency distribution. If you successfully add (accumulate) the number of frequencies within each class interval from lowest to highest, you obtain what is called a *cumulative frequency distribution*, illustrated in the medial right-hand column of Table 16-3. A cumulative frequency distribution enables you to consider the occurrences of each scoring interval in terms of the total number of persons who participated in providing the data (n = 20).

Cumulative percentages. A further extension of this idea of accumulated frequencies considers the cumulative frequencies in relation to the total number of persons taking the test, given as a percentage. The far right column of Table 16-3 designates these *cumulative percentages*, obtained by simply dividing the cumulative frequency by the total number of frequencies (n =

20) and then multiplying by 100%. This provides helpful information relating to what percent of the learners attained scores within each scoring or class interval. Just as the cumulative frequencies must total N (20), the cumulative percentages must total 100% (all 20 entries). As shown later, these percentages can assist in deriving other features of group performance.

A frequency distribution is an extremely helpful vehicle for organizing test data to see more readily where scores fell and how they were distributed. It visually indicates the highest, lowest, and all intermediate scores obtained, as well as the scores and scoring intervals achieved most often or not at all, in a fairly economical and readily comprehensible manner.

Measures of central tendency. As helpful as frequency distributions may be in summarizing a large number of test scores, they still involve a moderate amount of data manipulation and time to derive, and fail to yield a clear picture of overall group performance. In any test situation wherein a large number of scores are produced, you could reasonably expect that a few people would score low, a few high, and most earn scores between these two extremes. Even without knowing the tests or the examinees, then, you could reasonably predict that scores would be distributed in a customary bell-shaped or normal distribution curve (Fig. 7).

As the size of the group diminishes, the likelihood that scores will be distributed in this manner also diminishes, yet the scores still usually cluster around some central point and diminish in frequency toward peripheral areas on either side. This tendency of scores to pile up in the middle of a distribution of scores and thin out at the periphery enables the evaluator to locate one average, middle, or typical score that may be used to characterize concisely the entire distribution and compare it with other distributions of scores. The determinations that represent the central or pivotal scores are called *measures of central tendency*.

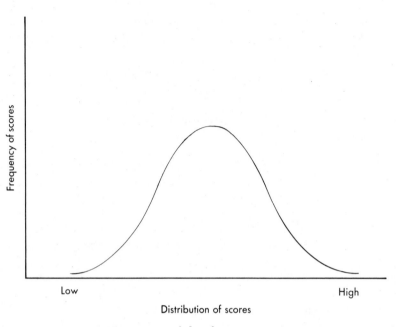

Fig. 7. Normal distribution curve.

Example 16-1

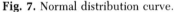

Nurse	Score
A	34
B	59
C	39
D	58
E	42
F	41
G	57
H	45
I	54
J	45
K	52
L	46
M	52
N	47
O	52
P	47
Q	51
R	49
S	51
T	49
	$\Sigma = \overline{970}$

$$\overline{X} = \frac{\Sigma X}{N}$$

$$= \frac{970}{20}$$

$$\overline{X} = 48.5$$

where $\overline{X}$ = Mean
Σ = The sum of
X = Scores
N = Total number of scores

The three different measures of central tendency are the mean, median, and mode. Each refers to a different aspect of centrality, whereas all three attempt to characterize concisely the entire distribution of scores.

Mean. The *mean* refers to the average score of a group of scores. It is determined by finding the sum of all scores and dividing this sum by the number of scores. If you added all 20 of the scores indicated in Table 16-1, you would get a sum total of 970. When this sum (970) is then divided by the number of scores (N = 20), the average or mean score is 48.5.

The abbreviation or symbol for mean score is "$\overline{X}$". Example 16-1 illustrates how to calculate a mean score.

The mean (also called an arithmetic mean) is the most widely used measure of central tendency because it considers the weight of each score and balances the total weight of the scores with how many scores contributed to that weight. As long as scores follow a pattern of normal (bell-shaped) distribution, the mean is the single most valid representation of any set of scores. In general, the less symmetrical the distribution of the scores, the less valid the mean is for characterizing that set of scores.

Because the mean considers the relative weights of scores, it is susceptible to influence by any extreme score. An extremely high score will usually deviate the mean upward, whereas an extremely low score will usually deviate the mean downward. Either way, the mean would then be a less accurate characterization of all of the scores. For example, suppose three groups of nurses took an ECG pretest. All of the nurses in group I had about the same amount of experience in interpreting ECGs, whereas a single member of group II was excellent in her ECG interpretation and a single member in group III had no experience in ECG interpretation.

	Group I	Group II	Group III
	45	45	45
	51	51	51
	43	43	43
	44	44	44
	52	92	07
TOTAL	235	275	190
MEAN	47	55	38

As you can see, despite four of the five scores being identical across the groups, the extreme scores of groups II and III significantly alter the mean and make it a less accurate indicator of overall group performance. Barring these two instances (lack of a normal distribution or the presence of extreme scores) the mean is the single best value to characterize a distribution of scores.

Median. Whereas the mean indicates the average of a group of scores, the *median* indicates the middle in a distribution of scores. It can be variously defined as the score that divides the top half from the bottom half of the scores, the score that divides the distribution of scores into halves, the score below which 50% of scores lie, or the score at the 50th percentile. With an uneven number (N = odd number) of scores, the median is the middle score; with an even number of scores (N = equal number), the median lies between the middle two scores.

To calculate a median, you must first rank order the scores; that is, list them from the highest to the lowest. The preceding example would show the following distributions after rank ordering: group I (52-51-45-44-43), group II (92-51-45-44-43), and group III (51-45-44-43-07). Because N = 5, an odd number of scores, the median can be determined by merely identifying the middle (in this case, the third) score of each: group I = 45, group II = 45, group III = 44.

As you can see in this example, the median is nearly the same across all three groups of nurses and is not affected significantly by the extreme scores of groups II and III that markedly affected the mean. Because it is less influenced by extreme scores, the median is the preferred measure of central tendency for characterizing sets of scores that do not follow a normal distribution or that contain extreme scores. It is also the most valid summary statistic when rating scale categories are given numerical values, as when excellent = 5, very good = 4, good = 3, fair = 2, and poor = 1. These numbers are not strictly arithmetic values, but numerical symbols that represent qualitative values.

The earlier example of 20 nurses has an even number of scores. Using Example 16-1 to obtain the rank ordering of scores, the first 10 scores are 59-58-57-54-52-52-52-51-51-49, whereas the second 10 scores are 49-47-47-46-45-45-42-41-39-34. The two middle scores are both 49, so the median is 49. If the two middle scores had been different numbers, the median would have been the midpoint between them. For example, if the two middle numbers had been 49 and 48, the median would have been 48.5; if they had been 52 and 48, the median would have been 50—again the midpoint between the middle scores.

Mode. The remaining measure of central tendency, the *mode*, represents the most frequently occurring score. The mode is the easiest of all measures of central tendency to determine because it only requires a visual scanning of frequencies (Table 16-2) to identify the score attained most often. Whereas the mean represents the average score and the median represents the middle score, the mode represents the most typical score.

From the earlier example of 20 nurses, the most commonly occurring score, the mode, is 52. The other example of three groups of nurses contained no score that was obtained more than once. In this case, there is no mode. Other sets of scores could conceivably contain more than one score obtained with an equally high frequency. A distribution of scores, then, may be without any mode, have a single mode, or be bimodal, trimodal, and so on.

Types of distributions. In a perfectly symmetrical normal distribution of scores, all three measures of central tendency would fall on the same value (Fig. 8, *A*). When scores predominate at either end of the distribution rather than in the middle, the distribution is said to be *skewed*. A *positively skewed distribution* (Fig. 8, *B*) shows most scores at the lower end of the distribution, whereas a *negatively skewed distribution* (Fig. 8, *C*) shows most scores at the high end of the distribution. Positively skewed distributions (skewed to the right) have a mean displaced higher than the median and mode, whereas negatively skewed distributions (skewed to the left) have a mean lower than the median and the mode. These findings underline the vulnerability of the mean to influence by the presence of asymmetrical distributions of scores.

Measures of variability. As you examine sets of test scores, you will find that they not only usu-

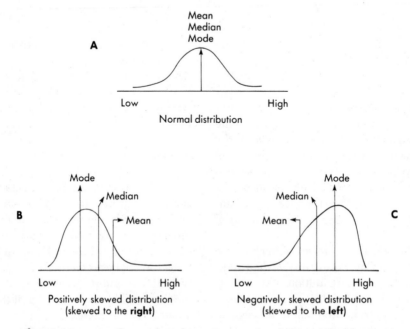

Fig. 8. Measures of central tendency in normal and skewed distributions.

ally cluster around some central value, but that they also extend to varying degrees in either direction from the central point. In addition to central tendency, then, the other major feature to derive from a set of scores is the extent to which they spread, disperse, or vary from their central values. This is the property of *variability* or *dispersion*.

Range. The easiest way to determine the spread of scores is by simply subtracting the lowest score from the highest score. This is known as the *range* of scores and is the crudest yet quickest measure of variability. In the example of 20 nurses who took the critical care pretest, the highest score was 59 and the lowest was 34, so the range was 59 minus 34, or 25.

The ranges for the three groups of nurses taking the ECG test would be as follows: group I: 52 minus 43 = 9; group II: 92 minus 43 = 49; group III: 51 minus 7 = 44.

Remember that in groups II and III, each had one very extreme score (group II had a very high score of 92 and group III a very low score of 7), whereas the other four scores in all groups were exactly the same. Group I's range of 9 indicates little variability or spread of scores within the group of scores; the drastic differences in range found in groups II and III reflect the instability of the range as a measure of dispersion because it can be markedly altered by only a single score value.

Another problem with the range that this example illustrates is the insensitivity of the range to the actual amount of proximity between scores. Remember that all three groups had four of five scores that were exactly the same. Because the range is so vulnerable to representing only the extreme scores of a distribution, it fails to appreciate that except for the extreme scores in groups II and III the remaining scores form a fairly compact distribution.

When calculating the range for rating categories assigned numerical values (excellent = 5, very good = 4), the range is always one less than the difference between the highest and lowest number of categories.

Although the range is easy to determine, its vulnerability to influence by extreme scores and its insensitivity to the true amount of actual dispersion limit its usefulness to being a rather crude estimate of variability.

Interquartile range. A second measure of variability of scores is the *interquartile range*. One definition of the median was that it was the score at the 50th percentile. After counting down (or up) half the total number (20) of pretest scores, you see that the score at the 50th percentile is 49. The interquartile range is determined by subtracting the score at the 25th percentile (Q_1) from the score at the 75th percentile (Q_3). Because the total number of scores was 20, you can find the scores at the 25th and 75th percentiles by counting up to the first quarter of all scores (¼ of 20 = first 5 scores out of 20) and include the top three quarters of scores (¾ of 20 = the first 15 scores out of 20) to determine Q_1 and Q_3. In the example, the first quartile of scores is approximately located at 45 and the third quartile is approximately located at 52, meaning that the first quarter of all scores fall below 45 and the first three quarters of all scores fall below 52. This is an admittedly cursory description of how interquartile range is calculated, so the values given here are truly only approximations. The reader interested in calculating true values will need to consult a text on descriptive statistics.

Standard deviation. The third measure of variability is the *standard deviation*. The standard deviation is the best and most widely used measure of dispersion and is most appropriately employed when values are normally distributed.

As a measure of variability, the standard deviation (abbreviated as "s") recognizes the mean of a set of scores as the measure of central tendency appropriate for a normal distribution and then considers how far each separate score deviates

Table 16-4. Calculation of standard deviation of 20 critical care pretest scores (mean $(\overline{X}) = 48.5$)

X	$X - \overline{X}$	$(X - \overline{X})^2$
59	10.5	110.25
58	9.5	90.25
57	8.5	72.25
54	5.5	30.25
52	3.5	12.25
52	3.5	12.25
52	3.5	12.25
51	2.5	6.25
51	2.5	6.25
49	0.5	0.25
49	0.5	0.25
47	−1.5	2.25
47	−1.5	2.25
46	−2.5	6.25
45	−3.5	12.25
45	−3.5	12.25
42	−6.5	42.25
41	−7.5	56.25
39	−9.5	90.25
34	−14.5	210.25
$\Sigma = 970$	$\Sigma = 0.0$	$\Sigma = 787.00$

$$s = \sqrt{\frac{\Sigma(x - \overline{x})^2}{N}}$$

$$s = \sqrt{\frac{787}{20}}$$

$$s = \sqrt{39.35}$$

$$s = 6.27$$

from this mean. By calculating each score's deviation from the mean, an average or standard deviation from the mean is identified to characterize how the scores are usually dispersed around the mean.

Calculating a standard deviation is a relatively simple process, but requires a fuller understanding than this brief mention to perform it accurately. The essence of calculating a standard deviation for raw data such as in the example here may be appreciated by noting that the formula for standard deviation is that standard deviation is equivalent to the square root of the sum of squared deviations from the mean divided by the total number of scores. Table 16-4 illustrates that the calculation of a standard deviation is by no means an impossible task. Table 16-4 uses the data obtained from the example of

20 critical care pretest scores used earlier.

Knowing only the mean and standard deviation of a normally distributed set of scores, you have the ability to describe the entire distribution of a set of scores and to compare one group of scores to another. The details of how to accomplish this are beyond the intentions of this book, and fall within the realm of descriptive statistics.

One of the values of knowing the standard deviation of a set of scores is that this information enables you to view scores on a normal distribution curve that contain the standard deviation about the mean of that set of scores. This constructs a *standard normal distribution curve* (Fig. 9) that tells you information such as the following:

1. Of all scores 68.26% will fall within plus or minus 1 standard deviation from the mean (34.13% plus 1 standard deviation and 34.13% minus 1 standard deviation).
2. Of all scores 95.44% will fall within plus or minus 2 standard deviations from the mean (47.72% plus 2 standard deviations and 47.72% minus 2 standard deviations).
3. Nearly all scores (greater then 99.7%) will fall within plus or minus 3 standard deviations from the mean.

In a later discussion of grading systems used with evaluating relative achievement, you will see how the use of standard deviations also has a very practical value.

Item analysis. When cognitive learning is assessed by means of a written test, the performance levels observed are a function of both learner performance and test performance. Test performance refers to how effective the test items are as individual measuring devices. If test items are poorly formulated, the test will be inherently ineffective in its ability to measure learning.

Item analysis consists of procedures for determining how well achievement test items function as testing vehicles. It is used primarily with

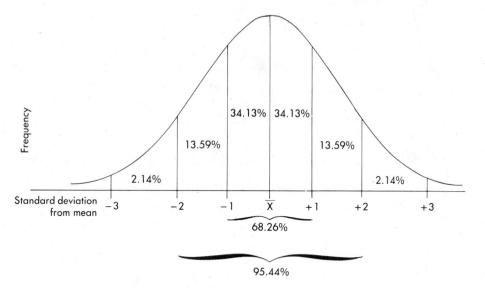

Fig. 9. Standard normal distribution curve.

multiple-choice tests, but may also be employed for other items. In item analysis, a norm-referenced approach is used to examine each test item in terms of how many and which learners marked it correctly or incorrectly.

The primary reason for subjecting a test to item analysis is to derive three pieces of information:

1. How difficult the item was for this group of examinees
2. How well the item discriminated between more and less knowledgable learners
3. How effectively the distractors functioned within each item

Beyond these immediate gains, item analysis may also reveal unsuspected flaws in item construction, clarity, and form that would diminish the validity and usefulness of a test. It lays the groundwork for improved item writing and assists in differentiating between learning defects and testing defects.

Item difficulty. Item difficulty is defined as the percentage of examinees who answer an item correctly. In reality, as the percentage of correct answers increases, the difficulty of the

item decreases; the percentage of correct responses is then inversely proportional to the item's difficulty.

Item difficulty may be determined by simply counting how many examinees marked that item correctly and then dividing the number of correct responses by the total number of persons tested. If left as a proportion (of examinees answering the item correctly to total number of examinees), this figure may be referred to as a *difficulty index*. If converted into a percentage, it is called the *difficulty level* or *difficulty percentage*. Either term carries the same implications because a difficulty level may range from 0% (all answered the item incorrectly) to 100% (all answered the item correctly), whereas a difficulty index may range from 0.0 (all answered the item incorrectly) to 1.0 (all answered the item correctly). Table 16-5 illustrates the calculation of item difficulty for a 10-item test involving 30 nurses.

The preceding section discussed the notion of a skewed distribution. If a test had a large number of very difficult items, few learners would likely get them correct and most scores would

Table 16-5. Calculation of item difficulty (n = 30)

Item	Number of correct responses (out of 30)	Proportion of correct responses	Item difficulty (%)
1	18	0.600	60.0
2	15	0.500	50.0
3	11	0.367	36.7
4	14	0.467	46.7
5	14	0.467	46.7
6	13	0.433	43.3
7	15	0.500	50.0
8	11	0.367	36.7
9	8	0.267	26.7
10	10	0.333	33.3

accumulate at the low end of the distribution curve, producing a positively skewed distribution. If a test had a large number of very easy items, scores would accumulate at the high end, producing a negatively skewed distribution.

Item difficulty is similarly applied to an individual test item. When it is necessary or desirable to differentiate between high and low achievers (competitive situations such as screening tests or tests for advancement), having some moderately difficult items may be useful. In general, however, items that no one answers correctly and items that everyone answers correctly are not very helpful in differentiating among varying levels of achievement. Most classroom achievement tests, therefore, attempt to avoid these extremes of difficulty and aim more at an intervening difficulty range of 45% to 85%.

The optimal difficulty level is partly a function of how many options the examinee must choose among in responding to the item. Because the likelihood of answering an item correctly is to some extent inversely proportional to the number of options available, the best difficulty level is often adjusted in light of how prevalent chance and guessing factors could be. In an alternate response item such as a true-false item, chance alone gives the item a 50% likeli-hood of being correctly answered, so that the difficulty level for two option items should probably be set at a moderately higher level. Multiple-choice items having three or four option choices, when chance and guessing correctly are less likely, could have proportionately lower acceptable levels of difficulty. Overall, a test item should have a difficulty level somewhere between chance (50% chance for two options, 33.3% for three options, 25% for four options) and the maximum of 100%.

As mentioned earlier, if an item is either very easy or very difficult, it does not allow for differentiating well between the better and the less well-informed learner. Theoretically, a moderate item difficulty level of 50% (index of 0.5) provides the best possible differentiation between the knowing and the unknowing. In achievement testing, item difficulty must be tempered so that it does not preclude that item's ability to discriminate between the knowing and the unknowing. Item discrimination, discussed next, is likely the *sine qua non* of all achievement testing, the bottom line of norm-referenced evaluation.

Item discrimination. The discrimination index (level, power) is a statistical measure of an item's ability to discriminate between those who scored highest and those who scored lowest on the entire test. If an item discriminates well, the high scorers usually answer it correctly, whereas the low scorers usually answer it incorrectly. Knowing how well an item discriminates is useful in supplementing instruction during test review and in indicating when improvement is necessary in item writing.

Discrimination levels are expressed as a ratio:

$$\text{Discrimination level} = \frac{\text{Proportion of high scorers answering item correctly}}{} \text{ To } \frac{\text{Proportion of low scorers answering item incorrectly}}{}$$

Discrimination levels can range from a maximum of + 1.0 when all high scorers answer it correctly and all low scorers answer it incorrectly to -1.0 when all high scorers answer it incorrectly and all low scorers answer it correctly (negative or reverse discrimination). The more closely a positive discrimination level approaches a value of 1.0, the more effectively the item functions in differentiating between high and low achievers in the test and the less likely the item needs any revision. As positive values fall closer to 0.0, the less discriminating it is and the more the item is likely to require revision or rejection as a test item. Negative or 0.0 discrimination levels indicate that either the answer key is incorrect or that the item as written is ambiguous or structurally unsound; in either case, the item needs to be revised effectively or deleted.

The optimal discrimination level, like the optimal difficulty level, falls within a moderate range because of the interrelatedness of these two item attributes. Most classroom tests aim at a discrimination level between 0.35 and 0.60; items with higher discrimination levels are usually proportionately more difficult, whereas items with lesser discrimination levels are usually too easy. Again, highly discriminating items that are very difficult and less discriminating items that are very easy fail to provide the distribution or spread of scores sought in achievement testing.

Determining a discrimination level requires that you do the following:

1. Identify the total number of examinees (N).
2. Decide how you wish to divide the total number of examinees into separate groups that constitute high, middle, and low scorers. Some options available here include the following:
   a. Dividing the total number of examinees into upper, middle, and lower thirds.
   b. Dividing the total number of examinees into an upper quarter, middle half, and lower quarter.
   c. Dividing the total number of examinees into an upper 27%, middle 46%, and lower 27%. The smaller the fraction of people contained in the upper and lower groups, the more refined the discrimination analysis because the high and low scorers become increasingly more select groups.
3. Arrange the answer sheets or tests so that the highest score is the top paper and the lowest score the bottom paper.
4. From the fraction selected for the highest and lowest groups, pull the top and bottom 33.3%, 27%, or 25% of scores and put the middle group aside, leaving separate stacks of highest and lowest scores.
5. For each test item, separately tabulate how many high scorers answered it correctly and how many low scorers answered it correctly.
6. Calculate the proportion of high scorers who answered it correctly from the total number of high scorers; do the same for the low scorers.
7. Subtract the proportion of low scorers who answered it correctly from the proportion of high scorers who answered it correctly. The resulting net proportion is the discrimination level.

Table 16-6 illustrates how to determine item discrimination for a 10-item test taken by 30 nurse examinees. The top one-third (10) constitutes the high scorers, whereas the lowest one-third (10) constitutes the low scorers.

Item evaluation. Once item difficulty and discrimination are known, the item should be evaluated in light of each to determine if the item is functioning well as written or if it needs revision. If subsequent revision of the item does not improve item performance, the item should be discarded or replaced entirely. Table 16-7 illustrates how the data from item analysis (Tables 16-5 and 16-6) can be used as a basis for overall evaluation of a test item.

Effectiveness of distractors. With multiple-

Table 16-6. Calculation of item discrimination for a 10-item test taken by 30 nurses

Item		Number of correct responses	Fraction of correct responses	Proportion of correct responses	Discrimination
1	H	10	$10/10$	1.00	
	L	8	$8/10$	0.80	0.20
2	H	9	$9/10$	0.90	
	L	6	$6/10$	0.60	0.30
3	H	7	$7/10$	0.70	
	L	4	$4/10$	0.40	0.30
4	H	7	$7/10$	0.70	
	L	7	$7/10$	0.70	0.00
5	H	10	$10/10$	1.00	
	L	4	$4/10$	0.40	0.60
6	H	8	$8/10$	0.80	
	L	5	$5/10$	0.50	0.30
7	H	10	$10/10$	1.00	
	L	5	$5/10$	0.50	0.50
8	H	9	$9/10$	0.90	
	L	2	$2/10$	0.20	0.70
9	H	6	$6/10$	0.60	
	L	2	$2/10$	0.20	0.40
10	H	8	$8/10$	0.80	
	L	2	$2/10$	0.20	0.60

Table 16-7. Item evaluation

Item	Item difficulty (%)	Item discrimination (proportion)	Item evaluation
1	60	0.20	Discriminates poorly. Difficulty falls within acceptable upper limits. Needs much improvement to retain it.
2	50	0.30	Discriminates only fairly well, while difficulty very good. Revise and retain.
3	36.7	0.30	Too difficult at this discriminating level; revise to reduce difficulty— perhaps reword.
4	46.7	0.00	Fails to discriminate, although possesses good difficulty. Would probably reject it.
5	46.7	0.60	Item discrimination and difficulty very good; retain as is.
6	43.3	0.30	Discrimination needs improvement and is too difficult for its discriminatory power; revise to retain.
7	50.0	0.50	Discriminatory power could be improved, but difficulty is excellent. Modify slightly or retain as is.
8	36.7	0.70	Discriminates very well, although it is rather difficult; a challenger. Retain at end of test.
9	26.7	0.40	Discriminates only reasonably well and is much too difficult. Revise and reduce difficulty to retain.
10	33.3	0.60	Discriminates very well, but is too difficult. Try rewording to reduce difficulty level.

Table 16-8. Effectiveness and evaluation of distractors (options)

Item	Groups	Options (asterisk indicates key)				Evaluation of distractors
		A	B	C	D	
1	H	10*	0	0	0	All distractors functioning well.
	L	2	3	4	1	
2	H	1	1	8*	0	Option D not functioning at all.
	L	2	2	6	0	D needs replacement.
3	H	3	1	2	4*	Options A and C are ineffective; need revision.
	L	1	3	0	6	Options A and D may be too fine for even high scorers to distinguish between.
4	H	3	2*	2	3	Spread of high scorer responses indicates ambiguous or poorly constructed item; revise entirely or discard; check accuracy of key.
	L	1	7	2	0	
5	H	1	1	7*	1	Distractors A and B are functioning well, but option D less well.
	L	2	2	5	1	
6	H	5*	0	5	0	Option C ineffective and may be too close a distinction from key.
	L	5	3	1	1	
7	H	0	0	1	9*	Options A and B are nonfunctional; replace.
	L	0	0	3	7	
8	H	2	6*	1	1	All distractors function at marginal level and do not assist in discrimination between learners.
	L	2	6	1	1	
9	H	0	10*	0	0	All distractors functioning well.
	L	3	4	2	1	
10	H	0	0	7*	3	Option A nonfunctional; replace.
	L	0	4	6	1	Option D ineffective; revise.

choice items, item discrimination may be taken a step further to check how effective distractors are as plausible alternatives to the correct (key) answer. Instead of merely indicating how many of the high and low scorers answered an item correctly, the specific options chosen (key or distractors) by members of each group are isolated and differentiated. This distractor analysis assists in identifying the following:

1. *Effective distractors* that are selected more often by low scorers than by high scorers.

2. *Ineffective distractors* that are selected more often by high scorers than by low scorers.

3. *Nonfunctioning distractors* that are not selected by anyone.

Table 16-8 illustrates how the effectiveness of an item's distractors may be determined and evaluated.

Grading achievement tests. The preceding sections have focused on how to design, construct, score, and analyze achievement test items used in evaluating cognitive learning. This section considers the terminal segment in evaluating achievement, assigning a grade to a learner's demonstrated performance level. Just as the approaches to performance and test item analyses were norm referenced, a norm-referenced approach is used for grade designation.

Grading the results of testing is a quasi-objective process at best, ideally preceded by valid measurements. A *grade* or mark is a symbol that represents an evaluation in a very condensed form. Grades may be derived and symbolized in various ways, depending on how that grade or mark will be used.

Traditional grading systems are norm referenced in that the grades assigned are determined by comparing one learner's performance to that of others. Such grading systems use either numerical or letter symbols to represent the relative evaluation of a learner's performance.

Numerical grading systems assign grades as either absolute raw scores or percentages. Raw scores typically constitute the absolute number of scoring units that a learner accumulated, whereas percentages convert the portion of correct responses into a percentage of correct items.

Letter grading systems, using the traditional letter grades of A, B, C, D, F, are usually slightly more complicated than numerical systems. They may incorporate one of three basic approaches to assignment of a letter grade:

1. *Direct conversion of a raw score or percentage to a letter grade.* For example, if scores were converted as follows for a 100-item test:

Score of less than 60 = 0% to 59% correct = F
Score of 60 to 69 = 60% to 69% correct = D
Score of 70 to 79 = 70% to 79% correct = C
Score of 80 to 89 = 80% to 89% correct = B
Score of 90 to 100 = 90% to 100% correct = A

2. *System of natural breaks.* This system may be used as a basis for assigning letter grades when a frequency distribution of grades reveals the absence of a normal distribution together

Example 16-2.

Test scores: *(out of possible score of 40)*

28	39	27
20	35	20
25	33	34
32	26	35
28	33	

Frequency distribution of scores using the grading system of natural breaks

Scores	f	Number of examinees	Grade
39	1	(1)	A
38	0	Natural Break	
37	0		
36	0		
35	2		
34	1		
33	2		
32	1	(6)	B
31	0	Natural Break	
30	0		
29	0		
28	2		
27	1		
26	1		
25	1	(5)	C
24	0	Natural Break	
23	0		
22	0		
21	0		
20	2	(2)	D

with the presence of breaks of more than one consecutive score. These breaks create clusters of scores at well-demarcated levels. Visual inspection down such a frequency distribution will indicate whether the system of natural breaks will be appropriate for that set of scores. Example 16-2 illustrates this system.

3. *Standard letter grade system.* When a large number (as least 30) of scores fall into a pattern of normal distribution, letter grades may be assigned on the basis of the location of the

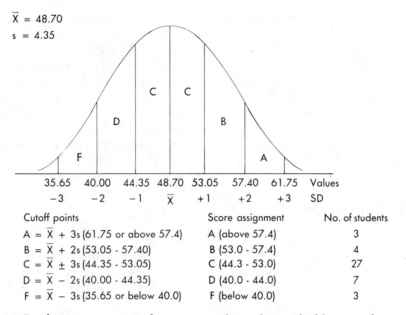

$\overline{X} = 48.70$
$s = 4.35$

35.65	40.00	44.35	48.70	53.05	57.40	61.75	Values
−3	−2	−1	$\overline{X}$	+1	+2	+3	SD

Cutoff points	Score assignment	No. of students
A = $\overline{X}$ + 3s (61.75 or above 57.4)	A (above 57.4)	3
B = $\overline{X}$ + 2s (53.05 - 57.40)	B (53.0 - 57.4)	4
C = $\overline{X}$ ± 3s (44.35 - 53.05)	C (44.3 - 53.0)	27
D = $\overline{X}$ − 2s (40.00 - 44.35)	D (40.0 - 44.0)	7
F = $\overline{X}$ − 3s (35.65 or below 40.0)	F (below 40.0)	3

Fig. 10. Graphic representation of test scores utilizing the standard letter grade system.

numerical grade under the normal curve. This is the pure form of grading on a curve that is performed without adding or subtracting any factor that supposedly corrects the curve for grading purposes.

In the unadulterated form of this system, the mean test score is used as the reference point for the middle range of a "C" grade, and the ranges of other letter grades are assigned according to the limits set by plus or minus 1, 2, or 3 standard deviations from the mean:

A = +3 standard deviations greater than the mean

B = +2 standard deviations from the mean

C = + or −1 standard deviation from the mean

D = −2 standard deviations from the mean

F = −3 standard deviations from the mean

Fig. 10 illustrates an example of how this standard letter grade system would work for a 60-item test administered to 44 examinees when the mean score was 48.70 (out of 60) and the standard deviation was 4.35. In addition to the full letter grades illustrated here, variously finer cutoffs for plus and minus letter grades could also be made if differentiation of C− from a C+, for example, were desired.

Contract grading system. Certain nontraditional grading systems should be briefly mentioned here following this discussion of traditional systems. One of these is *contract grading*.

A learning contract is a written agreement made between a learner and an instructor, signed by each at the initiation of a course study. A learning contract delineates the terms under which a specific grade (letter or numerical) is awarded to the learner. As with any other contract, a learning contract is a two-way agreement; the instructor agrees to award a specific grade if the learner meets all of the terms agreed on for that grade.

The terms of a learning contract generally include the following areas:

1. Period of time the contract is in effect (due dates, time limits, extension options)
2. Enumeration of the learning objectives that must be met
3. Sequence of learning activities the learner will undertake
4. Outcomes the learner must provide as evidence of learning
5. Criteria that instructor will use to evaluate learning

Some learning contracts are entirely fixed by the instructor, who determines all of the terms of the contract and options (if any) available to the learner, others are entirely learner determined, and in still others the terms are mutually negotiated. The degree of flexibility for the learner may vary widely.

Some educational settings in nursing, both formal and continuing, have found that contract grading promotes the philosophy of adult education by increasing the learner's active participation, responsibility, and motivation for learning, while reducing competition and anxiety, lessening preoccupation with grades rather than learning, and lessening the likelihood of subjective grading practices. By clarifying the instructor's expectations of the learner at the beginning of a learning experience, the learner does not need to wait until a grade is assigned to know what the instructor expected in performance.

Contracting has been used in both classrooms and clinical settings, but appears to be more commonly employed in clinical areas where the issue of instructor subjectivity in evaluation becomes more problematic.

While extolling its virtues, the educator should also be aware of some of the criticisms levied against using learning contracts. Some learners have found that their motivation for learning was actually reduced without the threat of not knowing what grade they would receive. Some felt they learned less because this approach to learning was too easy, whereas others felt that it did not bear any relation to what they actually derived from the learning situation. Learners who found they later had to contract for a lower grade experienced feelings of personal failure, whereas others who contracted for higher grades felt that the amount of time they had available was a more influential factor than how much they had learned. One common fault found with contracting for a grade was that the extra margin of work required to fulfill the requirement for a higher grade emphasized quantity more than quality of work. This approach to grading, while predicated on principles of adult education, may potentially only formalize the usual games that learners and instructors play.

Another nontraditional grading system is discussed in the next section when criterion-referenced evaluation procedures—their design, scoring, analysis, and grading—are addressed.

Criterion-referenced evaluation

The primary feature that distinguishes criterion-referenced evaluation from norm-referenced evaluation is its purpose: the former is conducted to evaluate mastery, whereas the latter is conducted to evaluate achievement. To evaluate achievement, norm-referenced testing devices are constructed to elicit the degree of learning attained. They ideally produce a spread of scores that can ultimately be used to grade the relative amount of learning attained. To evaluate mastery, criterion-referenced testing devices are constructed to determine whether mastery was attained or not, ideally produce little or no spread of scores, and grade on an absolute system that bears no relationship to group performance. Although norm- and criterion-referenced evaluations share many features, their differences are sufficient to merit some consideration here.

Purpose. As emphasized, purpose is the major distinguishing feature between these two evaluations. Criterion-referenced evaluation is only concerned with whether or not a learner can demonstrate a predetermined level of performance. Performance levels less or greater than the criterion level are irrelevant. When the educator needs to verify that all learners demonstrate a common set of essential abilities (cognitive, affective, or psychomotor) that constitute safe and competent practice, criterion-referenced evaluation should be used.

Instructional objectives. Both approaches to evaluation originate with instructional objectives. Norm-referenced evaluation is typically based on objectives derived from content area and instruction experts, whereas criterion-referenced evaluation is based on objectives derived from standards agreed on and established by practice experts.

The content areas and behaviors contained in objectives for evaluating achievement can sample from a nearly infinite range of instances within an instructional domain where the relative importance of meeting some objectives can vary widely. The evaluation of mastery, conversely, necessitates that the instructional domain be finite, that is, limited to those behaviors and content areas deemed essential (mandatory, critical, reflective of minimal required competencies), dictated by standards of competent and safe practice. Only those behaviors specified in the objectives are open to evaluative scrutiny. Because all evaluation in this approach hinges on determining whether the prescribed or criterion level of performance was demonstrated or not, criterion-referenced evaluation procedures make the need to define performance criteria clearly and unambiguously an absolute necessity.

Test construction. The process of designing a test blueprint and a table of specifications would be comparable with either evaluation approach, except that the behaviors and content areas contained within them would reflect the varying origin and nature of the objectives. In like manner, decisions on the type of test items would still be dictated by the nature of the instructional objectives.

Criterion-referenced evaluation devices may vary somewhat from norm-referenced devices in the number of items and relative emphases allotted to certain objectives. The only limiting factor of test length with criterion-referenced evaluation is in assuring that all essential abilities be evaluated and, if a competency-based model is used, that all behaviors necessary to constitute evaluating an encompassing competency be included. Rather than using apportioned amounts of instructional time to weigh emphases in evaluation, criterion-referenced evaluation uses the centrality or importance of a given behavior to determine the weights allotted. If all behaviors evaluated were equally important, variable emphases would be a moot issue.

Timetable for evaluation. Criterion-referenced evaluations are generally less restricted by the time available for testing. Theoretically, the amount of time required for the evaluation period should not be limited; the learner should have a virtually unlimited or extremely liberal amount of time available for the evaluation process.

Both formative and summative evaluation may be used and, in criterion-referenced evaluation, the learner can often repeat the evaluation procedure as often as necessary until she attains mastery.

Benchmarks of measurement. Although usefulness remains an integral attribute of any measuring device, the customary approaches to evaluating the validity and reliability of testing instruments are largely inappropriate and irrelevant in criterion-referenced evaluation.

Because criterion-referenced evaluation is predicated on standards of performance as consensually validated by expert practitioners (rather than content or curriculum experts), content validity appraised by comparable practice experts would seem to be the only plausible approach to assuring the validity of criterion-referenced tests. Concurrent and predictive forms of criterion-related validity appear to be clearly inappropriate as do attempts to establish construct validity when agreed standards are frequently lacking for even the definition and interpretation of these intangible qualities.

Traditional appraisals for reliability with criterion-referenced evaluation tools are similarly inappropriate on the whole because demonstrating mastery is a more or less static activity focused on a single learner. The only reliability estimates that may be helpful with criterion-referenced evaluation devices are those used for subjectively scored devices, intra-rater and inter-rater reliability coefficients. In general, criterion-referenced evaluation is more concerned with the validity of what is measured in the here and now and less concerned with maintaining the stability of measurements over time or other test instruments.

Measures of central tendency and variability. Because criterion-referenced evaluation is not concerned with establishing standards of group performance, measures of central tendency and variability are largely irrelevant. They may be determined for informative purposes, but play no role in the grading or evaluation processes.

Typically, mastery learning produces little if any spread between marks because learners are expected to attain near perfect scores. The anticipated distribution of scores in a criterion-referenced evaluation test, then, would be a negatively skewed distribution, characterized by an accumulation of high scores (Fig. 8, *B*). The range of scores would likely be very small and the lack of a normal distribution precludes using standard deviations.

Item analysis. In achievement tests, item difficulty is usually varied in degree to allow learners with differing capabilities to demonstrate their degree of learning. Some items will be very easy, others moderately difficult, and a few very difficult.

In criterion-referenced evaluation, when testing is limited to only the most important elements, all examinees should attain near perfect scores. Limiting the instructional and evaluative domain to the essentials and anticipating near perfect scores combine to diminish the difficulty of most criterion-referenced tests. Most difficulty indexes would be in the range of at least 85%. In items such as drug dosages or the interpretation of lethal dysrhythmias, where complete mastery would be required, the difficulty level is set at 100%, meaning all learners must answer these items correctly.

Criterion-referenced tests should likewise demonstrate virtually no discrimination between learners because all scores should fall at the criterion level set for proficiency. This type of evaluation has no need for differentiating among learners and, in actuality, typically produces no polarization of high and low scorers—all scores should be high at the mastery level.

Scoring. If behaviors and content areas have been clearly defined and test items are accurate correlates of these, scoring should be very straightforward in criterion-referenced evaluation. As previously discussed, scores will all usually be high, clustered at the criterion level, and negatively skewed in a compact distribution. Ideally, criterion-referenced evaluations are scored on a yes or no, demonstrated or not demonstrated basis. Scoring is based solely on determining whether the established standard or criterion level of performance was met.

Grading. Any grading system based on relative group performance is inappropriate to use with criterion-referenced evaluation. In this evaluation either the demonstrated performance was at the criterion level or it was not. The grading system used in criterion-referenced evaluation is, for consistency, as absolute as the scoring process it uses.

The usual grading system employed in criterion-referenced evaluation is the pass-fail (credit-no credit, satisfactory-unsatisfactory) system. To pass, a learner must demonstrate the specified behaviors at the prescribed or criterion level established. Passing standards are usually set high (90 to 100%) to constitute mastery.

Sometimes used in conjunction with contract grading or percentile grades, the pass-fail grading system has been credited with a number of potential attributes that make it an attractive evaluation mechanism. In addition to its inherent ability to complement the evaluation of mastery learning, the pass-fail system may be useful in reducing learners' anxiety about evaluation and competition for grades, fostering creativity and self-direction for learning, clarifying mutual expectations for the learning situation, and reducing the subjective nature of grading.

Because the pass-fail grading system only has two potential ways to categorize performance, the system is inherently insensitive to recognizing any differences in achievement between learners who barely pass and those who far exceed the minimal passing requirements. Often used in conjunction with contract grading, the pass-fail system shares in many of contract grading's strengths and weaknesses.

Norm- and criterion-referenced approaches to evaluation may be used singly or in combination. Neither possesses all of the attributes of the perfect evaluation remedy nor the antidotes for all of the problems encountered in evaluating cognitive learning. But each, when applied appropriately as prescribed, enables the educator to make more sound decisions about cognitive learning and teaching.

EVALUATING AFFECTIVE LEARNING

Affective behavior embraces the expression of a complex variety of attitudes, beliefs, and values that incline individuals to respond toward specific situations or things in characteristic ways. The affective realm focuses not so much on the behavior displayed as it does on the disposition from which that behavior emanates.

Individuals acquire their beliefs and values through both experience and education. Whereas educators cannot readily influence the experiential environment of others, they do seek to imbue learners with certain attitudes regarded as desirable, consistent, or appropriate for roles learners undertake.

Nursing has a substantial number of largely unwritten expectations for the deportment and demeanor of its practitioners. Formal and continuing nursing educators often find themselves responsible for facilitating the acquisition, internalization, and expression of many of these expectations as they affect patients (caring, empathy, acceptance, respect, trust, confidentiality, sensitivity) or how a nurse interacts with others in performing her role (organization of work, integrity, reliability, commitment, cooperation, sincerity, enthusiasm, initiative).

As much as certain dispositions and beliefs are clearly more therapeutic or desirable than others, the affective domain is fraught with many difficulties that make teaching and evaluating this area truly problematic. Some of the reasons contributing to this situation are that affective behaviors are inherently:

1. *Difficult to define* precisely in behavioral terms. Even when definitions are available for these abstract qualities, frequently a concomitant lack of consensus on the definitions exists.

2. *Difficult to measure* because of their lack of precision and clarity in definition. If an attribute cannot be clearly defined or if its expression is modified by an awareness of its being scored or graded, attempts to measure the attribute with any degree of reliability and validity are open to question. We are limited in our knowledge of how to measure these behaviors. The number and types of valid instruments available for evaluating attitudes is very limited.

3. *Complex and difficult to isolate.* Apart from the context in which they occur,

beliefs and attitudes have no independent focus that can serve as a basis for isolating them as discrete entities. For affective behaviors to be evaluated, learners must have an opportunity to experience a value-related issue, examine beliefs about that value, consider alternative courses of action and the consequences of each, and select the most appropriate course of action.

4. *Inaccessible*. Only the nurse can know what her true feelings and attitudes are; the behavior a nurse demonstrates may arise out of genuine beliefs, out of what she anticipates others expect of her, or even out of what is perceived as necessary behavior to obtain a good grade, positive evaluation, or praise. Because educators must infer that overt behaviors correspond to a given set of convictions, and because even the nurse may not be consciously aware of all of the influences governing her behavior, inferences made concerning that behavior may often be wholly inaccurate. Unlike other learning behaviors that are more or less directly attributable to specific causes, the genesis of affective behaviors may be less accurately inferred or may even be inaccessible to direct inference.

5. *Unstable*. Even if the measurement of affective behaviors were not problematic, the instability of these attributes makes them less than amenable to reliable measurement. Unlike cognitive or psychomotor behaviors, affective behaviors may not always be developed in a clearly linear fashion.

6. *Open to questions of propriety* with respect to their assessment and evaluation. For the most part, educators are reluctant to judge the attitudes and value systems of others and are resistent to the notion that these can be mandated in time or degree by the threat of grades. The demonstration of a newly acquired attitude or belief cannot be programmed as readily as other types of learning nor scheduled for integration within specific time periods. This lag time between providing instruction in affective areas and demonstrating its acquisition is a particularly thorny problem. Because of many concerns such as these, affective objectives are often clothed as concomitant or serendipitous components to more tangible and conventional aims of learning.

While acknowledging each of these limitations and considerations, attempts should be made to facilitate and to evaluate affective learning. Some of the methods that have been reported as useful in evaluating affective learning include the following:

1. Videotape of a nurse's spontaneous performance, supplemented by self, peer, and instructor critique

2. Direct observation of a nurse's performance supplemented by a checklist or rating scale for structured observation to detect tendencies to use sweeping generalizations, to label patient types, to assume judgmental postures, or to use absolutes

3. Process recordings or informal and serendipitous observations of nurse-patient interactions and interpersonal dynamics to detect patterns of value reflected behavior

4. Simulated patients and situations, presented by means of written simulations, audiovisual vignettes, audiotapes, role-playing, pictorial stimuli, or self-paced modules

5. Group discussions and patient care conferences with nurses to elicit how their beliefs influence the interventions they provide

6. Group process workshops involving identification of necessary traits, self-evalua-

tion of areas of weakness, contracting with peers to develop identified areas of need with peers, and instructor feedback

7. Interactional analysis and debates
8. Survey of attitudes with an attitude scale
9. Staff conferences on selected patient situations, management of conflict, problem solving, and patient care
10. Review of nursing care plans to identify value systems

It seems reasonable to question whether the more subtle dynamics of human behavior can be objectively assessed and evaluated in the same manner as other types of learning behavior. The continuing difficulty of this pursuit is not sufficient cause to deter people from attempting to persist in these endeavors. As anyone who practices or receives the ministrations of nursing can attest, there is more to being a competent nurse than merely knowing the science of nursing or performing the technical skills. Expertise in both of these is too often inadequate. A balance struck between the art and the science of nursing remains a necessity rather than a compromise.

EVALUATING PSYCHOMOTOR AND INTEGRATED LEARNING

If knowing were a sufficient condition for doing, evaluating the former would suffice for appraising the latter. If nursing were only a science, there would be no need to evaluate the integration of its art. If nursing were practiced in a classroom, evaluating education for its practitioners could be confined there. But theoretical competence is not the same as clinical competence, nursing is an art and a science, and nursing is practiced in a clinical setting rather than in a classroom. These assertions imply that educational evaluation in nursing cannot be limited to cognitive evaluation, theoretical considerations, or written examinations alone. Other forms of

evaluation are necessary to assure that knowing the science and performing the art are complementary processes to produce a truly competent practitioner.

Of the three types of learning described in Chapter 2, evaluating the cognitive and affective types has already been discussed. The third type, the psychomotor, is traditionally evaluated in terms of the myriad of tasks, procedures, and techniques that nurses must be able to perform. Although this is surely its major focus, a broadened interpretation of the term *psychomotor* reminds educators that the focus of clinical evaluation is not restricted to the motor aspect, that is, verifying a nurse's mechanical, technical, or automaton capabilities. Competency in practice involves a complex interplay among knowing, feeling, and doing—an interweaving of threads that is often difficult to unravel and evaluate separately. For this reason, you will note that this section addresses the evaluation of "integrated" rather than merely psychomotor learning. In every learning experience are cognitive, affective, and psychomotor components.

Once outside the more familiar and sheltered harbor of the classroom, the evaluation process takes a decidedly less steady course. Perhaps a consideration of some of the more common problems associated with clinical evaluation will help in arriving at some more effective means to navigate these waters.

One perennial problem is a lack of clarity and precision in identifying the intended destination for clinical learning. "Competent clinical performance" is a terribly encompassing phrase; unless it is defined in discernible, behavioral terms understood by both the instructor and the learner, it is not likely ever to be reached.

The second problem is identifying what landmarks will be used to indicate the educational process is staying on course. If subcomponent behaviors (cognitive, affective, psychomotor) have not been fully defined, the instructor and the learners will never know if the current process needs correction or what expectations to anticipate in the future. Major problems in clinical evaluation emanate from a poorly constructed or amorphous set of clinical objectives. Insofar as the instructor and the learners have the objectives within their purview, then evaluation of performance can be made.

The inherent complexity, breadth, and range of behaviors required of nursing practitioners is a third source of difficulty, compounded in critical care units by the additional expanse of skills required of staff nurses. Evaluating all of these areas is a weighty and time-consuming task in itself, aggravated by the lack of standardized procedures, policies, and criteria for each of these functions, and the high instructor to learner ratio.

Definitions of competent performance vary with time, agency, individual instructors, and local and regional norms. Only very recently have standards of practice been set for critical care nursing practice, and it will likely be some time before they are fully implemented nationally. Before that time, the unit's or preceptor's standards of practice were the only criteria against which performance could realistically be evaluated. Not all preceptors are equally adept at their role, yet a virtual cadre of them is often necessary to sample adequately a nurse's performance.

From both the instructor's and learner's viewpoints, assigning clinical grades is often an obscure process at best. Limited time for observing the performance of each learner, inequities in the types and numbers of learning experiences that can be provided, the paucity of valid instruments to measure integrated forms of learning, and irreconcilable problems with reducing a learner's performance to a single grade based largely on subjective accounting practices often cause even seasoned instructors to lose sight of the objectives. The influences precipitated by an observer's presence raise questions concerning the validity of clinical observations: learner anxiety over being watched may preclude and inhibit established practices, whereas putting on a show for the instructor is always an alternative course of action. Approaches to clinical evaluation may range from the nearly reflex level of specificity to such general glimpses that the entire process can become unwieldy, useless, and nearly ludicrous.

Each of the methods available for evaluating integrated learning attempts to resolve one or more of these recognized problems. Some are more promising than others, although none is a panacea for problems in appraising clinical performance. By considering the virtues and vicissitudes of each, you may find the combination most suitable for your situation.

Psychomotor and other forms of integrated learning are most readily evaluated in either the laboratory or the actual clinic. The advantages of each setting for the instructional process have already been cited and are equally applicable to the evaluation process.

The laboratory is a convenient setting for both formally and informally evaluating integrated clinical behaviors. Simulated patients and patient situations, written simulations, role-playing, and training manikins can all be effective for formal evaluation and for instruction. Demonstration with return demonstration of procedures has long been used as an evaluation device, whereas simulation gaming is only emerging. Many of these evaluation devices require the demonstration of higher level cognitive functioning together with affective and psychomotor skills. The more nearly these forms of simulation mimic the expectations and reality of the practice setting, the more validly they may evaluate proficiency without compromising patient safety or the reliability of measurements.

When high levels of specific technical performance and rapid critical thinking are required, training stations such as those used in the American Heart Association's Advance Cardiac Life Support (ACLS) Megacode may be constructed. Using actual equipment and simulated situations (cardiac or respiratory arrest, airway establishment and maintenance, definitive drug, oxygen and circulation assistance, intubation, defibrillation, cardioversion, ECG monitoring, and dysrhythmia recognition) and patients, the nurse can progress from one assigned role to another until all of the skills required for proficiency in life-threatening situations have been demonstrated to mastery levels. Criterion-referenced evaluation tools evaluate mastery, and at times also impose time limits.

In the clinical setting, too, many of the methods used for instruction can be used for evaluating learning. Learners' participation in nursing care conferences, team conferences, and case presentations can be an informal forum for evaluating the ability to assess and to implement effectively appropriate plans of nursing care. For an in-depth assessment of individual performance, periodic and unscheduled bedside nursing rounds on a one-to-one or small group basis can elicit a wealth of data useful in evaluation. Through a systematic approach to evaluation, one can determine a nurse's ability to obtain a comprehensive patient data base effectively and accurately, formulate an appropriate and rational plan of care based on these data, provide effective and timely nursing interventions, and verify the efficacy of these interactions by means of a valid and thorough reevaluation of the patient's status. Working directly with a learner, attending change of shift reports and staff meetings, or auditing charts can offer many insights for appraising a staff nurse's clinical abilities. Devices such as dual-headed stethoscopes, sound simulators, and recorded tapes can be used to evaluate assessment skills and to estimate the effect of various instructional programs.

Written forms of evaluation such as care plans, process recordings, clinical diaries, and written care reports are commonly used in formal educational settings to provide written samples of the learner's ability to transfer, integrate, and apply learning to complex patient care situations. Whereas many of these devices are useful in academic settings, the adult population of continuing education programs in nursing is generally more responsive to forms of evaluation that are more interactive and participatory.

Self-evaluations of clinical performance are becoming increasingly popular now, even in formal academic settings. If they are to be constructive evaluation devices, self-evaluations should be used from the onset of the program and frequently thereafter rather than merely at the end of a course of study. Strengths and weaknesses should be searched for to reinforce the former and remediate the latter.

When both the instructor and the learner use the same device for evaluating clinical competency, the outcomes of these separate appraisals should be compared and a mutually agreed on assessment reached. Television film, video trainers, and audiotapes can provide the instant replay of actual performance necessary for stimulating both self-awareness and peer analysis of learner performance. As you might anticipate, an adult's self-appraisal is frequently closely correlated with that of a preceptor or instructor. Because behavioral change, learning, is mediated initially by the learner's awareness of the need for change, gaining insight into one's performance can be extremely helpful in motivating a correction of deficiencies, while fostering greater personal and professional growth.

Peer and staff evaluations constitute another avenue for evaluating clinical performance. Whether employed in a multiple assignment or in one of many group discussion formats, peer practitioners can offer sensitive, honest, and constructive critiques of another's performance. Comments and suggestions may be more readily accepted when they originate from a member of one's peer or colleague group rather than from an instructor.

Of all the methods available for evaluating integrated learning, the most commonly employed is observing clinical performance. *Direct observation* involves the physical presence of an observer during a demonstrated performance. Whereas this seems to offer the most natural setting for observation, the presence of an individual "to observe" interjects an unnatural element into the situation that may interfere or artificially augment the resulting performance. Despite its potential for affecting the dynamics of the interaction, direct observation may be the only feasible way to evaluate the totality of a complex situation, especially when nonverbal communication and a multitude of subtle and highly specific variables are working in the situation. Many of these variables may not be fully appreciated through filmed or taped accounts, and the context and circumstances may not be reproducible by other means, except by using such devices as two-way mirrors. Although it is time-consuming and requires training persons for the observer role, first-hand witnessing of a performance may frequently be the most reasonable and expedient way to measure clinical competency.

Indirect observation entails using means such as videotape or audiotape to preserve observations for later review and comparison. By providing a permanent and retrievable record of performance, learners, peers, and instructors can all participate in the evaluation process as often as desired or necessary. Whereas the biasing effect of the observer's physical presence is removed with indirect observation, learners may also become preoccupied with being taped and again fail to provide natural behaviors in that situation. Recordings are also limited in their failure to convey the emotional overlay of an interaction and in their restricted sensory mode (camera distance and angle, adequacy of lighting, sensitivity of microphone).

Observations made casually and spontaneously usually provide no more than serendipitous information related to a nurse's clinical performance. For observation to be useful and valid in educational evaluation, it must be focused, systematically organized, and standardized.

Observations are focused by clarifying to both learners and observers what will be attended to in the observation and what criteria will be applied in judging the observations. The elements selected for evaluation by observation should consist of those facets of performance considered crucial and essential indexes of clinical competency. Extraneous aspects clutter the minds and eyes of observers and should be sifted out before the observation experience.

Once the procedures, skills, or techniques to be observed have been identified and their components specified, some means for recording and later analyzing observations must be devised. The purpose of this recording device may be either to judge or simply to tabulate observations as they are made. Rating scales are typically used for judging and performance checklists for tabulating. Both tools enable the observer to minimize the subjectivity and memory bias of the observation to afford a greater reliability to the measurement process. Because no way to completely eliminate the subjectivity of an observation exists, the checklist or rating scale merely attempts to circumscribe the amount of perceptual selectivity and bias of the observer. Recording observations as they occur also provides marks in the form of numerical, coded, or verbal data to analyze and evaluate later.

Crucial to the validity of observation as an evaluative device is providing an adequate training program for would-be observers. Their preparation should include practice in gaining familiarity and facility in using the tool for guided observation. Practice sessions may include simultaneously observing and rating a series of videotapes of selected procedures. By repetition and comparison of their observations with those of other observers, intra-rater and inter-rater reliability can be established to substantiate the consistency of these findings. This type of observer preparation more readily assures standards of uniformity and consistency in applying the measuring device and reinforces the essential elements for observers.

Observers must learn to function effectively while remaining as unobtrusive as possible to minimize the effect of their presence on the learner's performance. Except to protect the patient from harm, observers should be able to demonstrate that they can refrain from physically, verbally, or nonverbally influencing the outcome of observer performances or interfering with its natural occurrence. Learning to be invisible is no easy matter. Many nurse preceptors are adroit at consciously or unconsciously helping out while observing and fail to appreciate the degree to which their hands-on participation precludes even quasi-objective observation. Ways to get over the awkwardness of being an observer exist; they primarily consist of experience and self-reminders of the purpose of their presence at the bedside.

Because virtually all observations entail using either a rating scale or a checklist, the following section discusses each in further detail.

Rating scales

A rating scale is a device used to record and evaluate observations. The dimension being rated constitutes some type of behavior such as a skill, procedure, technique, trait, or attitude. Unlike a checklist, which has an all-or-nothing quality, a rating scale enables an observer to measure the degree to which a behavior is present or the frequency, relative nature, or quality of its occurrence.

Constructing a rating scale involves developing one or more rating categories for each pertinent aspect of an instructional objective. Rating categories consist of a range of distinguishable, nonoverlapping, or equidistant degrees or levels

of performance, typically arranged as three or more points along a continuum. Categories may be posed as descriptive words, phrases, or paragraphs that indicate relative quality or degree of possession such as the following:

Below average	Average	Above average
Unsatisfactory	Satisfactory	Satisfactory plus
Minimally acceptable	Acceptable plus	Outstanding

Poor → Fair → Good → Very Good → Excellent

Categories may also indicate the extent of success, consistency, or independence of the demonstrated performance:

Rarely successful	Usually successful	Always successful
Usually inconsistent	Usually consistent	Consistent
Performed only with assistance	Performed with minimal assistance	Independently performed

Ratings such as these produce qualitative data that can be tabulated and evaluated. At times, ratings are converted or more fully differentiated into numerical ratings that provide a means for quantifying and analyzing ratings. A specific number of points may be alloted to each rating category (excellent = 5, very good = 4, good = 3, fair = 2, poor = 1) or numerical ratings may merely constitute intermediate points between and within rating categories. At other times, a rating scale may only consist of a numerical scale with descriptions provided only at the extreme ends of the continuum:

1	2	3	4	5
Unable to initiate without assistance				Able to initiate and complete without assistance

Example 16-3 illustrates a three-category rating scale constructed on a five-point continuum to allow for finer discriminations among performance levels. Appendix C contains a comprehensive set of qualitative rating scales designed to prepare practitioners for their management and practice roles within critical care units.

Regardless of the format adopted, rating consists of designating the location along the scale where the number, words, or description most closely coincides with the observed performance. By standardizing the focus of observations and facilitating their immediate and efficient recording, rating scales help minimize the breadth of an observer's evaluation, improve its accuracy, and diminish its dependence on the observer's memory of events.

To be useful and valid evaluation tools, rating scales should be pilot tested for their objectivity, sensitivity, ambiguity, and consistency of ratings. Well-constructed scales may be tedious and time-consuming to design. Even with a well-designed rating scale, the ratings provided may be invalid or spurious if the rater or observer has an aversion to assigning extreme scores, is unwilling to take the time necessary to observe and rate carefully, or has a vested interest in the outcome of the ratings.

Example 16-3. Three-category rating scale

OBJECTIVE: Demonstrates ability to synthesize anatomical, physiological, and psychosocial data to arrive at decisions for planning appropriate nursing interventions.

	Minimally acceptable	Acceptable plus	Outstanding
1	Occasionally approaches patient problems without a problem-solving frame of reference or reaches conclusions without thoughtful consideration. Data base occasionally lacks both depth and breadth; judgments at times impulsive.	Usually approaches patient problems with problem-solving frame of reference, but occasionally reaches conclusions prematurely; in these instances, data base may be lacking in either depth or breadth, but usually not both; judgments not always wholly sound.	Consistently approaches patient problems with problem-solving frame of reference; arrives at conclusions only after thorough consideration of all relevant data, and describes conclusions as tentative. Judgments are sound within available knowledge base.
	(1) ☐ (2) ☐	(3) ☐ (4) ☐	(5) ☐
2	Usually able to identify verbally a mass of data related to specific patient problems; usually requires some assistance in clarifying precise nature of patient's problem. Initially presents data in disorganized fashion and on the basis of principles derived from common rather than scientific knowledge. Frequently requires assistance in organizing and identifying all principles of even general knowledge inherent in patient problems and in translating these into language of scientific principles.	Is able to express her perception of precise nature of patient's problem with minimal assistance from instructor. Usually uses the patient's problem as the initial step in determining a relevant data base. Data base presented is a mixture of common knowledge and valid scientific principles. Data base mixture initially presented in some organized fashion, reflective of recognition of all principles of common knowledge and integration of valid scientific principles.	Consistently able to identify specific nature of patient's problem without assistance of instructor. Initial presentation of data flows sequentially and logically from identified problems. Categorizes and describes data systematically on the basis of scientific principles involved and in professional terminology. Organization of data flows from principles identified and is inclusive of all or nearly all relevant factors. Occasionally requires minimal assistance, but generally accomplishes above on own resources.
	(1) ☐ (2) ☐	(3) ☐ (4) ☐	(5) ☐

Example 16-3, cont'd

Minimally acceptable	Acceptable plus	Outstanding

3 Usually able to state broader principles underlying patient's problem, but generally needs assistance in recalling more detailed facts related to specific principles involved; recognizes obvious physiologic and psychosocial factors, but discussions of these evidence gaps in details of knowledge base that limit student's ability to integrate data; frequently requires moderate assistance and information in translating data from specific situation into abstract principles; frequently requires assistance in interpreting data in light of identified principles. Theoretical and conceptual bases lacking or superficial in depth and breadth. Knowledge expressed in concrete, situation-based terms.

Able to specify broad principles underlying particular patient problem and can usually specify sufficient detail of principles to relate data factors in logical fashion. With assistance, is then able to integrate more fully factors in data base on her own and begin to identify alternative courses of action. Occasionally lacks knowledge of minor details: usually able to explain concrete situations with abstract principles involved and, with help, can then independently integrate numerous factors in data base. Theoretical and conceptual bases generally present in sufficient detail to relate various factors meaningfully.

Consistently able to explain the factors in a concrete patient situation in both abstracted principles and concepts and the details of these principles. Explains concrete situations as instances of principles involved, rather than as isolated, unrelated factors. Comprehension of principles goes beyond explaining concrete data to include potential changes in patient situations; evidences knowledge of detailed elements of principles by ability to cite alternative courses of action and their probable outcomes. Usually requires little if any assistance from instructor in supplementing or relating factors in data base.

(1) ☐   (2) ☐   (3) ☐   (4) ☐   (5) ☐

4 Frequently needs assistance in identifying gaps in data base; usually requires additional information to relate meaningfully needed data to data already available. Does not seek out all relevant data on her own initiative. Often not effective in eliciting needed data once its relevance has been determined; usually needs supervision and guidance to complete data base. Occasionally does not recognize need for direction when unsure of resources to collect data.

Usually can identify major gaps in data base and takes initiative to determine these on limited basis. Usually requires assistance and guidance in recognizing smaller gaps in information; usually recognizes need for and seeks out limited though appropriate resources when in doubt. Once gaps in data are determined, is usually effective in eliciting these and incorporating them meaningfully among other data.

Identifies both obvious and subtle gaps in data base; exercises self-direction in eliciting these from a wide variety of appropriate resources. Is able to explain importance of this needed information. Requires minimal guidance in completing data base except for validating findings. When in doubt, recognizes self-limitations and seeks appropriate resources and direction.

(1) ☐   (2) ☐   (3) ☐   (4) ☐   (5) ☐

5 Usually requires assistance in differentiating among facts, opinions, perceptions, inferences, principles, hypotheses, and theories in data base. Generally requires assistance in correctly identifying and appropriately weighing these differentially in analyzing data.

Generally can differentiate between facts, derivatives of facts, and more theoretical levels in data base. With assistance, can usually identify factual versus theoretical nature of data. Can usually identify factors carrying greatest weight in their relevance, but typically requires assistance in placing other factors within suitable perspective.

Explanations of various factors in data base reflect a valid and self-determined evaluation of their relative importance before instructor's request for clarification. Consistently identifies full hierarchy of important data elements and can place even hypothetical or potential data within this hierarchy.

(1) ☐   (2) ☐   (3) ☐   (4) ☐   (5) ☐

Continued.

Example 16-3, cont'd

Minimally acceptable		Acceptable plus		Outstanding
6 In general, nursing intervention alternatives follow from data analysis and hierarchy of importance, but frequently are stereotypical, reflecting textbook orientation rather than approach to specific situation and principles involved. Proposed alternatives are usually broad and vague; usually requires assistance in setting priorities of interventions.		Proposed nursing interventions usually follow logically from broad principles identified with some specific details incorporated. Can usually identify highest priorities of care on her own, but requires assistance with sorting out elements of lesser overall importance. Proposed interventions are usually individualized and reflect direct awareness of patient's situation.		Proposed nursing interventions consistently follow in systematic sequence from analysis of nature and hierarchy of data base elements. Generalizations are used only as the broader source of specific proposals whereby proposed interventions are validated. Proposed interventions are individualized for specific patient situations. Able to order nursing interventions on basis of their priority placement and validity of data source.
(1) ☐	(2) ☐	(3) ☐	(4) ☐	(5) ☐
7 Occasionally fails to recognize need for reevaluating intervention; usually requires assistance in incorporating results of interventions into prior data base for reassessment of appropriateness and effectiveness of actions. Frequently requires guidance and direction in subsequent selection of alternative courses of action and hesitates to do this on her own.		Usually recognizes need for evaluating nursing interventions, but occasionally requires assistance in evaluating the nature of the patient's response to her intervention. Usually able to identify subsequent courses of action, but may require minimal assistance. Occasionally uses self-initiative in attempting alternative courses of action; seeks instructor validation of these.		Consistently demonstrates clear awareness of need to evaluate her interventions in light of patient responses. Uses sound judgment in determining and validating patient responses; is able to speculate what alternative responses would have appeared as. Consistently able to specify what next most appropriate recourse would be and exercises self-direction in accomplishing and reevaluating these subsequent responses in a cyclic process. Seeks appropriate instructor validation when in doubt of her own evaluation of patient responses.
(1) ☐	(2) ☐	(3) ☐	(4) ☐	(5) ☐

In addition to rating the relative nature of a performance, observations may also be evaluated in a more rigid, all-or-nothing approach, using a performance checklist.

Performance checklists

A performance checklist (Example 16-4) provides a concise delineation of all behaviors required for satisfactorily completing a procedure or skill. When checklists were initially introduced for evaluating clinical performance, they merely enumerated all skills the nurse needed to acquire. Whereas these may provide an all-inclusive listing, they fail to specify to either the observer or to the learner what level or criteria of performance constitutes a satisfactory performance or a successful performance.

The emergence of mastery learning methods stimulated the construction of performance checklists that specified and differentiated

Example 16-4. Performance checklist (records a 12-lead ECG)

Instructions: As part of your orientation to this unit, you must learn to properly record a 12-lead ECG. The checklist that follows delineates the steps necessary to perform this clinical skill. You may use the checklist for learning how to acquire this skill; the unit inservice instructor will use the *same* form to evaluate your performance of the skill. Steps marked with an asterisk are "essential steps" that must all be included for your performance to be rated as "successfully completed."

	Done	Not done
1. Prepares patient and equipment		
a. Verifies patient's name	☐	☐
b. Introduces self and explains purpose and elements of procedure to patient	☐	☐
c. Plugs in grounded single-channel ECG recorder	☐	☐
d. Turns power switch to "on"	☐	☐
e. Checks that there is sufficient amount of ECG paper to complete recording; replaces paper roll if necessary	☐	☐
f. Draws curtain around patient's bed	☐	☐
g. Places patient in supine position at (45 degree) semi-Fowler's angle	☐	☐
h. Exposes patient's distal limbs and chest	☐	☐
*i. Prepares skin surfaces on limbs and chest by cleansing with alcohol pad and mildly abrading friction	☐	☐
*j. Applies conductive material (alcohol pad, electrode gel) to underside of each of four electrode plates without allowing leakage of material when plate is secured	☐	☐
*k. Securely attaches each designated electrode plate to its appropriate limb without straining or kinking cable wires	☐	☐
*l. Records patient's name, date, and time on ECG paper	☐	☐
2. Standardizes ECG for time and voltage		
a. Turns control knob to "run"	☐	☐
b. Centers stylus on ECG paper	☐	☐
c. Verifies paper speed is 25 mm/sec	☐	☐
d. Turns lead selector switch to "STD"	☐	☐
e. Presses STD button (1 mV) and verifies presence of a 10 mm boxed deflection; adjusts to 10 mm deflection if necessary	☐	☐
f. Verifies sensitivity swtich is on "on"	☐	☐
g. Verifies all waveforms are observable; if voltage inadequate, increases sensitivity to "2"; if voltage excessive, decreases sensitivity to "½"	☐	☐
3. Records six frontal plane leads		
*a. Records at least five ECG complex cycles for each of the six frontal plane leads	☐	☐
*b. Records frontal plane leads in standard order: I, II, III, AVR, AVL, AVF	☐	☐
c. Identifies each frontal plane lead by its respective code marking:	☐	☐

        I -   AVR ----
        II --   AVL -----
        III ---   AVF ------

	Done	Not done
If marking button does not operate properly, writes lead on ECG paper by hand	☐	☐
4. Records six horizontal plane leads		
a. Turns control knob to "on"	☐	☐
b. Attaches small suction cup to chest lead cable	☐	☐
c. Applies small amount of electrode gel to each of six chest lead locations:	☐	☐

        V_1 = Fourth ICS, RSB V_4 = Fifth ICS, MCL
        V_2 = Fourth ICS, LSB V_5 = Same level as V_4, A AXL
        V_3 = midway between V_2 and V_4 V_6 = Same level as V_4, Mid AXL

Continued.

Example 16-4. Performance checklist (records a 12-lead ECG)—cont'd

	Done	Not done
d. Applies suction cup to each V position	☐	☐
e. Turns lead selector to V position and power switch to "run"	☐	☐
*f. Records at least five ECG complex cycles for each of the six horizontal plane leads	☐	☐
g. Records chest leads in standard order: V_1 to V_6	☐	☐
h. Identifies each horizontal plane lead by its respective code marking:	☐	☐

V_1 ———— -

V_2 ———— --

V_3 ———— ---

V_4 ———— ----

V_5 ———— -----

V_6 ———— ------

	Done	Not done
5. Concludes ECG recording		
a. Turns power switch to "off"	☐	☐
b. Unplugs ECG recorder	☐	☐
c. Detaches electrodes from patient	☐	☐
d. Removes all conductive material from patient's skin	☐	☐

among crucial or essential elements of a procedure and elements that were only desirable or recommended. In their ideal form, such checklists enumerate each necessary step in a sequence, arrange it in its naturally encountered order, and include sufficient detail that commonly occurring errors or omissions would be detected by the observer.

Performance checklists can be useful for evaluating a wide variety of integrated behaviors, especially those readily dissociated into separate and identifiable component behaviors.

Checklists share the same general advantages and disadvantages as rating scales, but are more appropriately applied when the evaluation is for mastery rather than for achievement. Scoring a performance checklist does not then involve rating the degree to which a behavior is present, but rather merely indicating whether or not the criterion level of performance was met. Thus only two categories are available for scoring a checklist: satisfactory or unsatisfactory (pass or fail, successful or unsuccessful, met or not met).

Two differing approaches may be employed for determining mastery of a skill. Satisfactory performance may require the satisfactory performance of all essential (critical, crucial) elements of a procedure, when the omission or unsatisfactory performance of any one essential element precludes attaining satisfactory performance. A second approach is used when all behaviors are deemed to be of equal importance; here the score that must be attained to constitute mastery is specified (for example, satisfactory completion requires a score of at least 90 out of a possible 100, or satisfactory completion requires 100% mastery). Wherever the mastery or criterion level of performance is set, the final determination remains an either-or proposition: either mastery was attained or it was not.

REFERENCES

Educational evaluation

Chase, CI: Measurement for educational evaluation, ed 2, Reading, Mass., 1978, Addison-Wesley.

Ebel, RL: Essentials of educational measurement, ed 3, Englewood Cliffs, N.J., 1979, Prentice-Hall.

Erickson, RC, and Wentling, TL: Measuring student growth: techniques and procedures for higher education, Boston, 1976, Allyn and Bacon, Inc.

Nunnally, JC: Psychometric theory, New York, 1978, McGraw-Hill Book Co.

Stanley, JC, and Hopkins, KD: Educational and psychological measurement and evaluation, Englewood Cliffs, N.J., 1972, Prentice-Hall.

Thorndike, RL, editor: Educational measurement, ed 2, Washington, D.C., 1971, American Council on Education.

Westwick, CR: Item analysis, JNE 15:27, 1976.

Grading systems

Barritt, ER, and Irion, LA: Advantages and disadvantages of nongrading, Nurs Outlook 18:40, 1970.

Crancer, J, Maury-Hess, S, and Dunn, J: Contract systems and grading policies, JNE 16:29, 1977.

Dodd, MJ: A longitudinal study in the use of credit/no credit for grading of clinical course, JNE 17:14, 1978.

Ebel, RL: Measuring educational achievement, Englewood Cliffs, N.J., 1965, Prentice-Hall.

Gould, EO: Satisfactory/Unsatisfactory grading in the evaluation of clinical performance in nursing: its effect on student motivation as perceived by nursing students, JNE 17:36, 1978.

Kochman, AF: Are letter grades and modularized nursing programs compatible? JNE 15:25, 1976.

Kramer, MA, and Cowles, JT: Weighing and distributing course grades, Nurs Outlook 22:176, 1974.

Smania, MA, McClelland, MG, and McCloskey, JC: And still another look at clinical grading: minimal behaviors, Nurs Educ 3:6, 1978.

Ward, JA, and Griffin, JM: Improving instruction through computer-graded examinations, Nurs Outlook 25:524, 1977.

Woolley, AS: Reaching and teaching the older student, Nurs Outlook 21:37, 1973.

Learning contracts

Barrentine, MM: A contract for mastery learning. In National League for Nursing: Generating effective teaching, New York, 1978, National League for Nursing.

Becker, S: Learning contracts: helping adults educate themselves, Training HRD 15:57, 1978.

Crancer, J, Maury-Hess, S, and Dunn, J: Contracting systems and grading policies, JNE 16:29, 1977.

Dale, R: Contracting for student clinical experience, Nurs Educ 2:22, 1976.

Delaney, C, and Schoolcraft, V: Promoting autonomy: clinical contracts, JNE 16:22, 1977.

Homme, L: How to use contingency contracting in the classroom, Champaign, Ill., 1970, Research Press.

Marriner, A: The student and the contracted grade, Nurs Forum 8:31, 1974.

Paduano, MA: Introducing independent study into the nursing curriculum, JNE 18:34, 1979.

Rauen, K, and Waring, B: The teaching contract, Nurs Outlook 20:594, 1972.

Schmidt, MC, and Quaife, MC: Orientation by contract, Superv Nurs 5:38, 1974.

Woolley, AS: Reaching and teaching the older student, Nurs Outlook 21:37, 1973.

Evaluating affective learning

Curran, CL, and Mattis, AE: Construction of a reliable instrument to measure attitudes, Nurs Educ 3:6, 1978.

Davidson, ME, and McArdle, PE: Peer analysis of interpersonal responsiveness and plan for encouraging effective reshaping—pair/peer, JNE 19:8, 1980.

Lange, CM: Using media in evaluation, Nurs Outlook 25:241, 1977.

Rawnsley, MM: Toward a conceptual base for affective nursing, Nurs Outlook 28:244, 1980.

Reilly, DE: Teaching and evaluating the affective domain in nursing programs, Thorofare, N.J., 1978, Charles B. Slack.

Rogers, S: Testing the RN student's skills, Nurs Outlook 24:446, 1976.

Welch, C: Field research in interpersonal relations. In Popiel, ES, editor: Nursing and the process of continuing education, ed 2, St. Louis, 1977, The C.V. Mosby Co.

Evaluating psychomotor and integrated learning

Deets, CA: Evaluating CE programs, AORN J 26:152, 1977.

del Bueno, DJ: Performance evaluation: when all is said and done, more is said than done, J Nurs Admin 7:21, 1977.

Forbes, E, and Nelson, PT: The clinical evaluation dilemma: a survey of problems encountered. In National League for Nursing: The challenge of clinical evaluation, New York, 1979, National League for Nursing.

Holland, J: Videotaping clinical experience, Nurs Outlook 25:337, 1977.

Lawrence, RM, and Lawrence, SA: Clinical evaluation of students of nursing: a step toward quality nursing practice, Image 12:46, 1980.

Lenburg, CB: Criteria for developing clinical performance evaluation, New York, 1976, National League for Nursing.

Litwack, LL: Meeting the challenge of clinical evaluation. In National League for Nursing: The challenge of clinical evaluation, New York, 1979, National League for Nursing.

Loustau, A, et al: Evaluating students' clinical performance: using videotape to establish rater reliability, JNE 19:10, 1980.

McCaffrey, C: Performance checklists: an effective method of teaching, learning and evaluating, Nurs Educ 3:11, 1978.

McIntyre, H, et al: A simulated clinical nursing test, Nurs Res 21:429, 1972.

Memmer, MK: Television replay: a tool for students to learn to evaluate their own proficiency in using sterile technique, JNE 18:35, 1979.

National League for Nursing: The challenge of clinical evaluation, New York, 1979, National League for Nursing.

National League for Nursing: Considerations in clinical evaluation: instructors-students-legal issues-data, New York, 1979, National League for Nursing.

Norman, AE, and Hoffman, KI: The benefits of direct performance tests, J Contin Educ Nurs 7:34, 1976.

O'Leary, MM, and Holzemer, WL: Evaluation of an inservice program, J Nurs Admin 10:21, 1980.

Schweer, JE, and Gebbie, KM: Creative teaching in clinical nursing, ed 3, St. Louis, 1976, The C. V. Mosby Co.

Shortridge, L, et al: Opportunity to learn physical assessment in a continuing education course, J Contin Educ Nurs 8:6, 1977.

Smania, MA, McClelland, MG, and McCloskey, JC: And still another look at clinical grading: minimal behaviors, Nurs Educ 3:6, 1978.

Voight, JW: Assessing clinical performance: a model for competency, JNE 18:30, 1979.

Woolley, AS: The long and tortured history of clinical evaluation, Nurs Outlook 25:308, 1977.

Wyman, J, and Ferneau, K: Developing a criterion-referenced tool, Nurs Outlook 25:584, 1977.

Chapter 17

Summarizing educational evaluations

Early in this unit a distinction was made between product and process evaluation. Because product evaluation is the primary concern of educators, the major portion of this unit has been devoted to a discussion of ways to evaluate learning. The educational and administrative processes that support and facilitate this product deserve some attention as well because the product of education depends largely on the processes that nurture it.

Process evaluation of an educational program can encompass a virtually infinite range of variables. Process evaluation seeks to determine whether the procedural design, planning, and implementation of an educational program—its logistical and operational aspects—need refinement, revision, or improvement.

A truly comprehensive process evaluation would incorporate reconsidering every conceivable aspect of the program's design, planning, implementation, and evaluation, inclusive of all administrative and educational aspects (Chapters 1 to 4 and 6). It would encompass a thorough reexamination and appraisal of each step in curriculum design and instruction (Chapters 5, 7, 9, and 10), implementation (Chapter 8), and the evaluation process itself (Chapters 13 to 16). Suggestions from all of the groups and individuals who should be involved in the evaluation process would be solicited both formatively and summatively.

The Overview of Hospital-Based Educational Evaluation (pp. 162-167) outlined the numerous dimensions of an evaluative scheme and suggested the most meaningful forms for obtaining data to make the decisions faced by the educator and agency. Because the program director must be the central communicator for soliciting and incorporating all of this information into a total evaluation of the program, one of the director's responsibilities is to compile this information into a written format to facilitate this decision-making process.

If you will be using a written device for some of your evaluations, some suggestions include designing a reporting form or questionnaire that would do the following:

1. Use simple, concise, and clear wording.
2. Solicit information directly and unambiguously.
3. If lengthy, use a variety of formats (rating scales, open-ended questions, ranking).
4. Have adequate spacing available for comments and suggestions.
5. Provide self-evident or clearly stated instructions for completing it.
6. Group information into logically related categories.
7. Provide anonymity if you desire candor.

Example 17-1 illustrates a suggested program evaluation device designed for eliciting feedback from program participants. Example 17-2 provides a summary program evaluation form that could be used for compiling evaluative

235

Example 17-1. Program evaluation form

	Ratings					Comments	Suggestions
	Poor	Fair	Satis	Very good	Excellent		
1. Learning environment a. Classroom							
b. Use of AV aids							
c. Clinical units							

2. Curriculum and instruc-
  tion
  a. Relevance of topics							

b. Adequacy of time allot- ted to topics							
c. Relevance of articles							
d. Textbooks							
(1) Pulmonary text							
(2) Cardiovascular text							
(3) ECG workbooks							
(4) Core curriculum							

e. Overall quality of in-
   struction (clarity, orga-
   nization preparation,
   knowledge of topic)							

(1) Classroom instruc- tion							
(2) Clinical instruction							
f. Appropriateness of in- structional level							

3. Evaluations
  a. Fairness and validity of
   written tests							

b. Adequacy of time allot- ted to written testing							

c. Relevance and inclu-
   siveness of clinical skills
   Inventory							

d. Adequacy of time for
   completion of clinical
   skills inventory							

e. Performance evalua-
   tions
   (1) Relevance							

(2) Fairness and con- structiveness							
(3) Frequency and ad- equacy of time							

Example 17-1. Program evaluation form—cont'd

Please list (if any apply):

Topics best covered	Topics inadequately covered	Irrelevant topics that were covered	Topics that should have been covered

Areas of growth	Self-evaluation						
	Estimated degree of growth					Comments	Suggestions
	None	Minimal	Moderate	Significant	Exceptional		
1. Knowledge a. Psychosocial							
b. Pulmonary							
c. GI							
d. Cardiovascular							
e. Metabolic							
f. Neurological							
g. Renal							
h. Burns							
2. Skills a. Psychosocial							
b. Pulmonary							
c. GI							
d. Cardiovascular							
e. Metabolic							
f. Neurological							
g. Renal							
h. Burns							

Considering your initial reasons for entering this program and your expectations of the program, how well have we met your needs and expectations? ☐ Not met ☐ Minimally met ☐ Adequately met ☐ Very well met ☐ Met above expectations

Comments: _____
_____
_____
_____

What I liked best about the program	What I liked least about the program	Suggestions for improving the program

Would you recommend this program to other nurses new to critical care nursing? ☐ Yes ☐ No
Comments: _____

Miscellaneous comments: _____
_____
_____
_____

Example 17-2. Summary program evaluation form

Dimension	Aspect evaluated	Information source	Outcomes	Recommendations
A. Learning environment Classroom or laboratory	1. Adequacy of space, size			
	2. Availability			
	3. Lighting			
	4. Comfort			
	5. Utilities			
Clinical areas	1. Physical space			
	2. Patient population			
	3. Quality of learning experiences			
	4. Quantity of learning experiences			
B. Learning resources	1. Textbooks			
	2. Journal articles			

	3. Audiovisual media
	  a. Usefulness
	  b. Availability
	  c. Need for development
	  d. Hardware adequacy, compatibility			

C. Curriculum	1. Content relevance			
	2. Appropriate emphases			
	3. Organization			
	4. Sequencing			
	5. Omitted topics			
	6. Balance of theoretical and practical			

D. Instruction	1. Classroom
	  a. Teaching methods
	  b. Delivery quality
	  c. Faculty evaluation			

	2. Laboratory and clinical setting
	  a. Adequacy of facilities
	  b. Adequacy of equipment, aids
	  c. Adequacy of preceptor training
	  d. Availability of instructors
	  e. Correlation of theory with practice			

E. Evaluation process	1. Test instruments
	  a. Validity
	  b. Reliability
	  c. Usefulness
	  d. Variety			

	2. Appropriateness of grading systems employed			

Example 17-2. Summary program evaluation form—cont'd

Dimension	Aspect evaluated	Information source	Outcomes	Recommendations
E. Evaluation process—cont'd	3. Frequency and timing of evaluations			
	4. Fairness and constructiveness of evaluations			
F. Administrative	1. Cost-effectiveness of program a. Marketing, recruitment costs b. Number of participants c. Attrition rates during and after program d. Retention rates after program e. Cost of program provision f. Cost-benefit ratio per participant			
	2. Impact of program on nursing department and hospital a. Public relations value of program within community b. Effect of program on staffing (scheduling, mix, nurse-patient ratio, hours of care provided) c. Effect of program on staff morale d. Effect of program on standards of practice and performance appraisals e. Effect of program on time and cost of orientation			
G. Clients	1. Effect of program on care evidenced in chart audits: a. Retrospective b. Concurrent c. Process vs outcome			
	2. Effect of program on care provided through a. Direct observation b. Performance checklists			
H. Professional issues	1. Effect of program on fostering pursuit of a. Continuing education b. Formal degrees in nursing			
	2. Ability of program to meet requirements for CEU approval by state, national, and professional specialty accrediting bodies			
	3. Effect of program in stimulating pursuit of certification in critical care nursing (CCRN)			

information necessary for a final and total evaluation of an educational program. Each could initially be used to solicit formative and summative information and could later be used to summarize the information obtained into a final report. This summary report of the total program makes available the data needed for making decisions regarding subsequent educational programming and readies recycling the educational process within the agency.

The preceding pages of this book have shown that the hospital-based nurse educator's role is expansive and at various times incorporates elements of being a practitioner, administrator, educator, researcher, consultant, coordinator, statistician, and an agent for change. As a professional nurse, the clinically based educator looks beyond the local employing agency to reflect on how the clinical nurse educator role extends to incorporate the profession and the practice. The final chapter of this book is devoted to considering these extensions of the critical care educator's role.

Unit V

EXTENSION

Chapter 18

Extensions of the critical care educator's role

As a provider of continuing education for nurses, the critical care educator in a hospital-based setting is most directly responsible to the agency that employs her. As a professional nurse educator, she has an attendant responsibility to the profession that embraces her. In this regard, the critical care educator should be cognizant of the current professional issues surrounding continuing education, be knowledgeable concerning how to obtain professional approval for programs offered, and be capable of counseling staff nurses and administrators about the relative quality of continuing education programming available in nursing.

In addition to these monitoring, administrative, and consultant roles, the clinical educator assumes professional responsibility for assuring that a meaningful and direct relationship exists between continuing education and nursing practice. This chapter addresses each of these professional responsibilities.

MONITORING THE STATUS OF CONTINUING EDUCATION IN NURSING

There was a day when continuing education in nursing consisted of what a nurse managed to acquire by simply remaining in the profession. Completing a basic program of education, being in the right place at the right time for some on-the-job training, and surviving a variety of inci-

dental experiences constituted the sum of a nurse's professional education.

Today, the implications of being a professional nurse are much more far-reaching. They reach out to consumer advocacy groups who want assurances of consumer protection in health care, and to the federal government, which assists in financing nurse training. They reach out to state legislators who are elected to represent and legislate in favor of the public's right to be protected in health care, and who license professionals to practice within the state. They reach out to professional associations and organizations who posit that continuing education is essential for maintaining professional competency, and to individual nurses who practice under state nurse practice laws that mandate their professional accountability. They also reach out to nursing students who are being raised on these concepts in their early professional preparation.

As a result of the collective pressures exerted by governmental, legislative, private, and professional sectors, the confrontation of issues surrounding the continuing education of licensed professionals has gained both momentum and direction. Despite vigorous and laborious debate between professional and public interest groups, in spite of deferments, postponements, amendments, partial revocations, and lobbying

243

against proposed legislation, professional groups are coming to terms with the emergent reality that being relicensed to practice their profession will sooner than later require evidence of continuing education.

The issues surrounding continuing education for nurse relicensing are numerous, complex, and at times perplexing. Although a majority of professional nursing organizations ascribe to the belief that continuing education is essential for maintaining the competency of its practitioners, consensus among individual members of these organizations is by no means universal. Although none have espoused continuing education to be a bad thing, the degrees of good ascribed to it vary widely from negligible to superlative.

As a continuing educator in nursing, you have a responsibility to keep abreast of these issues and participate in their discussion and resolution. As a professional nurse, you, too, will be affected by their outcome. Regardless of your opinion of these issues, however, the present facts are that

1. Many states have already enacted legislation that mandates continuing education for relicensing nurses.
2. Such legislation is currently in effect in a few states, slated for the 1980s in a larger number, and impending in still others.
3. States that have not yet enacted legislation for continuing education of nurses are actively considering and debating these issues now.
4. States are currently at varying stages in revising their nurse practice acts as they affect RNs, LPNs, and nurses in extended roles.
5. Political, private, and professional groups are proceeding in their deliberations with an uncommon sense of urgency.

Few things emerge clearly from these current discussions. It does seem clear, however, that for nurses and many other licensed professionals, the days of being licensed for life and relicensed for a fee alone are gone. Beyond this, regulations, requirements, and decisions are so mutable they defy attempts at generalization.

If your state has already enacted legislation mandating continuing education as a requirement for relicensing nurses, or if this is imminent or even being considered, you should acquaint yourself with its implications by contacting your state board of nursing or state nurses' association. Either agency should be able to answer questions you or your staff nurses or administrators may have concerning the issue of continuing education for relicensing. The American Nurses' Association Council on Continuing Education has published *Standards of Continuing Education in Nursing, Continuing Education Guidelines for State Nurses' Associations,* and *Guidelines for State Voluntary and Mandatory Systems,* which you may use. Even if your state has not yet legislated mandatory continuing education for relicensing, you may be interested in obtaining voluntary approval of programs offered at your agency by contacting your state nurses' association concerning its Continuing Education Approval and Recognition Program (CEARP).

Another way the clinical nurse educator may participate in these initiatives is by becoming familiar with the procedures for obtaining continuing education approval for programs offered at the local agency.

OBTAINING APPROVAL FOR A CONTINUING EDUCATION PROGRAM OR OFFERING

A number of different professional agencies may grant approval for continuing education programs in nursing. Many educational institutions such as colleges or universities, federal nursing services, national specialty nursing organizations such as the American Association of Critical-Care Nurses or Emergency Department Nurses Association, state boards of nursing, state nurses' associations, and national nursing organizations such as the American Nurse's Association or the National League for Nursing are organizations that may be accredited to approve continuing education programs in nursing. Accredited groups may grant approval for an individual continuing education offering or related courses that constitute a continuing education program. Approval is granted to a specific sponsor or constituent for a specific program or offering; it is not granted to the individuals who apply for approval nor to the persons who provide the program or offering.

The application forms for obtaining approval for a continuing education program or offering from a state nursing association (Example 18-1) or a specialty nursing organization (Example 18-2) are the ones you will most likely be using as a critical care nursing educator. As you can see, each form requests that the individual completing the application provide specific information; as follows:

1. Sponsor. The sponsor is the agency or institution assuming responsibility for all aspects of the continuing education program: its planning, implementation, evaluation, financing, and recording.
2. Cosponsor. The cosponsor is another organization or institution jointly and equally sharing responsibility for all aspects of the program with the sponsor. Joint sponsorship may entail providing additional materials and a copy of the contractual agreement between the involved parties.
3. Title of the program or offering.
4. Dates the program will be presented.
5. Location or facility where the program will be held.
6. Level of instruction.
7. Number of contact hours. One contact hour is usually defined as being equivalent to 50 minutes of instruction in an approved and organized learning experience. The number of clinical hours that constitute 1 contact hour may vary; for some approvers, 2 supervised hours of clinical instruction are equivalent to 1 contact hour, whereas with others 3 clinical hours

are equivalent to 1 contact hour. The calculation of contact hours must be made exclusive of registration periods, coffee breaks, lunch, or any other noninstructional time.

The remaining portion of the application form typically specifies the support materials sponsors must submit with their application. Be sure to request these forms and the policies and procedures for application of approval for continuing education programs well ahead of your anticipated program dates; processing time may require 4 to 10 weeks before you are notified of the status of your application. Here are some hints for submitting these documents:

1. *Program description*. In clear, concise language, provide a brief synopsis of major program features. Include its overall purpose, relevance to specific target audience, format, and the instructional methods that will be employed. Delineate the major points that will be emphasized and specify how the program content will be useful for the target audience. You may develop the program description on the basis of the program objectives and overall goal or purpose of the program.

2. *Content outline*. All major headings and subheadings should be arranged in a standard outline format, indicating the amount of instructional time allotted for each segment. Enough specificity should be included so that the approval agency can clearly see the areas to be addressed. Lengthy programs (lasting weeks to months) need not include the degree of detailed breakdown that a 1-day offering might warrant; be reasonable in the amount of specificity you include. If you have questions related to how detailed this breakdown should be, request a clarification on policy from the accrediting agency. Most accreditors require that the content be directly related to the practice of nursing; be certain that the content described clearly indicates this intention and includes an emphasis on how this material will be applicable to nursing practice.

Example 18-1. MNA CEU application form

Maryland Nurses Association
Office Of Continuing Education

APPLICATION FOR OFFERING APPROVAL

1. This application is: (check appropriate box)
   - ☐ An initial submission
   - ☐ A renewal of a MNA Approved Offering
     Code No. _____
     Expiration date: _____
   - ☐ A resubmission of a disapproved application
   - ☐ Supplemental information for a deferred
     application Code no. _____

2. Sponsoring agency _____
   Address _____ Phone _____
     Street
   _____ _____ _____
   City   State   Zip
   Cosponsor (if applicable) _____

3. Title of offering _____

4. Contact hours requested: _____ Is there a clinical component? ☐ Yes ☐ No _____ Hours

5. Presentation dates: _____ MNA district: _____

6. Location: _____

7. Types, level, and numbers of participants expected: _____

8. Method of financing offering: _____
   _____
   _____
   _____

9. Planning committee: (Must include a registered nurse)

Name	**Discipline**	**Position**	**Organization**

10. Needs assessment: (Descriptive information and data that indicate a need for this offering)

11. Offering description: (state the purpose and provide an overview)

12. Course design: (see attached form)

Continued.

12. Course design

Objectives	Content	Teaching methods	Time allotment	Faculty	Evaluation
Specific, behavioral statements that describe what the learner (registered nurse) should be able to do following content presentation.	An outline of the subject matter to be presented in relation to *each* objective. The content must give evidence that the offering is designed for nurses to keep them abreast of recent trends, ideas, and developments as they are applicable to the practice of nursing. (Attach content *bibliography.*)	Specific instructional strategies that are consistent with the objectives, content, and learning needs of the participant.	Time frame in minutes necessary to achieve each objective and its related content. (Attach *program schedule.*)	Identify instructors for each specific content area. (Complete curriculum vita sheet for each instructor.)	Indicate method by which objective is measured. (Attach evaluation forms that permit participants to evaluate faculty, objectives, content, teaching methods, and facilities.)

Example 18-1. MNA CEU application form—cont'd

13. Contact person for offering information:
    Name: _____ Position: _____
    Address: _____ Phone: _____
    _____

Ten sets of the collated supporting documents and the $15.00 fee (made payable to MNA) should be mailed with this application at least *60 days prior* to the presentation date to:

Office of Continuing Education
Maryland Nurses Association
5820 Southwestern Boulevard
Baltimore, Maryland 21227

Do not forget to send:
Faculty C.V.s
Program schedule
Bibliography
Evaluation forms

_____   _____
Authorized signature   Please print name here

_____   _____
Title   Date

REV 9/80
CE #1
To be used in conjunction with criteria for approval of Continuing Education Offerings

Maryland Nurses Association
Continuing Education Program for Nursing

CURRICULUM VITAE

Name: _____

                First   Middle   Last   Titles

Present position: _____

Agency/program/facility: _____

Address: _____

Professional (relevant) experience or special preparation to participate in teaching this course offering:

Professional education:

Institution	Major	Degree	Year

Relevant publications and studies (past 5 years):

Example 18-2. AACN CEU program approval application

American Association of Critical-Care Nurses

AACN CEU PROGRAM APPROVAL APPLICATION

Applicant name _____   Relationship to program _____
(instructor, director, etc.)

Address _____   City _____

State _____ Zip _____ Telephone _____

Sponsor name _____
(individual/organization/agency)

Cosponsor _____

Cosponsor _____

Program title _____ Program date _____

Facility _____ City/state _____

Program Level: ☐ Basic   ☐ Intermediate   ☐ Advanced

Participant fee _____ Anticipated registrant number _____

Contact hours _____ (Not to include breaks, lunch, etc.)

Required documents

Submit one copy of each of the following documents with this application.
1. Complete program description
2. Program outline (include program content and hours of presentation)
3. Program objectives
4. Participant objectives
5. Evaluation tool
6. Bibliography of resource materials
7. Complete instructor/speaker list (include academic background, clinical experience, field of practice)

Also include:
1. Program review fee   (Check must accompany each program.)
2. Order form for CEU certificates   (if appropriate)
3. Cosponsorship financial agreement   (if appropriate)
4. AACN CEU program approval application

Signature _____
Applicant

Amount of fees enclosed $ _____   Signature _____
Sponsor

Date _____

---

3. *Behavioral objectives.* Behavioral objectives must be stated so that they are observable, measurable, and attainable within the time available. Objectives must be written in terms of what participants should be capable of doing as a result of the learning experience. Because these instructional objectives are the core of the entire offering or program of offerings, they are likely to be the most closely scrutinized portion of the application. Before you submit the application, then, double-check that the content outline, instructional methods, learning resources, evaluation tools, techniques, and faculty credentials are all consistent with what the program is intended to provide.

4. *Program objectives.* If program objectives

are requested, remember that they are not the equivalent of participant behavioral (instructional) objectives. Program objectives should indicate what the program is designed to provide (opportunity to exchange and share information, to practice new skills, to update or review information, to answer questions concerning current issues in nursing, and to provide hands-on experience and skill acquisition). These objectives are derived from the overall goal or purpose of the program.

5. *Teaching methods*. Include evidence that nurses have participated in designing teaching methods and techniques used in providing the learning experiences and that principles of adult education have been incorporated. This does not preclude using traditional teaching methods such as the lecture, but does suggest that the application will be examined for verification that learning experiences incorporate active participation and involvement of learners in various aspects of the learning situation. These may be provided with discussion or question and answer periods, practice sessions or workshops, group work, or participant evaluation.

6. *Instructional resources*. Suggested reading lists or bibliographies should be included for the adult learner's further study of program topics; these should be screened for currency, completeness, accuracy, and pertinence. If textbooks or other written or audiovisual references will be used or recommended, the full reference should be provided for each. Copies of all handouts and related learning materials distributed at the offering are also useful to include with the application because they reflect the sponsor's intention to reinforce and to supplement learning experiences.

7. *Evaluation devices*. In the early days of continuing education approval, submitting the "reaction form" distributed to participants met the criteria of evaluation devices. More recently, accrediting agencies are looking less toward how participants responded to the learning experience and more toward how the sponsor will be able to verify that the instructional objectives were met. Again, be sure the program's evaluation device reflects a valid assessment that the objectives delineated were met by the participants. The evaluation tool may be in the form of a written test, self-assessment, study guide, performance checklist, or other device; it should indicate that learning has occurred. Ideally, a follow-up evaluation is also included for appraising long term learning retention.

8. *Faculty credentials*. You need not include a full curriculum vita for each member of the faculty. The accrediting agency will check to see that the faculty members possess the formal and experiential expertise for the learning experiences and content areas they are assigned to provide. Formal academic degrees and credentials should be verified for accuracy and spelling. In addition to the degree held, it may also be helpful to include the major area of study and the year the degree was obtained. You need to include only experience and accomplishments related to the content areas provided. You may also expect that approval agencies will check to see that faculty members responsible for applying the content to nursing practice are in fact nurses themselves. It may be difficult to rationalize with the agency how a physician or allied health professional can validly speak to nursing practice. Even joint or team approaches to learning call for a balanced faculty background. Besides formal credentials, certifications, and related work experiences and accomplishments, the present position and previous experience as an instructor are useful supportive information to include in the application. In short, the approval agency is looking for what makes a particular faculty member qualified to teach in the area assigned.

Once the application and its support materials are readied and signed by the appropriate authorities in the employing agency, review all of these for their inclusiveness and accuracy. Be sure you have allowed adequate time for the following:

1. Obtaining payment of the required application fee.
2. Duplicating the specified number of copies of documents.
3. Remembering to retain at least one copy of all records for your own files.
4. Obtaining all necessary local signatures and approvals.
5. Mailing all documents to their necessary destination within the time required for the approval process.
6. Printing that includes mention of the program's approval for brochures, and advertising and marketing of the program. Because it may take 1 to 2 months before you are notified of the decision on your application, and further documentation, clarification, or revision may be required by the approval agency, you should allow a lead time for submitting these materials of at least 3 to 4 months ahead of the intended starting dates of the program. Retrospective approval is usually not obtainable, so avoid the time problems that leave the sponsor and participants very dissatisfied. Advertising that the program "has been approved" says much more about your efforts to potential attendants than only being able to say that "approval is pending" or that "approval has been applied for."Remember that you cannot advertise CEU approval until you have received the notification of approval.

The approval agency will then acknowledge receipt of the application and support materials. The decision on the application may be any one of the following:

1. *Approval*. When a program or offering is approved for continuing education, a specified number of continuing education units is awarded for participation in the program. One continuing education unit is equivalent to 10 contact hours of participation in a continuing education program that is organized and has responsible sponsorship, capable direction, and qualified instruction. Remember that program approval is contingent on the sponsor who applied for approval of the program and is applicable only for the dates specified in the application.

2. *Deferral of action*. The approval agency may defer action on an application if the information is incomplete, or is in need of revision, refinement, or clarification. If deferral is deemed the appropriate action, the approval agency will contact the program's sponsor or co-sponsors to obtain the necessary information or modifications. Until such information has been supplied or refined, program approval will not be granted. If the sponsor or co-sponsors desire program approval, they will need to supply the requested information within a specified time before presenting the program.

3. *Denial*. When an application for approval of continuing education offering falls far short of the criteria required for program approval, the application for approval will likely be denied. In this case, the approval agency will usually delineate the major areas of discrepency and suggest ways for bringing the application in line with these criteria. Sponsors who wish to obtain approval for the continuing education offering will need to communicate closely with the approval agency to accomplish this.

Prior approval of a program does not assure its continued approval; subsequent actions may include reaffirmation, deferral, or denial of the approval previously granted. Application for approval may also be withdrawn by the sponsor and approval status may be revoked by the accrediting agency. The sponsors of programs or offerings that fail to be approved may also seek methods to appeal these decisions. The procedures for appeal of an approval agency decision are usually outlined in the brochure that describes the policies and procedures for program approval.

If you are ever uncertain about any facet of the approval process, call or write the approval agency with which you are working. You will typically find individuals there who are most helpful in answering your questions and in facilitating the approval process. Do this early so that later diappointments and frustrations are averted and sponsors, providers, and participants are equally pleased with the outcome.

Being informed about the approval process for continuing education in nursing and being able to obtain this approval for your own offerings are two important facets of the educator's expanded role. A third emerges with the reality that staff and administrators are likely to seek your guidance in assisting them to determine which continuing education activities outside of your institution are a worthwhile investment of their time, money, and effort.

SELECTING AMONG PROGRAMS FOR CONTINUING EDUCATION IN NURSING

The momentum toward mandatory continuing education for relicensing nurses has precipitated a plethora of continuing education programs and groups participating in providing these. Brochures, flyers, booklets, posters, and catalogs glut the in boxes of nurse educators in a seemingly endless stream. As the announcements of continuing education programs pile up on administrative desks and get lost amongst their competitors on bulletin boards, nurses face the task of having to make rational choices amidst this bombardment. It is an unfortunate truism that although the brochures clothe continuing education in excellence, program quality and relevance to an individual practitioner are often provided in mediocrity. Another extension of the nurse educator's role is in discerning which programs are the most relevant, appropriate, and cost-effective for the nurses' individual learning needs and the needs of the employing institution.

The sophistication and attractiveness of an announcement bears no necessary relationship to the quality or usefulness of the program it describes. The fees charged for continuing education escalate to nearly prohibitive levels at times and do not generally fall in commensurate degree with agency budget cuts. No direct and positive correlation exists between the cost or length of a continuing education program and its merit. Unfortunately, not all continuing education providers are reputable individuals or organizations interested in providing high-quality programming for nurses.

Some ways to wade through this proliferation of continuing education offerings exist to determine which can survive a critical preevaluation by their potential consumers. Before endorsing or condemning any continuing education program, you should verify the nature of nurses' learning needs. Regardless of how interesting, intriguing, or compelling the topic, if nurses have no learning needs in this area, there is not much reason for further evaluation of the program.

Example 18-3 provides a checklist you can use to evaluate the major aspects of any continuing education program. Each area addressed requires a response of "not applicable," "yes," "no," or "unknown." The greater the number of "yes" responses, the more confidence you can have that the program will be worthwhile. The greater the number of "no" responses, the less confidence you should place in the offering's potential as a good learning experience. The greater the number of "unknowns," the less basis you have for being assured concerning any aspect of the program and the more you will need to investigate further to obtain relevant information necessary for determining whether enrollment is worthwhile.

Do not be misled into assuming that approval of a program for continuing education units assures you of its excellence or relevance; approval only means that the criteria for approval from a given approval agency have been met.

Example 18-3. Checklist for evaluating and selecting among continuing education programs in nursing

	N/A	Yes	No	Unk	Comments
Program sponsors					
1. Does the sponsor already have an established reputation for providing high quality programs for CE in nursing?	☐	☐	☐	☐	
2. Is this sponsor's past record commendable?	☐	☐	☐	☐	
3. Is the sponsor associated with an accredited educational or professional institution or organization?	☐	☐	☐	☐	
4. Is the education of nurses the primary function and motive of the sponsor?	☐	☐	☐	☐	
5. Is there evidence that nursing educators were involved in program planning with the sponsor?	☐	☐	☐	☐	
6. Do potential participants or others express favorable opinions regarding this sponsor?	☐	☐	☐	☐	
Program planning					
7. Is there evidence of nursing participation in program planning (design, implementation, and evaluation)?	☐	☐	☐	☐	
8. Is there evidence that the program is derived from an assessment of learning needs?	☐	☐	☐	☐	
9. Is the program designed specifically for professional nurses? Specific categories of nurses?	☐	☐	☐	☐	
Program level					
10. Can the program level be clearly identified?	☐	☐	☐	☐	
11. Are variable instructional levels provided for accommodating individual differences?	☐	☐	☐	☐	
12. Are prerequisite skills participants should possess clearly identifiable?	☐	☐	☐	☐	
13. Is the program level appropriate for staff nurses who are interested in the program?	☐	☐	☐	☐	
Program audience					
14. Is the program designed for critical care nurses?	☐	☐	☐	☐	
15. Have upper and lower limits been set for attendance?	☐	☐	☐	☐	
16. Are enrollment limits congruent with teaching format and methods?	☐	☐	☐	☐	
Program objectives					
17. Are the purpose and objectives of the program clearly stated in behavioral terms?	☐	☐	☐	☐	
18. Are the objectives congruent with the proposed content, teaching methods, format, and evaluation devices?	☐	☐	☐	☐	
19. Are the objectives meaningful and feasible?	☐	☐	☐	☐	
Program content					
20. Is the content relevant and applicable to nursing practice?	☐	☐	☐	☐	
21. Will the program offer more than basic nursing information?	☐	☐	☐	☐	
22. Is the content immediately applicable in the employing agency?	☐	☐	☐	☐	
Program faculty					
23. Are faculty qualified to teach their designated topics?	☐	☐	☐	☐	
24. Is there a congruence between an instructor's formal credentials and work experience and the topics to be addressed?	☐	☐	☐	☐	
25. Are faculty known to be skilled as teachers and practitioners?	☐	☐	☐	☐	
26. Are faculty credentials relevant and adequate for the content level of the program?	☐	☐	☐	☐	
27. Are faculty knowledgeable in the teaching methods to be employed?	☐	☐	☐	☐	
28. Are faculty who will speak to nursing practice known to be current practitioners in nursing?	☐	☐	☐	☐	

Example 18-3. Checklist for evaluating and selecting among continuing education programs in nursing—cont'd

Teaching strategies

29. Are a variety of teaching methods used? ☐ ☐ ☐ ☐
30. Are teaching methods compatible with principles of adult education? ☐ ☐ ☐ ☐
31. Are teaching methods consistent with the objectives and content? ☐ ☐ ☐ ☐
32. Is the program format satisfactory for those interested in attending? ☐ ☐ ☐ ☐
33. Are the program format and teaching strategies compatible with the preferred learning style of those interested in attending? ☐ ☐ ☐ ☐
34. Will audiovisual aids be used to enhance the learning experiences? ☐ ☐ ☐ ☐
35. If appropriate, will an interdisciplinary approach be used? ☐ ☐ ☐ ☐
36. Will hands-on practice of nursing skills be supervised and provided for? ☐ ☐ ☐ ☐
37. Will additional learning materials (worksheets, study guides, lists of references) be provided? ☐ ☐ ☐ ☐
38. Are learners prepared for the offering by the availability of suggested reading lists or outlines? ☐ ☐ ☐ ☐
39. Will materials be provided so learners are able to pursue continued learning in this area? ☐ ☐ ☐ ☐

Program duration

40. Has a sufficient amount of time been allotted to meet the objectives? ☐ ☐ ☐ ☐
41. Will segments of the program be brief enough to minimize fatigue yet long enough to cover the topic adequately? ☐ ☐ ☐ ☐
42. Has adequate time been allocated to practice skills? ☐ ☐ ☐ ☐

Program evaluation

43. Will there be provision for evaluating the overall program, faculty, facilities? ☐ ☐ ☐ ☐
44. Will there be provision for evaluating the attainment of personal and course objectives? ☐ ☐ ☐ ☐
45. Will long-term retention or transfer of learning to practice be evaluated? ☐ ☐ ☐ ☐
46. How valid are evaluation instruments? ☐ ☐ ☐ ☐

Program cost

47. Are costs (registration, lodging, travel, incidentals) reasonable and comparable to similar programs? ☐ ☐ ☐ ☐
48. Are expenses justified in relation to benefits gained by participants? ☐ ☐ ☐ ☐
49. Is a comparable program unavailable locally or within the employing agency? ☐ ☐ ☐ ☐
50. Is the total cost affordable for either the employing agency or the employee? ☐ ☐ ☐ ☐
51. Is this program the most cost-effective means for providing this type of learning experience? ☐ ☐ ☐ ☐

Program location

52. Will the physical facilities enhance the learning experience? ☐ ☐ ☐ ☐
53. Will the physical facilities provide comfort, good acoustics, and visibility? ☐ ☐ ☐ ☐
54. Does location afford accessibility, travel convenience, and adequate parking space? ☐ ☐ ☐ ☐
55. Is the sponsor approved as a provider of continuing education in nursing? ☐ ☐ ☐ ☐
56. Has the program otherwise been approved for CEUs by a nationally recognized professional specialty nursing organization? ☐ ☐ ☐ ☐

Continued.

Example 18-3. Checklist for evaluating and selecting among continuing education programs in nursing—cont'd

Program approval—cont'd					
57. Has the state nursing association approved this program?	☐	☐	☐	☐	
58. In states having mandatory continuing education for relicensing, does the offering meet the criteria for approval?	☐	☐	☐	☐	
59. Will some certificate attesting to participation or successful completion of the program be provided?	☐	☐	☐	☐	
60. Is an identified number of CEUs or contact hours awarded to the program?	☐	☐	☐	☐	
Program relevance to nursing practice					
61. Will the program enhance the participants' nursing practice?	☐	☐	☐	☐	
62. Will participants be able to demonstrate how their practice has been improved by the program?	☐	☐	☐	☐	
63. Does the program directly relate to the nurse's current responsibilities and position?	☐	☐	☐	☐	

Sometimes the criteria are less than they could and should be. Relevance is a highly personal and relative commodity. Program quality is sometimes only superficial. Because all of these points may not be relevant for every potential continuing educational offering, there is also a space to indicate "not appropriate."

There are no foolproof or magic formulas in this survey. Your professional judgment and ability to weigh the relative importance of various factors must be used to guide your decision. But as nurses gain awareness that they, too, are consumers and have rights to competency and quality in return for their investments of time, money, and effort, they will become more discriminating in their choices of continuing education programming.

This checklist (Example 18-3) may be used to provide information to use as a basis for supporting or advising against participation in a given continuing education program. It includes the major areas consumers of continuing education should consider in deciding the potential merit of a program: its sponsors, planning, instruction-al level, target audience, behavioral objectives, content, faculty, format, teaching strategies, duration, evaluation, cost, location, approval by a legitimate accrediting agency, and relevance to nursing practice.

The sequence of aspects is not intended to imply the necessary order of importance. This priority varies with participants and local circumstances. In fact, the most important aspect for determining the essential attributes of a worthwhile continuing education program in nursing is the last, its relevance in nursing practice. Because of the centrality of this point to the entire field of continuing education in nursing and to the issue of mandatory continuing education for relicensing nurses, the relationship between continuing education and nursing practice has been reserved for the end of this chapter and book. Because our awareness of the relationship between continuing education and nursing practice has seemingly been little, late, and as yet, very limited, virtually no facts are available to substantiate its location at the beginning of this book. Rather, the issue is presented here not as an afterthought, but as a parting thought to consider as you view the full perspective of your role.

RELATING CONTINUING EDUCATION TO NURSING PRACTICE

The most meaningful extension of any form of nursing education—formal or continuing—is its influence on nursing practice. Saying you ascribe to this belief is very common. Meaning what you say may well be less prevalent. Putting into operation this conviction is a curiously rare event often viewed as a somewhat heroic venture that clearly extends above and beyond the call of educational duty.

Extending your role to the setting of nursing practice is not an infringement on territoriality. You need not fight for the right to be there; you have an obligation to be there. Nursing service and nursing administration would like to know where you are and why you are not there more often. Opponents of mandatory continuing education for relicensing nurses are there and would like to know how what you do makes a difference in patient care. An earlier generation of nurses would like to know why, all of a sudden, they have to attend your programs to retain their licenses. And a more recent generation of nurses is demanding your presence.

The legislation mandating continuing education for relicensing has opened a Pandora's box of accountability for providers of continuing education in nursing. No longer is it ludicrous to ask whether continuing education improves nursing practice, or whether continuing education makes a difference at all. The assumption, "Given a continuing education experience, the participant's practice of nursing will improve" is no longer dismissed as easily as the class.

The unification of nursing education and practice should be more than a contemporary buzzword of nursespeak, that rhetoric we feed one another so often and in such large portions. No one seems to question that continuing education

should improve patient care, but a growing number of nurses are questioning that it does. But since their separation a few decades ago, the disaffections between nursing education and nursing practice have grown to a point where it seems that visitation rights have to be legislated to reunite the two.

The expectations that continuing education should have a discernible effect on patient care are not unreasonable. Nor are the questions posed by these various groups of nurses. Unless some basis exists for knowing that continuing education makes a difference—an improvement—in nursing practice, then mandating continuing education for relicensing is a dubious process at best and a waste of a lot of time, money, and resources at worst.

Discussion of the pros and cons of mandatory continuing education for relicensing continues and likely will for some time. The issue at hand is not finding a culprit or scapegoat for this dilemma; the list of excuses is well known and generates no useful information for action. Rather, it would seem more productive at this point to identify the responsibility of providers of hospital-based continuing education in nursing and suggest some potential ways in which they may reconcile the parties involved.

If what you do every day has no discernible impact on nursing practice, it is time to reexamine what you are doing. The first issue to confront is why you are in an educator position at all. Providing for the educational needs of the critical care staff is your most immediate responsibility, but there is no point to it if the quality of practice is not simultaneously or ultimately enhanced.

Some things you can do at this point to better assure that continuing education has a measurable effect on nursing practice include the following:

1. Being available to staff nurses to follow through and reinforce previous learning
2. Organizing and sequencing programs so

that they lead to recognizable outcomes in practice

3. Involving staff nurses in critiquing selected nursing practices, procedures, and skills to identify ways to improve and validate them

4. Including a clinical practicum that complements any didactic learning experiences

5. Emphasizing transferring, integrating, and applying learning to the clinical setting rather than only evaluating cognitive abilities

6. Fostering a climate where reasoned inquiry and application of research findings are the norm

7. Assisting staff nurses to identify ways to verify and apply research findings in practice

8. Planning continuing education programs around a valid and comprehensive learning needs assessment derived in large part from staff nurses

9. Suggesting that release for staff nurses' attendance at continuing education programs be dependent on their attendant responsibility to share the program's information with peers and to translate it into changes in practice

10. Participating in establishing, revising, or implementing pre-established standards of critical care nursing practices in your agency

11. Pursuing your own continuing education and experience to maintain clinical skills and currency in practice

12. Initiating or facilitating practice-oriented clinical research studies

13. Experimenting with developing tools to evaluate clinical performance based on patient outcomes and standards of nursing practice

14. Reexamining instructional objectives and revising them as necessary so that they emphasize relevance to nursing practice

15. Calculating where most of your time is spent in allocating the majority of that time to the clinical setting

16. Participating in quality assurance programs in critical care and in follow-through from the results

17. Soliciting staff nurses' suggestions about how continuing education may be made more meaningful to nursing practice

18. Arranging for evaluation of continuing education programs for the units, including head nurse and staff nurse critiques

19. Suggesting to nursing administrators that university faculty be brought in to practice, conduct research, and participate in a more collaborative role with nursing practitioners

The issues confronting hospital-based nurse educators have national dimensions. To see only what is before you is short-sighted. The paucity of data to substantiate the effect of continuing education on nursing practice should not deter you from attempting to generate such information. Knowing the issues confronting continuing education in nursing and keeping informed of their bearing on nursing practice and the role of clinical educators is a necessary responsibility. This can be done by participating in efforts to substantiate the quality of continuing education and its influence on nursing practice, and by guiding others in the pursuit of quality continuing education with the potential to improve practice. Remembering why you do all of these things is the most important element of all.

REFERENCES

The status of continuing education in nursing

American Association of Critical-Care Nurses: Position paper on continuing education in critical care nursing, Heart Lung 6:935, 1977.

Brault, GL, and Pflaum, SS: Planning and development of a masters degree program in critical care, Heart Lung 8:933, 1979.

Cantor, M: The roles and responsibilities of continuing education in nursing, J Contin Educ Nurs 8:16, 1977.

Cantor, M: Staff development: what about the CEU? J Nurs Admin 4:8, 1974.

Clark, KM, and Dickinson, G: Self-directed and other-directed continuing education: a study of nurses' participation, J Contin Educ Nurs 7:16, 1976.

Cooper, SS: A brief history of continuing education in nursing in the United States, J Contin Educ Nurs 4:5, 1973.

Cooper, SS: Continuing education: yesterday and today, Nurs Educ 3:25, 1978.

Cooper, SS: Trends in continuing education in the United States, Intern Nurs Rev 22:117, 1975.

Edelstein, RRG, and Bunnell, M: Determinants of continuing nursing education, J Contin Educ Nurs 9:19, 1978.

France, J: The implementation of mandatory continuing education through planning. In National League for Nursing: Implementation of continuing education in nursing, New York, 1978, National League for Nursing.

Matthews, AE, and Schumacher, S: A survey of registered nurses' conceptions of and participation factors in professional continuing education, J Contin Educ Nurs 10:21, 1979.

Mundinger, M: CE: current contradictions in inservice, Nurs Admin Q 2:65, 1978.

National League for Nursing: Implementation of continuing education in nursing, New York, 1978, National League for Nursing.

O'Connor, AB: The continuing nurse learner: who and why, Nurs Educ 5:24, 1980.

Popiel, ES: Continuing education. In Williamson, JA, editor: Current perspectives in nursing education, vol 1, St. Louis, 1976, The C. V. Mosby Co.

Welch, D: The real issues behind providing continuing education in nursing, J Contin Educ Nurs 11:17, 1980.

Selecting among programs for continuing education in nursing

Curran, C: Let the buyer beware, J Contin Educ Nurs 9:11, 1978.

Deets, C, and Blume, D: Evaluating the effectiveness of selected continuing education offerings, J Contin Educ Nurs 8:63, 1977.

del Bueno, DJ: How to get your money's worth out of continuing education, RN 41:37, 1978.

Gaston, S: Nursing faculty evaluation of continuing education offerings in nursing, J Contin Educ Nurs 11:10, 1980.

Hochman, G: Continuing education: how can you make the most of it? Nurs 78 8:81, 1978.

O'Conner, AB: Diagnosing your needs for continuing education, Am J Nurs 78:405, 1978.

O'Neal, EA: Maximize the return on your investment, J Contin Educ Nurs 9:21, 1978.

The impact of continuing education on nursing practice

Cantor, M: Education for quality care, J Nurs Admin 3:49, 1973.

Cantor, M: Staff development: what about the CEU? J Nurs Admin 4:8, 1974.

Cox, CL, and Baker, MG: Evaluation: the key to accountability in continuing education, J Contin Educ Nurs 12:11, 1981.

del Bueno, DJ: The effect of continuing education on on-the-job behavior, Proceedings of the National Conference, Kansas City, 1976, American Nurses' Association.

del Bueno, DJ: Viewpoint: CE: treatment for outdatedness, Nurs Admin Q 2:59, 1978.

Forni, PR, and Overman, RT: Does continuing education have an effect on the practice of nursing? J Contin Educ Nurs 5:44, 1974.

Griffin, JK: Perspectives and Concerns on Continuing Education. In National League for Nursing: Implementation of continuing education in nursing, New York, 1978, National League for Nursing.

Konefal, MM: continuing education pays off in the care of high risk infants, J Contin Educ Nurs 8:22, 1977.

Levine, ME: Does continuing education improve nursing practice? Hospitals 52:138, 1978.

Puetz, BE, and Rytting, MB: Evaluation of the effect of continuing education in nursing on health care, J Contin Educ Nurs 10:22, 1979.

Rufo, KL: Guidelines for inservice education for registered nurses, J Contin Educ Nurs 12:26, 1981.

Schlotfeldt, RM: Continuing education: no proof of competency, AORN J 22:770, 1975.

Stetler, CB, and Marram, G: Evaluating research findings for applicability in practice, Nurs Outlook 24:559, 1976.

Valencius, J: Impact of a continuing education program in cancer nursing, part I: results affecting patient care, J Contin Educ Nurs 11:14, 1980.

Wolanin, MO: Continuing educational approval committee works toward evaluation of nurse outcomes, J Contin Educ Nurs 10:31, 1979.

APPENDIXES

Appendix A

Critical care nurse training program
content syllabus

I. PSYCHOSOCIAL COMPONENT

Topic	Participant objectives	Teaching method	Instructional media	Method of evaluation
Introduction to critical care nursing	A. Given the AACN definition, define critical care nursing in terms of its essential elements:		Handouts Program goal, objectives, participant objectives.	Informally group and individual discussions and conferences
	1. Holistic, open systems approach 2. Acutely ill target population 3. Using nursing process 4. Professional accountability for practice 5. Collaborative, team effort 6. Need for continuing education	Lecture Discussion	American Association of Critical-Care Nurses position papers on critical care nursing theory for professional nursing and scope of practice.	Formally Clinical skills inventory
	B. To specify the distinguishing features of critical care nursing practice:			

	1. To describe the role of the critical care nurse
	2. To identify the distinguishing features of critical care nursing:
	  a. Knowledge required
	  b. Number and kind of skills required
		Group discussion
		Group discussion
			Programs
			Hospital policies for ICU, CCU, PCU.
			Readings
			Hudak, CM, Gallo, BM, and Lohr, T.: Critical care nursing, chapters 1, 3.
			Meltzer, LE, Abdellah, FG, and Kitchell, JR: Concepts and practices of intensive care for nurse specialists.
				Team conference

	c. Degree of illness of patients
	  d. Complexity of care required
	  e. Degree of collaboration required
	  f. Level and frequency of independent decision making required
	  g. Nature and amount of equipment used
	  h. Nature and stress of work situation
		Lecture
		Discussion
			Whipple, GH, et al: Acute coronary care, Chapters 7, 8.	

Continued.

I. PSYCHOSOCIAL COMPONENT—cont'd

Topic	Participant objectives	Teaching method	Instructional media	Method of evaluation
Introduction to critical care nursing—cont'd	3. To identify the distinguishing features of patients appropriately admitted to critical care units: a. Level and type of care required b. Life support, monitoring equipment, and techniques required c. Salvageability	Lecture Discussion	Benoliel, JD, and Van De Velde, S: As the patient views the intensive care unit and the coronary care unit.	Group and individual clinical conferences
	C. To describe the primary features of various types of critical care units: 1. Critical care units as part of the hospital social system a. Hospitals as social systems b. Members of critical care team 2. Critical care units: their purposes, philosophies, primary features a. critical care units (in general) b. Coronary care unit c. Intensive care unit d. Progressive and intermediate care unit e. Emergency room and trauma center 3. Physical characteristics of critical care areas a. Physical design b. Equipment	Lecture Discussion Discussion Discussion Clinical tour of facilities		Clinical conference Team conference
	D. Given a summary of its historical evolution, identify the present developmental status of critical care nursing	Lecture Discussion		
■ **Orientation to the psychosocial component: an overview** A. Yourself and influencing factors B. The patient and influencing factors C. The family of the patient and influencing factors	To describe how the nurse's personality and demeanor influence her nursing practice. Describe social factors influencing the patient's response to illness. Describe how the family influences the patient's response to illness.	Lecture Group discussion	Handouts Michaels, DR: Too much in need of support to give any? Cassem, N: The nurse in the coronary care unit. Bilideau, CB: Nurses' reaction to critical care nursing.	Videotape
■ **The emotional impact of**	To describe nurse's emotional response to: 1. The critical care environment 2. Critical care nursing responsibilities 3. The critically ill patient 4. The family of the critically ill patient	Discussion Lecture Team conference	Pelletier, IO: Patients' predicament and nursing functions. Cassem, NH, and Hackett, TP: Stress on the nurse and therapist in the ICU and CCU.	Clinical conference Role-playing
■ **Stress: the tone of the critical care area** A. Effects of	To recognize the manifestations of stress and identify the effects of stress on all concerned in the critical care area	Lecture Discussion Critical incident		Clinical conference Interviews with patients and family members

Content	Objectives	Teaching method	Resources	Evaluation
B. Past experiences				
C. Potentially stressful situations in critical care areas				Simulated situation
■ An introduction to dealing with stress	To relate and apply principles of dealing with stress to themselves and to others	Lecture Inquiry Role-playing		Return demonstration Clinical conference Clinical performance
■ Previously conceived ideas and fantasies about critical care nursing	To differentiate between realistic and unrealistic expectations of critical care nursing	Inquiry Discussion Conex lab	Readings West, ND: Stresses associated with ICU's effect on patients, families and staff.	Clinical performance Essay item
■ The function of nursing (Orlando)	To define and describe the function of nursing service, using both conceptual and practical frameworks	Lecture	Lazarus, RS: Psychological stress and the coping process.	Clinical performance Written testing
■ Positive aspects of critical care nursing	To identify the positive aspects of critical care nursing			Clinical conference List of individual goals
Physiological effects of stress	A. To define "stress" as a stimulus and as a response: 1. To define "stress," "stressor," "stress response," "general adaptation syndrome (GAS)," "anxiety" 2. To interrelate the concepts of stress and the stress response	Lecture Discussion	Handouts AACN: Anxiety, FOCUS. Readings Kopin, IJ: Catecholamines, adrenal hormones, and stress. Robinson, AM: Stress can make you—or break you.	Short essay item True-False item
	B. To describe the different types of stress: physiological, psychological	Group discussion		Short essay item
	C. To identify the major functions of the central nervous system's neurobiological defense systems activated with stress: 1. Limbic system 2. Hypothalamus 3. Reticular formation	Lecture		Completion item
	D. To differentiate between the hormonal responses involved in the "fight or flight" stress response and those involved in the "conserve-withdraw" stress response	Lecture		Multiple-choice item
	E. To identify the potential clinical problems or complications associated with the patient's response to stress	Case study		Case study
	F. To describe appropriate nursing interventions aimed at minimizing the adverse responses to stress	Case study		Case study
■ Maxim: All behavior has meaning	To describe own reactions to the critical care environment	Lecture	Handouts Williams, F: The crisis of hospitalization.	

Continued.

I. PSYCHOSOCIAL COMPONENT—cont'd

Physiological effects of stress—cont'd

Topic	Participant objectives	Teaching method	Instructional media	Method of evaluation
■ Adaptive reactions to stress seen in nursing personnel A. Identification of usual coping mechanisms B. Resources available	Describe own adaptive responses to stress from past experiences	Small sharing groups Conex lab	Janken, JK: The nurse in crisis. Versteeg, RI: If I could hold your hand.	Clinical conference
■ An existential perspective on critical care nursing: the need for openness in the process of becoming	To list own strengths and weaknesses as beginning critical care nurses	Group discussion	Kornfeld, DS, et al: Psychological hazards of the ICU.	Self evaluation list
■ Potential problems (occupational hazards) common to critical care nursing	To state two problem areas on which they are working to improve abilities to cope with stress and describe the plan created for improvement. Identify resources available when encountering occupational hazards	Discussion Role-playing	Readings Hay, D, and O'Ken, D: The psychological stress of ICU nursing.	Written assignment
A. Feelings of fear, anger, depression B. Scape goating and death-watching C. Competition among staff vs cooperation			Holscow, PR: Nursing in high emotional risk areas.	Team conference
D. Feeling "new" E. Authority struggles with doctors	To identify ways of adapting to new job To recognize how to manage conflicts	Role-playing Role-playing		Team conference
F. Vulnerability when caring for people with irreversable health problems	To identify adaptive coping mechanisms	Simulated situation		
■ Some qualities helpful for critical care nurses to develop	To demonstrate some degree of trust and openness with peers and colleagues.	Conex lab		Clinical performance Observation
■ Critically ill patients' reactions to stress, and common attempts to cope with stress A. Coronary care patients:	To identify common reactions to stress associated with hospitalization	Lecture Case presentations	Handouts Royle, J: Coronary patients and their families receive incomplete care. Gould, EP: The emotional effects of surgical illness. Pranulis, M: Coping with an acute M.I., In Gentry, WD, and Williams, RB, editors: Psychological aspects of myocardial infarction and coronary care.	
1. Type A and B personality stereotypes	1. To differentiate between stereotypes of type A and B personalities	Simulated situation		Written testing
2. Post-MI behavioral syndromes	2. To predict behavior patterns common in post-MI patients	Group discussion	Readings Benson, H: the relaxation response.	Written testing

Content	Objectives	Learning Experiences	References	Evaluation
3. Coping mechanisms used	3. To identify the coping mechanisms of specific post-MI patients, and evaluate their effectiveness	Team conference		Clinical performance
4. Criteria for assessing the adequacy of patient's coping mechanisms	4. To distinguish between adaptive and maladaptive coping mechanisms	Team conference		Clinical conference
5. Suggestions for nursing interventions	5. To deal with the behavior of specific post-MI patients, and evaluate their effectiveness		Gentry, WD, and Williams, RB, editors: Psychological aspects.	Clinical conference
■ Behavioral effects of pathophysiological alterations involving:	To describe the usual emotional effects of common cardiovascular, pulmonary, neurological, renal, and metabolic diseases	Lecture; Group discussion		Written testing; Multiple-choice item
A. Cardiovascular disease	A. To describe emotional response to an MI	Team conferences	Kieley, W: Critical care psychiatric syndrome.	Team conference
B. Pulmonary disease	B. To identify coping methods of COPD patients		Scalzi, C: Nursing management of behavioral responses following an acute MI.	
C. Nervous system disease	C. To describe emotional responses to spinal cord injuries			
D. Renal disease	D. To describe psychosocial responses to need for chronic hemodialysis or insulin therapy			
E. Metabolic disease				
■ Nursing interventions that are usually helpful to patients suffering emotional reactions to critical illness	To relate and apply principles of psychological assessment and comfort when caring for patients with critical illness	Lecture; Case presentation	Roberts, SL: Behavioral concepts and the critically ill patient.	Clinical performance
■ Pain				
A. Influencing factors	A. To assess accurately factors contributing toward an individual patient's pain level and tolerance	Lecture; Discussion		Completion item; Clinical conference
B. Helping the patient minimize pain 1. Relaxation exercises 2. Therapeutic use of placebos	B. To use two methods of helping a patient work toward minimizing pain	Multiple assignment		
■ Maxim: We respond to whatever is going on around us	To identify environmental forces affecting critical care patients	Use of tape recording of bedside sounds in the ICU	Handouts Miller, J: Cognitive dissonance in modifying families' perceptions.	
■ The effects of personalized and depersonalized care on patients	To differentiate between personalized and depersonalized approaches to care	Simulated situation	Foster, S, and Andreoli, K: Behavior following an acute M.I.	Clinical conference
■ Suggestions for personalizing and humanizing critical nursing care	To apply principles of personalized nursing care in at least one situation	Role-playing; Performance checklist	Griffin, J: Family decision . . . a crucial factor in terminating life.	Clinical performance

Continued.

I. PSYCHOSOCIAL COMPONENT—cont'd

Topic	Participant objectives	Teaching method	Instructional media	Method of evaluation
Physiological effects of stress— cont'd				
■ Assessing behavior in critical care	To assess the following in one patient or family member: behavior; emotional level; response to the environment	Multiple assignment	Maron, L, et al: Toward a unified approach to psychological factors in the ICU.	Written interview with one patient or family member
■ Assessing emotional levels in critical care	To assess the following in one patient or family member: behavior; emotional level; response to the environment	Multiple assignment	Storlie, F: Double entendre in a CCU.	Written interview with one patient or family member
■ Assessing the patients' response to the critical care environment (to include sensory deprivation and overload and sleep deprivation)	To assess the following in one patient or family member: behavior; emotional level; response to the environment	Multiple assignment		Written inverview with one patient or family member
■ Recommendations for improving the patient's environment	To plan and implement therapeutic interventions for one patient experiencing sensory overload	Simulated patient	Readings Martin, AW, and Prange, AJ: Human adaptations: a conceptual approach to understanding patients. Maslow, AH: Toward a psychology of being.	Written plan of care on kardex Clinical performance
■ The emotional impact of an atmosphere of competency vs incompetency as reflected in nurses	To assess patient's feeling of security or insecurity	Multiple assignment		Clinical conference
■ Behaviors of family members frequently seen in critical care areas	To identify behaviors that may indicate anxiety, anger, helplessness, hopelessness	Incident process		Written testing
■ Nursing responsibilities toward the families of patients in a critical care unit	To plan and implement therapeutic interventions for the family of one patient	Multiple assignment		Clinical performance Observation
■ Ways to accomplish the work of nursing comprehensively		Role-playing Lecture	Handouts Benoliel, JQ, and Van De Velde, S: As the patient views the intensive care unit and the coronary care unit.	
A. Organizing the work of the nurse: the nursing process	To use the components of the nursing process with at least a minimum degree of competency			Written nursing assessment

268

Content	Objectives	Teaching methods	Readings/Resources	Evaluation
B. A tool to assist with the assessment phase: the disciplined nursing process (Orlando)			Readings Orlando, IJ: The dynamic nurse-patient relationship, G.P. Putnam's Sons. Orlando, IJ: The discipline and teaching of nursing process, G.P. Putnam's Sons.	Formulate a nursing care plan Clinical conferences to evaluate the effectiveness of planned interventions
■ Practicum on effective assessment and intervention	To demonstrate own disciplined nursing process, using the principles of Ida Orlando, and to describe at least a beginning level of familiarity with own process	Role-playing Discussion Analysis of interactions Process recording		Review of process recordings
A. Role reversal: acting out an immediate need for help				
B. Using the assessment tool in role plays and planning intervention		Role-play of silent lady pacing		Written testing
		Short role-plays "Nurse, where have you been?" "Get out of my room . . . you're giving me another heart attack!" "Difficult patient."		Role-playing Role-playing
	To demonstrate how effectively to manage the "difficult patient"			Role-playing
■ Human body image	To explain the derivation of human body image	Lecture	Slide presentation of patient's facial expressions depicting Lee's 4 phases.	Essay item
■ Body image changes A. Lee's phases of alteration in body image B. The emotional effects of body image changes	To list the four usual phases people experience when body image is altered	Case presentation	Handouts Tierney, E: Accepting disfigurement when death is the alternative. Sanopietro, MC: Meeting the emotional needs of hemodialysis patients and their spouses. D'Afflitti, J, and Swanson, D: Group sessions for the wives of home-hemodialysis patients.	Completion item
■ Nursing interventions when caring for patients experiencing body image changes	To state and apply two principles underlying nursing interventions in caring for patient's experiencing recent body image changes	Lecture Discussion		

Continued.

269

I. PSYCHOSOCIAL COMPONENT—cont'd

Topic	Participant objectives	Teaching method	Instructional media	Method of evaluation
Physiological effects of stress— cont'd			Readings Wylie, RC: The self concept. Murray, R: Symposium on the concepts of body image. Gallagher, AM: Body image changes in the patient with a colostomy.	Essay item Clinical performance Observation
■ Addictive personalities A. Characteristics	To identify two characteristics of addictive personalities	Lecture	Handouts Lewis, LW: The hidden alcoholic: a nursing dilemma. Nursing grand rounds: Confronting alcoholism.	Completion item
■ Nursing care of patients recovering from ingestion of toxic levels of drugs (including alcohol) A. Behavior during acute withdrawl phase B. Nursing interventions that may be helpful	To formulate and implement a plan of nursing care for an individual withdrawing from a drug	Case presentation Bedside rounds	Readings Heinemann, E, and Estes, N: Assessing alcoholic patients	Clinical conference
■ Family reactions to addicts	To provide support to family members of a patient with an addiction problem during initial phase of withdrawal	Case presentation Role-modeling	Reed, SW: Assessing the patient with an alcohol problem.	Clinical performance
■ Middle age identity and adjustments	To list the developmental tasks of middle age and identify how acute illness may affect these	Lecture Case study	Handouts Reading Die Kelmann, N, and Galloway, K: The middle years: a time of change.	Completion item
■ Old age identity and adjustments	To list the developmental tasks of old age	Lecture		Completion item
■ Crisis intervention	To describe the crises that can occur with illness	Lecture Discussion	Mazzola, R, and Jacobs, GB: Helping the patient and family deal with a crisis situation.	Written testing Clinical performance
A. Principles	A. To state the principles of crisis intervention			

Content	Objective	Teaching/Learning Activity	Readings/Handouts	Evaluation
B. Practicum	B. To demonstrate the application of the principles of crisis intervention	Role-playing	Ryan, M: Helping the family cope with a cardiac arrest.	Role-playing
C. Role plays ■ Suicide as crisis			Handouts	
A. Factors seen with depression	A. To list three behaviors commonly seen in people who are depressed	Lecture Case presentation	His own executioner. Renshaw, DC: Suicide and depression in children.	Completion item
B. Previous experiences with suicidal persons	B. To list three behaviors commonly seen in people who are actively suicidal	Discussion		Written testing
C. The emotional impact of suicidal gestures and attempts	C. To predict usual behaviors often seen in persons who have attempted suicide and in those close to someone who has attempted suicide	Case study	Readings Dealing with rage.	Clinical conference
■ Crisis intervention as it relates to significant others involved with someone who has attempted suicide	To demonstrate the steps of crisis intervention when working with people close to one who has attempted suicide	Role-playing	Robischon, P: The challenge of crisis theory for nursing.	Simulated situation
■ Nursing care of alert persons who have attempted suicide	To prepare a general nursing care plan appropriate for most patients who have attempted suicide	Multiple assignment		Care plan criteria Multiple assignment
■ Feelings about death	To describe some of own thoughts and feelings about death	Poster-making Discussion of posters	Handouts	Ability to illustrate and speak about some aspect of death
■ The phenomenon of dying	To describe various feelings involved in the dying process, as described in the literature (to include the research done on near-death experiences)	Lecture Discussion	Ross, EK: What is it like to be dying? Northrup, FC: The dying child. Lacasse, C: A dying adolescent.	Clinical conferences on dying patients
■ Nursing interventions that may be useful when working with alert people who are dying	To list three nursing interventions that are usually helpful to people who are dying	Team conference		Completion item
■ Bereavement	To describe two behaviors characteristically seen in people who have recently experienced bereavement	Team conference		Written testing
■ Nursing interventions useful when working with recently bereaved people	To list three nursing interventions that are useful when working with the loved ones of a patient who has died	Case presentation Team conference	Readings Moody, R: Life after life. Popoff, D: What are your feelings about death and dying?	Clinical performance Conference

Continued.

II. PULMONARY COMPONENT

Topic	Participant objectives	Teaching method	Instructional media	Method of evaluation
Physiological effects of stress—cont'd				
■ Functional anatomy of the respiratory system	To describe the primary functional characteristics of pulmonary anatomy as they relate to patient management	Lecture, group discussion	Slides Chalkboard Text Bushnell, SS: Respiratory intensive care nursing.	
	1. To identify the primary functions of major pulmonary structures and the clinical implications of bypassing each	Clinical instruction at bedside		Clinical conferences at bedside Written testing Clinical skills inventory
	2. To specify the clinical implications of key anatomical features of pulmonary structure	Group discussion	Handout Pulmonary anatomy. Chest films: malposition of ET tube in RMB.	
	3. To delineate the sequential layers traversed in respiratory gas diffusion	Lecture	Readings Bushnell, pp. 1-14. Turner, HG: The anatomy and physiology of normal respiration.	Written testing
	4. To compare and contrast the functional anatomy of pulmonary circulation and systemic circulation	Lecture		Matching item Completion item Nursing care plans
	5. To describe how the accessory muscles of respiration enhance the efficiency of ventilation	Bedside rounds		
■ Pulmonary physiology A. Ventilation	A. To describe pulmonary ventilation in terms of normal physiology, effect of pathophysiology, and clinical implications for nursing care:	Discussion Clinical instruction		

	1. To define:
	  a. Ventilation
	  b. Bulk flow
	  c. Pressure gradient
	  d. Compliance
		Lecture, discussion	Readings
			Bushnell, pp. 15-20.
			Secor, J: Ventilation: concepts essential to comprehensive nursing care.
				Written testing
				True-False item

	2. To describe the changes in atmospheric, intra-alveolar, and intrapleural pressures that occur during the inspiratory and expiratory phases of the respiratory cycle	Lecture	Slides	Multiple-choice item
	3. To identify the factors influencing intrapleural pressures during the respiratory cycle	Group discussion	Slides	Multiple-choice item
	4. To specify the relationship between pulmonary compliance and ventilation	Bedside rounds		Clinical conference
	5. To identify the factors influencing airway resistance	Lecture	Handouts Pulmonary volumes & capacities.	
	6. To define the pulmonary volumes and capacities and specify their normal adult values and abbreviations	Lecture	Symbols and abbreviations used by pulmonary physiologist.	Matching item

	7. To define and accurately calculate:
	  a. Minute ventilation
	  b. Dead space ventilation
	  c. Alveolar ventilation
		Demonstration
		Performance check-list
			Wright respirometer
			Respiratory therapy flow sheet
				Written and clinical testing worksheets

Content	Objectives	Learning activities	Resources	Evaluation
	8. To describe the relationship between alveolar ventilation and $PaCO_2$	Lecture, Written simulation	Slides	Multiple-choice item
	9. To identify the function of surfactant	Lecture, Cast study	Chalkboard	Multiple-choice item
B. Respiration	To describe respiration in terms of normal physiology, effects of pathophysiology, and clinical implications for nursing care	Lecture	Handout, Pulmonary physiology.	Written testing
	1. To define: a. External respiration b. Internal respiration c. diffusion d. Concentration gradient e. Pressure gradient f. Partial pressure g. Solubility of a gas	Lecture		Completion item
	2. To explain the physiology of external and internal respiration in terms of the relative pressure gradients of the respiratory gases	Lecture, Discussion	Chalkboard, Slides	True-false item
	3. To describe how the efficiency of respiration can be evaluated clinically	Role modeling, Examing charts (lab-work), Patient assessment rounds	Charts, Selected patients	Clinical conference, Clinical skills inventory, Return demonstration
C. Transport of O_2 and CO_2 in blood	C. To describe the mechanism by which oxygen and carbon dioxide are transported in the bloodstream.	Lecture, Discussion	Handouts, Summary of partial pressures. Pulmonary physiology.	Written testing
	1. To define: a. PO_2 b. PCO_2 c. Percent saturation of hemoglobin d. Oxyhemoglobin dissociation curve e. 2-3 DPG f. Chloride shift	Lecture	Readings Bushnell, pp. 21-24. Vander, pp. 313-322.	Multiple-choice item
	2. To specify the relationship between arterial oxygen and carbon dioxide tensions and the amount of these gases carried in a dissolved state	Lecture, discussion	Slides and charts	Written testing
	3. To identify the combined forms in which most of the oxygen and carbon dioxide in the blood are transported	Lecture	Chalkboard, Filmstrip ABG's	Matching item
	4. To list the functions of the hemoglobin molecule with respect to respiratory gas transport	Lecture	Filmstrip ABG's	Completion item
	5. To explain the relationship between arterial oxygen tension and percent saturation of hemoglobin in terms of the oxyhemoglobin dissociation curve	ABG lab reports review, Case study	Slides	Clinical interpretation of ABG results—worksheets
	6. To identify the clinical advantages of sigmoid shape of the oxyhemoglobin dissociation curve	Lecture, discussion	Slides	Multiple-choice item
	7. To specify the effects of 2-3 DPG, pH, PCO_2, and temperature on the affinity of O_2 for the hemoglobin molecule	Lecture	Chart	Completion item
	8. To identify the effect of abnormal hemoglobin levels on oxygen transport	Written simulation	Selected patients	Clinical discussion: interpretation of hemoglobin levels
	9. To describe the function of carbonic anhydrase in relation to respiratory gas transport	Lecture, discussion	Chalkboard	Multiple-choice item

Continued.

273

II. PULMONARY COMPONENT—cont'd

Topic	Participant objectives	Teaching method	Instructional media	Method of evaluation
Physiological effects of stress— cont'd				
D. Pulmonary circulation	D. To describe the major features of pulmonary circulatory dynamics in relation to their clinical implications	Lecture, discussion Nursing care conference	Slides	Care conference
	1. To identify the principal structural elements of pulmonary circulation	Lecture	Reading Bushnell, pp. 20-21. Slides	Multiple-choice item
	2. To specify normal PAP, mean PAP, and PAWP	Lecture Bedside rounds	Slides	Clinical skills inventory
	3. To define physiological shunting (2% to 3%) capillary shunt)	Lecture	Filmstrip ABG's	Completion item
	4. To relate the reservoir function of the lungs to pulmonary ventilation and perfusion ratios with changes in body position and gravity	Clinical conferences Simulated patient		Beside rounds and clinical conference
	5. To explain the clinical effects of abnormal pulmonary capillay hydrostatic and colloidal pressures on pulmonary capillary fluid exchange	Lecture Peer participatory conference	Chalkboard Slides Selected patients Handout Pulmonary edema of cardiac origin.	Multiple-choice item
E. Regulation of ventilation	E. To describe the physiological mechanisms involved in the production of normal and abnormal patterns of ventilation	Lecture, discussion Clinical instruction, discussion	Reading Bushnell, pp. 29-32.	Multiple-choice item Clinical conference
	1. To specify the anatomical location and functions of the following respiratory centers: a. Inspiratory center b. Expiratory center c. Apneustic center d. Pneumotaxic center e. Chemoreceptors (medullary, carotid, aortic arch, pulmonary arteriolar, bronchiolar) f. Stretch receptors	Lecture Physical simulation (model)	Transparencies Cerebral model	Written testing Clinical conference Matching item
	2. To describe the role of pH, PCO_2, and PO_2 in the regulation of ventilation	Lecture, discussion Nursing care conference	Slides	Multiple-choice item Clinical conference
	3. To explain the clinical significance of the Hering-Breuer reflex	Written simulation		True-false item
	4. To identify the primary (normal) stimulus to ventilation	Lecture	Selected patients having pulmonary obstructive defects.	Treu-false item
	5. To describe the local pulmonary mechanisms available for matching ventilation to perfusion	Lecture	Filmstrip ABG's	True-false item
	6. To define: a. Shunting b. Physiological dead space	Lecture	Filmstrip ABG's	True-false item
F. Physiology of acid-base balance	F. To recognize and interpret acid-base imbalances in terms of their underlying pathophysiology and ciinical implications	Lecture, discussion Preceptor reinforcement	Slides, chalkboard Readings (physiology of ABG's) Bushnell, pp. 24-26, 170-185.	Written testing Clinical conference Worksheets
	1. To define the following terms: a. Acid b. Base			

Continued.

275

II. PULMONARY COMPONENT—cont'd

Topic	Participant objectives	Teaching method	Instructional media	Method of evaluation
Physiological effects of stress—cont'd	10. To differentiate between the following acid-base abnormalities: a. "Compensated" and "uncompensated" b. "Compensated" and "corrected"	Lecture Practice sheets for interpreting Bedside rounds		Multiple-choice item Review of practice sheets
	11. To identify the signs and symptoms of the four major acid-base disturbances 12. To recognize the clinical implications of the four major acid-base disturbances	Lecture, discussion Clinical preceptor Class discussion Simulated situation	Reading (ABG's clinical implications) Lee, CA, et al: What to do when acid-base problems hang in the balance.	Clinical conference Written testing Clinical conference Written testing
	13. To demonstrate the procedure for obtaining arterial blood gas samples	Performance check-list Physical simulation (arm model) Demonstration	Handouts Procedure for drawing blood for arterial blood gas analysis. Arterial blood gas drawing. Equipment for ABG drawing.	Clinical conference Return demonstration Clinical skills
■ Clinical assessment of the pulmonary system	To formulate a valid clinical assessment of the pulmonary system	Performance checklist Role model's demonstration	Readings Bates, pp, 25-27, 73-78. Broughton, JO: Chest physical diagnosis for nurses and respiratory therapists. Sedlock, SA: Detection of chronic pulmonary disease. Traver, GA: Assessment of the thorax and lungs.	Performance checklist
A. Process of physical assessment	A. To describe the purpose of the four major components of physical assessment	Lecture, discussion Reinforcement in clinical area Bedside rounds	Chalkboard Slides	Written testing Return demonstration in clinical area
	1. To identify the data that may be obtained from each major component of physical assessment		Selected patients	Return demonstration in clinical area
	2. To demonstrate the technique of each component of physical assessment	Performance checklist Simulated patient	Selected patients	Performance checklist Rating scale
B. Health history of pulmonary system	B. To obtain a patient's respiratory health history	Lecture, discussion Clinical role model Role-playing	Handout Example of respiratory assessment tool.	Clinical demonstration of ability
	1. To specify the most pertinent parameters to assess in obtaining a health history of the respiratory system	Lecture, discussion Nursing care conference	Chalkboard	Multiple-choice item
	2. To produce a written record of a patient's respiratory health history	Demonstration Simulated patient	Nursing notes form	Clinical demonstration of ability: rating scale

Objective	Learning activities	Resources	Evaluation
3. To interpret how the patient's respiratory history relates to present respiratory status	Discussion	Markerboard	Clinical conference
4. To identify the most common presenting symptoms of pulmonary disease	Multiple assignment		Multiple-choice item
5. To differentiate between pleuritic chest pain and cardiac chest pain	Lecture, discussion; Simulated patient		Multiple-choice item
C. Inspection C. To perform satisfactorily a clinical assessment of the pulmonary system by inspecting the patient	Clinical role model; Performance checklist	Selected patients	Clinical demonstration of ability: performance checklist
1. To identify the parameters most relevant to inspecting the patient's pulmonary status	Lecture, discussion; Clinical reinforcement	Slides	Written testing; Clinical demonstration: clinical rating scale
2. To interpret appropriately and discuss normal and abnormal findings of inspection	Bedside rounds	A-V; Slides; Examination of the lungs and thorax (filmstrip and cassette).	
3. To differentiate between the appearance and clinical implications of central and peripheral cyanosis	Simulated situations; Bedside rounds	Chalkboard; Slides; Reading; Roberts, SL. Skin assessment for color and temperature.	Direct observation
4. To describe the additional functional benefits derived from using the accessory muscles of respiration	Lecture, discussion; Case study		Completion item; Clinical conference
5. To identify the distinguishing physical features of clubbing	Lecture, discussion; Preceptor demonstration		Written testing
D. Palpation D. To perform satisfactorily clinical assessment of the pulmonary system by palpating the chest	Clinical role model; Performance checklist	Selected patients; Filmstrip	Clinical demonstration of ability: checklist
1. To determine accurately whether tactile fremitus is present, absent, increased, or decreased.	Performance checklist	Selected patients; Filmstrip	Checklist
2. To specify the conditions under which tactile fremitus may be increased or decreased.	Lecture, discussion	Chalkboard	Multiple-choice item
3. To define and interpret the clinical significance of crepitance	Nursing care conference		
E. Percussion E. To perform satisfactorily clinical assessment of the pulmonary system by percussing the chest	Clinical instruction and role model; Performance checklist	Filmstrip	Clinical demonstration of ability: checklist
1. To recognize a description of the proper technique for percussion	Lecture; Clinical demonstration	Handouts; Percussion technique.	Written testing
2. To identify the chest surface locations representative of the five underlying lobes of the lungs	Performance checklist	Lobes of the lungs.	Clinical demonstration
3. To identify the five percussion notes and clinical significance of each	Bedside rounds; Clinical instruction	Selected patients	Matching item
F. Auscultation F. To perform satisfactorily clinical assessment of the pulmonary system by auscultating the chest	Clinical instruction and role model; Performance checklist	Selected patients; Stethoscope	Clinical demonstration
1. To indicate the rationale for auscultating breath sounds, stating examples	Lecture, discussion	Filmstrip, audiotape	Completion item

Continued.

Topic	Participant objectives	Teaching method	Instructional media	Method of evaluation
Physiological effects of stress— cont'd	2. To specify appropriate use of the stethoscope for auscultating breath sounds	Clinical instruction and demonstration Simulated patient	Reading Littmann, D: Stethoscopes and auscultation.	Return demonstration in clinical area
	3. To demonstrate a systematic approach to auscultation of breath sounds	Performance checklist	Filmstrip	
	4. To describe how the two components of breath sounds are produced	Lecture, discussion		Written testing
	5. To identify the location, characteristics, and schematic diagram of the four normal breath sounds	Lecture, discussion Clinical reinforcement	Selected patients Slides	Completion item
	6. To classify and relate the clinical significance of five abnormal breath sounds	Lecture, discussion Clinical rounds	Handout Pulmonary lobes.	Matching item Clinical conference
	7. To compare and contrast the auscultatory characteristics and clinical significance of fine, medium, and coarse rales	Lecture, discussion Clinical instruction	Tape Breath sounds.	Written testing Clinical demonstration of ability
	8. To differentiate between atelectatic and crepitant rales in terms of how to identify each and in terms of their respective clinical significance	Lecture, discussion Clinical rounds	Selected patients	Written testing Clinical demonstration of ability
	9. To identify the clinical implications of the two types of musical rales	Lecture, discussion Care conference		Written testing
	10. To differentiate between pleural and pericardial friction rubs	Lecture, discussion Tape simulations	Chalkboard	Written testing Clinical conference
	11. To identify the category and clinical significance of abnormally transmitted voice sounds	Lecture, discussion Clinical rounds	Chalkboard Tape Breath sounds.	Clinical conference
	12. To chart appropriately the findings made during auscultation of breath sounds	Clinical guidance and role model demonstration	Nursing notes form	Clinical demonstration of ability: rating scale
■ **Patients with pulmonary system dysfunction**	To demonstrate the knowledge and ability required for managing nursing care of patients with pulmonary system dysfunction based on a valid data base and rationale for care	Lecture, discussion Clinical instruction and demonstration	Selected patients Slides	Written testing Clinical demonstration of ability: performance checklists
A. Patients with acute respiratory failure (ARF) 1. Pathogenesis	A. To describe the rationale and provide for nursing management of the patient with ARF as determined by the: 1. Various pathophysiological processes involved in the pathogenesis of acute respiratory failure			
	a. To define respiratory failure in terms of its current clinical definition	Lecture, discussion Clinical conferences Lecture Clinical reinforcement	Readings (pathogenesis & pathophysiology) Bushnell, pp. 33-43. Seriff, NS, Khan, F, and Lazo, BJ: Acute respiratory failure: current concepts of pathophysiology and management.	Multiple-choice item Individual clinical conferences
	b. To recognize the potential clinical situations in which ARF may be precipitated	Group discussion		Individual clinical conferences
	c. To identify the most frequent cause of ARF	Lecture, discussion Clinical conferences		Multiple-choice item
	d. To deduce the common etiological factor present in all conditions that may lead to ARF	Lecture, discussion		Multiple-choice item
2. Pathophysiology	2. Common underlying pathophysiological features of the diverse causes responsible for producing ARF	Lecture, discussion Clinical reinforcement	See readings of previous section	

Objectives	Methods	Resources	Evaluation
a. To specify concisely how the major pathophysiological causes of ARF ultimately produce alveolar hypoventilation and hypoxemia	Bedside rounds; Brief case studies	Programmed instruction; ARF	Written testing; Individual clinical conferences
b. To identify the primary pathophysiological processes involved in ARF	Lecture, discussion	Selected patients	Written testing; Clinical conference
c. To describe the fundamental physiological defect present in ARF	Lecture, discussion	Chalkboard; Slides	Multiple-choice item
d. To identify the hallmarks of ARF	Lecture	Handout	Multiple-choice item
e. To define: (1) Regional ventilation (2) Closing volume (3) Shunting (venous admixture) (4) V/Q mismatching (5) Hypercapnia	Lecture, discussion	Shunting phenomena.	Completion item
3. Clinical assessment			
3. Clinical and laboratory evaluation of the patient with ARF			
a. To list the most important assessment parameters to be evaluated in a patient with ARF	Lecture, discussion; Bedside rounds	Refer to previous sections on Pulmonary physiology; Pulmonary circulation; Physiology of acid-base balance; Clinical assessment of the pulmonary system	Written testing; Clinical evaluation of performance; Written testing
b. To specify the single most valid determinant of the presence of ARF	Lecture		
c. To identify the clinical signs and symptoms of ARF in relation to the major pathophysiological defects	Lecture, discussion; Nursing care conference	Chalkboard	Written testing; Clinical correlation
d. To interpret the findings of clinical assessment in terms of their relevance to patient care	Lecture, discussion; Team conference	Reading Sitzman, J: Respiratory problems and the nurse's changing responsibilities.	Team conference
4. Clinical problems			
4. Priority of clinical problems associated with ARF		Readings Bushnell, pp. 193-216. Nett, LM, and Petty, TL: Acute respiratory failure: principles of care.	
a. From the clinical evaluation of the patient in ARF, to list the anticipated clinical problems	Lecture, discussion; Case presentation	Chalkboard	Completion item; Clinical demonstration of ability
b. To describe how the complications of ARF would potentially alter the priority of clinical problems	Case presentation	Chalkboard; Patient care plans (kardex)	Written testing with clinical examples; Review of written care plans
c. To explain how one could recognize and verify the existence of selected clinical problems and complications of ARF	Lecture, discussion; Clinical instruction	Selected patients	Clinical demonstration of ability; Written testing; Clinical conference
d. To specify the objectives of care for nursing management of the patient in ARF	Multiple assignment	Patient care plans (kardex)	Review of written care plans

Continued.

II. PULMONARY COMPONENT—cont'd

Topic	Participant objectives	Teaching method	Instructional media	Method of evaluation
Physiological effects of stress—cont'd				
5. Modes of therapy	5. Currently available modes of therapy for the patient in ARF		Reading Seriff, NS, Khan, F, and Lazo, BJ: Acute respiratory failure.	
a. Airway patency	a. To describe the rationale and techniques of alternative modes of care aimed at providing a patent airway	Lecture, discussion Clinical instruction		
(1) Suctioning	(1) Suctioning			
	(a) To perform correctly and effectively and to describe accurately the nursing responsibilities with tracheal suctioning	Clinical role model Class demonstration	Equipment necessary for suctioning Selected patients Reading Bushnell, pp. 197-199. Respiratory tract aspiration	Clinical demonstration of ability: checklist Written testing Clinical conference
	(b) To perform correctly and to describe the procedure for nasotracheal suctioning of secretions from nonintubated patients	Clinical role model Lecture with class demonstration	Equipment necessary for suctioning Selected patients	Clinical demonstration of ability: checklist Written testing Clinical conference
	(c) To differentiate between the appropriate instructions to the patient for (nonintubated) nasotracheal suctioning and patient instructions when inserting an NG tube	Group discussion Role-playing		Clinical demonstration of appropriateness of patient instruction Written testing
	(d) To perform correctly and effectively and to describe accurately the nursing responsibilities in suctioning secretions from intubated patients	Lecture, discussion Clinical instruction Performance checklist	Selected patients	Clinical demonstration of ability: checklist Written testing
	(e) To explain the rationale and alternative technique for "preoxygenation" with intubated and nonintubated patients	Lecture, discussion Preceptor	Readings Demers, RR, and Saklad, M: Minimizing the harmful effects of mechanical aspiration.	Completion item Clinical conference
	(f) To summarize the features of a safe and effective suction catheter as a rationale for catheter selection	Lecture, discussion	Sackner, MA, et al: Pathogenesis and prevention of tracheobronchial damage with suction procedures.	Multiple-choice item
	(g) To recognize the potential complications of tracheal suctioning and their predisposing pathophysiological conditions	Lecture, discussion Clinical reinforcement during suctioning	Chalkboard Variety of suction catheters available for use Videocassette Hazards of suctioning.	Demonstrated ability to cite advantages and disadvantages of various suction catheters

	Objectives	Teaching methods	Resources	Evaluation
(h)	To specify nursing interventions designed to prevent each complication of suctioning	Discussion in class Role model	Readings Demers, RR, and Saklad, M: Minimizing the harmful effects. Jacquette, G: To reduce the hazards of tracheal suctioning.	Clinical demonstration of ability Simulated situation
(i)	To describe the rationale and technique for suctioning with an angled tip catheter rather than with a straight tip catheter	Preceptor		Rounds

(2) Artificial airways

	Objectives	Teaching methods	Resources	Evaluation
(a)	To identify the general indications for using artificial airways	Lecture, discussion	Bushnell, pp. 45-67, 203-207. Trout, C: Artificial airways: tubes and trachs.	Multiple-choice item Clinical conference
(b)	To compare and contrast the clinical indications for using the following types of airway adjuncts: [1] Oropharyngeal airway [2] Nasopharyngeal airway [3] Orotracheal tube [4] Nasotracheal tube [5] Esophageal obturator airway [6] Tracheostomy	Lecture, discussion Clinical reinforcement by preceptor	Chalkboard Transparencies Samples of airways to be considered	
(c)	To insert correctly and to describe the procedure for inserting oro- and nasopharyngeal airways	Clinical demonstration of techniques Discussion	Airways indicated Selected patients Intubation manikins	Clinical demonstration of ability: checklist Written testing Skill stations
(d)	To specify how to evaluate the presence and quality of the four airway reflexes	Lecture Performance checklist	Selected patients	Clinical demonstration of ability: checklist Written testing
(e)	To differentiate between the order in which the airway reflexes are lost and the order in which they recover	Lecture, discussion Case study	Slides	Multiple-choice item
(f)	To identify the general hazards associated with using artificial airways	Lecture, discussion Incident process	Chalkboard	Multiple-choice item
(g)	To compare and contrast the advantages and disadvantages of orotracheal and nasotracheal tubes	Lecture, discussion Written simulations	Chalkboard Selected patients	Written testing Individual clinical conferences
(h)	To compare and contrast the advantages and disadvantages of endotracheal tubes and tracheostomy	Lecture, discussion	Chalkboard Selected patients	Written testing Individual clinical conferences
(i)	To recognize the complications of endotracheal intubation and how each may be averted	Case study	Readings Demers, RR, and Saklad, M: Intratracheal inflatable cuffs: a review.	True-false item

(2) Artificial airways

Continued.

281

II. PULMONARY COMPONENT—cont'd

Topic	Participant objectives	Teaching method	Instructional media	Method of evaluation
Physiological effects of stress—cont'd	(j) To describe the rationale for high volume, low pressure endotracheal tube cuffs	Class discussion	Lawless, CA: Helping patients with endotracheal and tracheostomy tubes communicate.	Multiple-choice item
	(k) To identify normal tracheal wall venous and arterial pressures		Weber, B: Eating with a trach.	Completion item
	(l) To specify the advantages of the minimal occluding volume (minimal leak) technique over periodic deflation of endotracheal tube cuffs	Lecture, discussion; Clinical reinforcement	Trout.	Multiple-choice item
	(m) To list the distinct advantages of the esophageal obturator airway	Lecture	Stone, EW, and Zuckerman, S: The esophageal obturator airway.	Completion item
	(n) To describe and administer a clinically acceptable form of tracheostomy care, inclusive of dressing change	Clinical demonstration; Performance checklist	Selected patients	Clinical demonstration of ability: videotape
(3) Breathing exercises, chest physiotherapy, and postural drainage	(3) Breathing exercises, chest physiotherapy, and postural drainage			
	(a) To describe the rationale and techniques for breathing exercises, chest physiotherapy, and postural drainage in the patient with ARF	Lecture, discussion; Clinical laboratory	Readings; Bushnell, pp. 71-80. Selected patients	Written testing; Clinical demonstration of ability: checklist
	(b) To demonstrate and describe the technique of deep breathing exercises	Performance checklist	Chalkboard; Slides	Return demonstration
	(c) To define and state the rationale for cupping, clapping, and vibrating the chest	Lecture, discussion	Readings; Kurihara, M: Postural drainage, clapping and vibrating.	Written testing; Clinical conference
	(d) To identify the appropriate positioning for draining specific lung segments	Role model; Discussion	Ungvarski, P: Mechanical stimulation of coughing. Videocassette; Postural drainage.	
	(e) To specify the rationale and techniques of mechanically stimulated coughing		Videocassette	Written testing; Clinical demonstration of ability: checklist
b. Adequate ventilation and oxygenation	b. To perform and describe how various modes of therapy provide for adequate ventilation and oxygenation of the patient in ARF			
(1) Mechanical ventilation	(1) Mechanical ventilation		Mechanical ventilation.	

Objective	Method	Resources/Readings	Evaluation
(a) To enumerate the clinical indications for mechanical ventilation	Lecture, discussion Care conference	Readings Bushnell, pp. 111-131, 199-203.	Multiple-choice item Clinical conference
(b) To explain the meaning of the following abbreviations: [1] IPPB [2] PEEP [3] CPAP [4] IMV	Lecture, discussion	Chusid, EL, and Bryan, H: Application of ventilators in acute respiratory failure. Fitzgerald, LM: Mechanical ventilation.	Matching item
(c) To identify the relative contraindications for IPPB	Class discussion		True-false item
(d) To specify the side effects and complications of mechanical ventilation	Lecture, discussion	Handout IPPB: indications, hazards, contraindications.	Clinical conference Written testing
(e) To explain the physiological principles underlying using the iron lung or cuirass ventilator	Lecture		Multiple-choice item
(f) To specify how positive pressure ventilators are classified	Lecture Clinical reinforcement		Multiple-choice item
(g) To categorize various types of ventilators as volume or pressure cycled	Clinical instruction Lecture	Various types of ventilators available	Clinical demonstration of ability Written testing
(h) To list the advantages of volume-cycled ventilators over pressure-cycled ventilators	Class discussion Clinical reinforcement	Chalkboard Selected patients on ventilators	Multiple-choice item Clinical conference
(i) To define "sensitivity" in relation to mechanical ventilation	Lecture, discussion Clinical demonstration of setting changes	Use of sensitivity setting on Bird and MA-1 ventilators	Multiple-choice item
(j) To relate the functions of each setting on an MA-1 ventilator	Performance checklist	MA-1 ventilator	Clinical demonstration of ability: checklist Written testing
(k) To compare and contrast the uses and rationales for humidification and nebulization	Lecture, discussion	Humidifier Nebulizer Chalkboard	Written testing
(l) To indicate how ABGs and V_T are used in initial ventilator settings	Lecture Clinical reinforcement		Clinical conference Written testing
(m) PEEP and CPAP			
(a) PEEP and CPAP [1] To identify the clinical indications for instituting PEEP and CPAP	Case study	Readings Ashbaugh, DG, and Petty, TC: Positive end expiratory pressure.	Multiple-choice item
[2] To specify the potential clinical complications of PEEP and CPAP and how to prevent these	Care conference		True-false item Clinical conference
[3] To demonstrate appropriate responses to ventilator alarms	Performance checklist		Clinical demonstration of ability: checklist Written testing

Continued.

II. PULMONARY COMPONENT—cont'd

Topic	Participant objectives	Teaching method	Instructional media	Method of evaluation
Physiological effects of stress— cont'd				
(b) Weaning	(n) Weaning			
	[1] To recognize the clinical indications for discontinuation of mechanical ventilation	Lecture, discussion	Bushnell, pp. 135-138. Downs, JB, et al: Intermittent mandatory ventilation: a new approach to weaning patients from mechanical ventilators.	Clinical conference
	[2] To compare and contrast the advantages and disadvantages of conventional weaning techniques and IMV technique	Class discussion Clinical reinforcement	Fitzgerald, LM: Weaning the patient from mechanical ventilation.	Written testing
	[3] To describe nursing responsibilities during a patient's weaning from mechanical ventilation	Class discussion Clinical reinforcement Case study		Clinical conference Essay item
	[4] To interpret accurately how well a patient is tolerating the weaning procedure and to indicate appropriate interventions for complications	Lecture, discussion Clinical instruction	Selected patients being weaned	Written testing Clinical demonstration of ability: checklist
(2) O₂ therapy	(2) O₂ therapy			
	(a) To enumerate the general indications for O₂ therapy	Lecture, discussion	Reading Bushnell, pp. 83-94.	True-false item
	(b) To identify the physical signs of O₂ need	Class discussion Clinical reinforcement		Clinical conference Written testing
	(c) To recognize the primary features and rationale for using various O₂ therapy devices	Lecture, discussion Bedside rounds	Chalkboard Variety of available O₂ therapy equipment Venti-masks Retard valves Selected patients	Written testing Clinical conference
	(d) To differentiate between using O₂ therapy for patients with and without COPD and describe the rationale for this distinction	Lecture, discussion		True-false item Case presentations
(a) O₂ toxicity	(e) O₂ toxicity			
	[1] To recognize the types of clinical situations in which O₂ toxicity is likely to develop	Lecture, class discussion Clinical conference Lecture	Reading Nett, L, and Petty, TI: Oxygen toxicity.	True-false item
	[2] To describe the pathophysiology of O₂ toxicity			Written testing
	[3] To identify the clinical indicators of O₂ toxicity	Lecture Case presentation	Chalkboard	Clinical conference Multiple-choice item
(b) Drug therapy	(f) To describe the indications, pharmacology, side effects, and therapeutic effects of the major classes of drugs used in respiratory therapy, citing a specific example of each	Lecture, discussion Clinical instruction	Selected patients receiving respiratory drugs Readings Bushnell, pp. 106-109, 129.	Matching item

284

Continued.

Content	Objective	Teaching methods	Resources	Evaluation
c. Monitoring and support of other systems; prevention of complications	c. To describe how to monitor other pertinent parameters, support patients' and families' psychological adaption, and prevent or minimize secondary complications	Class discussion	Pierson, DJ: Respiratory stimulants: review of the literature and assessment of current status. **Bushnell, pp. 193-216.**	Clinical conference / Essay item
B. Patients with adult respiratory distress syndrome (ARDS)	B. To describe the rationale and provide for nursing management of the patient with ARDS as determined by the:	Lecture, discussion / Clinical instruction	Nursing care plan (kardex)	Review of kardex
1. Pathogenesis	1. Spectrum of clinical situations and precipitating factors implicated in the pathogenesis of ARDS	Lecture, discussion	Readings / Cook, WA: Shock lung: etiology, prevention and treatment.	
	a. To identify the patient population at risk for developing ARDS	Team conference	Gracey, DR: Adult respiratory distress syndrome.	Written testing / Clinical conference
	b. To summarize the primary factors that precipitate the development of ARDS	Lecture	Petty, TL, and Ashbaugh, DG: Adult respiratory distress syndrome: clinical features, factors influencing prognosis and principles of management.	Written testing
	c. To recognize which types of ICU and ER patients are most predisposed to develop ARDS	Class discussion / Clinical reinforcement		Clinical conference / Written testing
2. Pathophysiology	2. Various theories proposed for the pathophysiology of ARDS			
	a. To classify the wide spectrum of the etiology of ARDS into major categories of associated clinical situations	Lecture, discussion	Slide-tape program on ARDS	Multiple-choice item
	b. To distinguish the major pulmonary lesions associated with ARDS	Lecture / Clinical reinforcement / Class discussion	Chalkboard / Slides	Written testing
	c. To indicate the result of surfactant loss in ARDS	Lecture		Multiple-choice item
	d. To discuss the rationale for the alternative characterizations of ARDS: (1) "Shock lung" (2) "Wet lung syndrome" (3) "Stiff lung syndrome" (4) "Noncardiac pulmonary edema"	Class discussion	Slides	Written testing
3. Clinical assessment	3. Clinical and laboratory evaluation of the patient with ARDS			
	a. To identify the clinical indicators of ARDS	Lecture	See readings above	True-false item / Clinical conference
	b. To recognize associated signs and symptoms of ARDS	Lecture / Case study		Written testing
	c. To calculate the ABG values anticipated in a patient with ARDS	Bedside rounds	Charts	Clinical conference / Simulated situations

II. PULMONARY COMPONENT—cont'd

Topic	Participant objectives	Teaching method	Instructional media	Method of evaluation
Physiological effects of stress—cont'd				
4. Clinical problems	d. To explain why refractoriness to usual ventilatory supports is characteristic of patients with ARDS	Bedside rounds		Essay item
	Priority of clinical problems associated with ARDS			
	a. To list the anticipated clinical problems of a patient with ARDS from data supplied by actual or theoretical clinical and laboratory evaluation of the patient	Discussion Lecture	Selected patients for case study Nursing care plans (kardex)	Group review of homework assignment Written testing
	b. To rank the anticipated clinical problems in order of their immediacy of treatment	Class discussion	Chalkboard	Review of assignment Written testing
	c. To describe how to verify and re-evaluate selected clinical problems and complications of ARDS	Lecture Clinical instruction	Selected patients	Clinical demonstration of ability Written testing
	d. To explain why complications of PEEP and CPAP are particular problems for the patient with ARDS	Class discussion	Chalkboard	Completion item
	e. From the priority list of clinical problems in ARDS, formulate a priority of objectives of care for nursing management of these patients	Multiple assignment	Nursing care plans (kardex)	Review of care plan objectives
5. Modes of therapy	Currently available modes of therapy for the patient having ARDS		See readings above	
	a. To compare and contrast the treatment regime for ARDS and ARF	Lecture, class discussion Clinical conference	Slides	Written testing
	b. To specify appropriate nursing management aimed at preventing further pulmonary damage for patients with ARDS	Lecture, discussion Clinical conference	Simulated patients	Clinical conference Completion item
C. Patients with chronic obstructive pulmonary disease (COPD)	C. To describe appropriately and provide for nursing management of patients with COPD as determined by the:			
1. Pathogenesis	1. Various forms and etiological factors involved in the pathogenesis of COPD			
	a. To distinguish among the clinical forms of COPD: (1) Bronchitis (2) Bronchiectasis (3) Asthma (4) Emphysema	Lecture, discussion Clinical reinforcement	Slides and tape on COPD Chalkboard Selected patients	Matching item Clinical conference
	b. To rank the precipitating or etiological factors of COPD according to their frequency of occurrence in these patients	Class discussion	Markerboard	Written testing Clinical conference

Content	Objectives	Teaching methods	Resources	Evaluation
	c. To identify the role of serum alpha, antitrypsin deficiency in COPD.	Lecture, discussion	COPD chart	Written testing
2. Pathophysiology	2. Pathophysiology of the various forms and precipitating circumstances involved in COPD			
	a. To summarize the major pathophysiological features of: (1) Bronchitis (2) Bronchiectasis (3) Asthma (4) Emphysema	Lecture, discussion	Handout Emphysema. Reading Fuhs, MF, and Stein, AM: Better ways to cope with COPD.	Written testing
	b. To differentiate between centrilobular and panlobular emphysema	Lecture, discussion	Slides and COPD tape	Matching item
	c. To define "air-trapping"	Class discussion	Chalkboard	Multiple-choice item
	d. To differentiate between obstructive and restrictive pulmonary lesions	Lecture	Transparencies	Clinical conference
	e. To identify the clinical significance of bullae formation in emphysema	Lecture	Chalkboard	Clinical conference
	f. To summarize the common pathophysiologic features in all types of COPD	Team conference		Completion item
3. Clinical assessment	3. Clinical and laboratory evaluation of the patient with COPD			
	a. To identify the primary and secondary signs of COPD	Lecture, discussion Bedside rounds	Readings Sedlock, SA: Detection of chronic pulmonary disease.	Written testing Clinical conference
	b. To describe how to verify clinically the presence of COPD	Class discussion Clinical demonstration		Clinical demonstration of ability
	c. To recognize typical ABG results for a patient with chronic COPD and for an acute phase of COPD	Bedside rounds	ABG practice results from selected patients Homework sheets on ABGs in COPD	Review of homework assignment
4. Clinical problems	4. Priority of clinical problems associated with COPD			
	a. To compare and contrast the priority of clinical problems of COPD and those of ARF	Group discussion	Reading Fuhs, MF, and Stein, AM: Better ways to cope with COPD.	Multiple-choice item

Continued.

II. PULMONARY COMPONENT—cont'd

Topic	Participant objectives	Teaching method	Instructional media	Method of evaluation
Physiological effects of stress—cont'd	b. To specify why mechanical ventilation, oxygen therapy, and PEEP become potential problems for the COPD patient	Class discussion Lecture Clinical reinforcement		
	c. To state the objectives of care for the COPD patient in order of importance	Kardex assignment	Nursing care plan (kardex)	Kardex
	d. To identify the signs, symptoms and clinical significance of CO₂ narcosis	Bedside rounds	Selected patients	Review of written objectives Clinical demonstration of ability
5. Modes of therapy	5. Currently available modes of therapy for the patient with COPD			
	a. To differentiate between how support of ventilation is managed with COPD patients and those with ARF	Lecture, discussion	Readings Lagerson, J: Nursing care of patients with chronic pulmonary insufficiency.	Written testing Clinical conference
	b. To identify the action, side effects, and rationale for drugs used by patients with COPD	Lecture, discussion Clinical reinforcement Peer participatory conference	Rodman, MJ: Drug therapy today.	Multiple-choice item
	c. To describe appropriate nursing interventions for managing the patients' and families' psychological adaptation to COPD		Dudley, DL, Wermuth, C: Aspects of care in the chronic obstructive pulmonary disease patient.	Clinical conference
D. Patients with pulmonary embolism	D. To describe the rationale and provide for nursing management of the patient with pulmonary embolism as determined by the:	Lecture, discussion Clinical preceptor		Written testing
1. Pathogenesis	1. Clinical situations and precipitating factors involved in the pathogenesis of pulmonary emboli		Baldwin, L: The problem of pulmonary embolism. Zschoche, pp. 158-162, 197-198.	
	a. To recognize which types of patients are most predisposed to pulmonary emboli	Lecture Class discussion Clinical reinforcement	Chalkboard Selected patients	Clinical conference True-false item
	b. To identify the most common etiological factor of pulmonary embolism	Class discussion	Blackboard	Multiple-choice item
	c. To list four precipitating factors of pulmonary embolism	Lecture Clinical instruction	Handout Pulmonary embolism. Chart	Clinical conference Completion item

2. Pathophysiology	2. Major pathophysiological features of pulmonary embolism			
	a. To differentiate between pulmonary embolism and pulmonary infarction	Lecture, discussion	Handouts Embolism and infarction. Pulmonary embolism.	Multiple-choice item
	b. To specify the pathophysiological features included in Virchow's Triad	Lecture, discussion	Readings Bloomfield, DA: Recognition and management of massive pulmonary embolism.	Multiple-choice item
	c. To describe two clinical situations that illustrate each of the three features in Virchow's Triad	Case presentations Clinical reinforcement Class discussion	Fitzmaurice, JB, and Sasahara, AA: Current concepts of pulmonary embolism: implications for nursing practice.	Multiple-choice item Clinical conference
	d. To differentiate among the clinical significance of the following: (1) Thrombophlebitis (2) Phlebothrombosis (3) Thromboembolism	Lecture, discussion	Transparencies	True-false item Clinical conference
	e. To identify the major pulmonary changes associated with pulmonary emboli	Lecture, discussion • Clinical reinforcement	Chalkboard Slides	Multiple-choice item
	f. To explain how intracardiac mural thrombi are formed and mobilized	Lecture, discussion Clinical reinforcement	Slides	Written testing Clinical conference Completion item
	g. To describe the causal relationship between pulmonary embolism and cor pulmonale	Lecture	Chalkboard Slides	
3. Clinical assessment	3. Clinical and laboratory evaluation of patient with pulmonary embolism			
	a. To characterize the general nature of signs, symptoms, and laboratory evaluation of patients with pulmonary embolism	Team conference	Readings Bloomfield. Fitzmaurice. Ryan, R: Thrombophlebitis assessment and prevention. Wyper, MA: Pulmonary embolism: fighting the silent killer.	Written testing

Continued.

Topic	Participant objectives	Teaching method	Instructional media	Method of evaluation
Physiological effects of stress—cont'd	b. To indicate what to expect to find for patients with acute pulmonary embolism in the following parameters: (1) ABGs (2) ECG (3) Type and character of pain (4) Respiratory pattern (5) Vital signs (6) PAWP, PAP, CVP (7) **Breath sounds** (8) **Heart sounds**	Lecture Class discussion Clinical instruction Multiple assignment	Chalkboard	Clinical conference Multiple-choice item Review of assignments
	c. To list the most common presenting findings of patients with pulmonary embolism	Lecture, discussion	Chalkboard	Completion item
	d. To identify the nursing responsibilities associated with lung scans and pulmonary angiography, in addition to stating the value of each test	Class discussion Lecture Clinical reinforcement	Videocassette Pulmonary arteriography.	Clinical conference Written testing
4. Clinical problems	4. Priority of clinical problems associated with acute pulmonary embolism			
	a. From the anticipated clinical problems identified above, formulate and rank order the priority of clinical problems to be anticipated for a patient with acute pulmonary embolism	Multiple assignment	Nursing care plans (kardex) Homework sheet	Review of assignments Written testing
	b. To describe how to detect the development of complications that patients with pulmonary embolism may develop	Class discussion Lecture Clinical instruction	Chalkboard Stethoscope	Clinical conference Written testing
	c. To explain how anticoagulant therapy influences the priority of clinical problems for the patient with acute pulmonary embolism	Class discussion Clinical instruction	Selected patients	Written testing Clinical conference
	d. To specify the objectives of care for nursing management of the patient with acute pulmonary embolism	Multiple assignment	Nursing care plans (kardex)	Review of written objectives Written testing
5. Modes of therapy	5. Currently available modes of therapy for the patient with acute pulmonary embolism	Lecture Class discussion Clinical reinforcement	Readings Bloomfield. Daly, CR, and Kelley, EA: Prevention of pulmonary embolism: intracaval devices. Fitzmaurice. Genton, E: Therapeutic aspects of pulmonary embolism.	Multiple-choice item
	a. From the stated objectives of care, to identify the rationale for using the following in managing patients with pulmonary embolism: (1) Heparin (2) Streptokinase, Urokinase (3) ASA, Persantin			

| | | | Written testing |
| | | | Clinical conference |

Content	Teaching Method	Resources	Evaluation Method
b. To specify the clinical circumstances under which vena caval and intracaval umbrella insertion would be warranted	Class discussion Case study		Written testing Clinical conference
c. To delineate the advantages of the intracaval umbrella over other caval interruption procedures in treating pulmonary embolism	Lecture Class discussion	Picture of intracaval umbrella (see Daly.)	Clinical conference Written testing
d. To recognize pharmacological agents that interfere with the action of warfarin	Lecture		True-false item
e. To identify appropriate patient education areas that require teaching for the patient and family before discharge from the hospital	Class discussion Case presentation by student	Selected patients	Clinical conference Review of case presentation Written testing Multiple-choice item
f. To describe the rationale for low dose heparin therapy in thrombosis prophylaxis	Lecture Discussion		
E. Patients with status asthmaticus			
E. To describe the rationale for nursing management of patients with status asthmaticus as determined by the:			
1. Pathogenesis		Handout Status asthmaticus.	
1. Variety of pathological, psychological, and environmental factors implicated in the pathogenesis of acute asthmatic episodes			
a. To identify the primary, secondary, and environmental stimuli responsible for asthmatic attacks	Lecture Class discussion Clinical instruction	Readings Moody, LE: Nursing care of patients with asthma.	Clinical conference Written testing
b. To classify the etiological or precipitating factors in asthma as preventable or nonpreventable	Class discussion	Segal, MS, and Weiss, EB: Current concepts in the management of the patient with status asthmaticus.	Written testing Clinical conference
c. To differentiate between extrinsic and intrinsic asthma, citing the incidence features of each	Lecture Discussion		Completion item
2. Pathophysiology			
2. Primary pathophysiological features involved in an acute, sustained asthmatic episode			
a. To define status asthmaticus according to its relationship to bronchial asthma	Lecture, discussion Clinical reinforcement	Bocles, C: Status asthmaticus.	Multiple-choice item
b. To specify the two main pathological features of status asthmaticus	Class discussion Clinical reinforcement	Moody, LE: Asthma: physiology and patient care.	Clinical conference Written testing
c. To recognize the pathological feature of asthma that is responsible for most of the clinical sequelae observed	Class discussion		Clinical conference
d. To describe the role of chemical mediators in the allergic pathophysiology of asthma, giving examples of mediators	Lecture	Handout Bronchial asthma.	Written testing
e. To identify the major pathophysiological events that occur during an acute asthmatic episode	Lecture, discussion	Slides	Written testing Clinical conference

Continued.

291

II. PULMONARY COMPONENT—cont'd

Physiological effects of stress— cont'd

Topic	Participant objectives	Teaching method	Instructional media	Method of evaluation
3. Clinical assessment	3. Clinical and laboratory evaluation of the patient with status asthmaticus			
	a. To delineate the anticipated patient history of symptoms and their duration before hospitalization	Class discussion Clinical rounds	Reading Moody.	Written testing
	b. To list the presenting signs and symptoms to expect to find in a patient newly admitted for status asthmaticus	Class discussion Case presentation	Chalkboard Selected patients	Clinical conference Written testing Simulated patient
	c. To explain the pathophysiological features responsible for producing the abnormal breath sounds characteristic of asthma	Lecture, discussion Clinical rounds	Chalkboard Selected patients	Clinical evaluation of ability to correlate Written testing
	d. To explain why to expect dehydration to be present in a patient with status asthmaticus	Class discussion Clinical reinforcement	Chalkboard	Essay item
	e. To use ABG results of an asthmatic patient to designate which of four sequential stages of asthma a patient is in	Clinical reinforcement Lecture Class discussion in small groups	Reading Bocles.	Clinical demonstration of ability Written testing Review of group findings
	f. To differentiate between "initial" and "late" symptomatology in an asthmatic episode	Case study	Chalkboard	Multiple-choice item
4. Clinical problems	4. Priority of clinical problems associated with status asthmaticus			
	a. To list the anticipated clinical problems of the patient with status asthmaticus from the clinical findings	Class discussion Lecture Clinical reinforcement	Programmed instruction	Written testing Clinical conference
	b. To rank the clinical problems of status asthmaticus according to their clinical priority	Clinical reinforcement	Nursing care plans (kardex)	Review of written problem lists Written testing Case study
	c. To correlate the clinical problems of status asthmaticus with the appropriate pathophysiological cause	Lecture, discussion Clinical instruction	Chalkboard	Written testing
	d. To identify the potential complications of status asthmaticus and the explanation for their possible occurrence	Lecture, discussion Clinical reinforcement	Chalkboard	
	e. From the priority of clinical problems listed for the patient with status asthmaticus, formulate a complementary listing of the objectives of care for nursing management of the patient	Clinical instruction Multiple assignment	Selected patients Nursing care plans (kardex)	Review of care plans
5. Modes of therapy	5. Currently available modes of therapy for the patient with status asthmaticus	Class discussion Lecture Clinical reinforcement	Readings Dewey, J: 18 ways to live with asthma.	Clinical conference Written testing
	a. To specify the rationale for the administration of aminophylline as the initial drug of choice in status asthmaticus			

Content	Teaching methods	Resources	Evaluation methods
b. To explain epinephrine resistance in patients with status asthmaticus and the agent used to offset it	Lecture, discussion	Spencer, R: Helping your asthmatic patient to breathe.	Clinical conference Multiple-choice item
c. To identify the rationale for corticosteroids in patients with status asthmaticus	Class discussion	Handout Pharmacology of drugs used in critical care-pulmonary diseases: asthma.	Multiple-choice item Review of care plans
d. To compare and contrast oxygen therapy for a patient with status asthmaticus as it is affected by a chronic and acute patient history	Lecture, discussion Clinical instruction Case presentation	Chalkboard Selected patients	Written testing Clinical conference Review of therapy and patients
e. To recognize the side effects, toxic effects, and contraindications of drugs used for patients with status asthmaticus	Lecture Class discussion Clinical instruction		Clinical review True-false item
f. To outline areas in need of predischarge teaching for the asthmatic patient and the family	Class discussion Clinical reinforcement		Clinical conference Completion item
g. To identify the types of medications the asthmatic patient should avoid taking	Class discussion		Clinical conference Multiple-choice item
F. Patients with acute thoracic trauma 1. Pathogenesis To describe the rationale for nursing management of patients with acute thoracic trauma as determined by the: 1. Various categories and types of acute thoracic trauma	Lecture	Readings Alspach, J: Chest trauma. Bushnell, pp. 247-255.	
a. To identify the two major categories of chest trauma and the general types of injury each causes	Lecture Class discussion	McCormack, KA, and Birnbaum, ML: Acute ventilatory failure following thoracic trauma.	Multiple-choice item
b. To specify the four primary types of chest trauma, giving an example of each 2. Pathophysiological features of the primary forms of acute thoracic trauma	Lecture	Slides	Written testing Clinical conference
2. Pathophysiology a. To describe how rib fractures may result in either pneumothorax or hemothorax	Lecture, discussion Case study	Chalkboard Slides Videocassette Chest trauma.	Clinical conference Written testing Clinical conference Multiple-choice item
b. To define the pathological features associated with: (1) Pneumomediastinum (2) Closed pneumothorax (3) Open pneumothorax (4) Tension pneumothorax (5) Hemothorax	Lecture, discussion Clinical instruction and reinforcement	Chalkboard Slides	

Continued.

II. PULMONARY COMPONENT—cont'd

Topic	Participant objectives	Teaching method	Instructional media	Method of evaluation
Physiological effects of stress— cont'd	c. To differentiate between the pathophysiology of a progressing closed pneumothorax and a tension pneumothorax	Lecture Class discussion	Chalkboard Slides	True-false item
	d. To specify the cardiovascular effects of a mediastinal shift	Class discussion Lecture	Slides	Clinical conference Completion item
	e. To analyze how subcutaneous emphysema may be produced in chest trauma	Case study	Chalkboard	Written testing Patient rounds
	f. To identify the pathological sequelae of esophageal tears or ruptures	Lecture Class discussion	Slides	Multiple-choice item
	g. To describe the progressive features of pneumothorax produced by penetrating thoracic trauma	Lecture Class discussion	Slides	Written testing
	h. To clinically define "simple pneumothorax" and "pulmonary contusion"	Lecture Clinical reinforcement		Clinical conference True-false item
	i. To differentiate among "minimal," "moderate," and "massive" hemothorax	Lecture		Clinical conference Multiple-choice item
	j. To describe the anticipated types of pathological conditions associated with "dashboard injuries"	Lecture, discussion	Videocassette	Completion item
3. Clinical assessment	Clinical and laboratory evaluation of a patient with acute thoracic trauma			
	a. To compare and contrast the types of respiratory chest wall motion associated with tension pneumothorax and flail chest	Lecture, discussion Clinical instruction	Handout Clinical features of chest wall injury which impair normal respiratory mechanics.	Clinical demonstration of ability to contrast Multiple-choice item
	b. To recognize which direction of tracheal displacement would be observed in various types of chest trauma	Class discussion Lecture	Slides	Clinical conference Written testing
	c. To explain the purpose and technique involved in the "plunger test" for tension pneumothorax	Class discussion Clinical demonstration	Equipment used for "plunger test" Chalkboard	Clinical conference Skill station—laboratory
	d. To identify the clinical significance of a Hamen's sign	Lecture	Slides Selected patient (if available)	Written testing
	e. To describe how to detect the presence of subcutaneous emphysema	Clinical rounds	Selected patient	Clinical demonstration of ability to detect: checklist
	f. To delineate the clinical parameters of primary importance in assessing a patient with possible esophageal laceration	Class discussion		Written testing
	g. To describe the alterations in assessment by palpation, percussion, and auscultation produced by various types of chest trauma	Lecture, discussion Clinical instruction	Reading Alspach, J. Chest trauma.	Written testing Clinical demonstration of ability to detect and describe alterations: rating scale

	Objectives	Teaching–learning methods	Resources	Evaluation
4. Clinical problems	**4. Priority of clinical problems associated with various types and degrees of thoracic trauma**			
	a. To compare and contrast the clinical problems associated with tension pneumothorax and flail chest.	Lecture Team conference Class discussion	Chalkboard	True-false item True-false item Clinical conference Clinical conference
	b. To identify the most frequent clinical problem associated with rib fractures	Lecture, discussion Clinical reinforcement	Slides Chalkboard	Matching item
	c. To recognize the primary clinical problems associated with hemothorax and pneumomediastinum	Lecture Written simulation	Slides Chalkboard	Multiple-choice item
	d. To differentiate between the clinical problems posed by tracheal or bronchial tear and esophageal laceration	Lecture, discussion	Reading Alspach, J: Chest trauma.	Multiple-choice item
	e. To specify the potential hemodynamic problem caused by subcutaneous emphysema	Lecture, discussion Clinical reinforcement		Multiple-choice item
	f. To identify the potential clinical problems associated with myocardial contusion	Class discussion		Clinical conference
	g. To formulate the objectives of care in nursing management of a patient with chest trauma	Multiple assignment	Nursing care plan (kardex)	Multiple-choice item
5. Modes of therapy	**5. Currently available modes of therapy for the patient having acute chest trauma**			
	a. To specify the degree of severity at which a chest tube is indicated for pneumothorax and hemothorax	Case study	Readings Bushnell, pp. 255-261. Morgan, CV, and Orcutt, TW: The care and feeding of chest tubes.	Multiple-choice item
	b. To differentiate between the rationale for inserting one or two chest tubes in a patient with chest trauma	Lecture Class discussion Clinical reinforcement	VanMeter, M: Chest tubes: basic techniques for better care.	Clinical conference True-false item
	c. To explain the rationale for administering antibiotics to a patient with esophageal rupture	Lecture, discussion	Alspach, J: Chest trauma.	Written testing
	d. To enumerate the problems that may follow taping the chest for fractured ribs	Class discussion	Chalkboard	Clinical conference Completion item
	e. To describe the nursing responsibilities during assistance with chest tube insertion, maintenance, and removal	Clinical instruction Clinical demonstration of techniques and procedures Lecture	Equipment required	Written testing Clinical return demonstration of abilities: rating scale
	f. To perform and explain the procedure and rationale for setting up waterseal drainage with and without suction	Clinical instruction and demonstration Performance checklist	Equipment for various chest tube drainage systems	Clinical return demonstration of ability to set up drainage systems: checklist Written testing
	g. To recognize the initial mode of therapy sought for a patient with flail chest	Class discussion Lecture		True-false item

Continued.

III. CARDIOVASCULAR COMPONENT

Topic	Participant objectives	Teaching method	Instructional media	Method of evaluation
Physiological effects of stress—cont'd				
■ Functional anatomy of the cardiovascular system	To describe the functional anatomy of the cardiovascular system as it relates to nursing management of patient care		Text Andreoli, KG, et al: Comprehensive cardiac care.	
	1. To identify the position of the heart within the thoracic cavity	Lecture, discussion Clinical reinforcement		Written testing Demonstration with model
	2. To specify the cardiac chambers and valves on each surface and border of the heart	Class discussion Lecture Clinical reinforcement	Readings Andreoli, pp. 1-7. Warner, HF, Russell, MN, and Spann, JF: Heart muscle: clinical applications of basic physiology and cellular anatomy.	Diagram labels
	3. To delineate the four layers of the heart and the primary function of each layer	Lecture, discussion		Matching item
	4. To relate the proposed functions of the pericardium	Class discussion		Written testing
	5. To describe each of four cardiac chambers in terms of its:	Lecture, discussion	Handouts Cardiac anatomy (myocardial, vascular).	Multiple-choice item
	a. General anatomical features b. Characteristics of contraction c. Inflow tract d. Outflow tract e. Normal pressure		AHA diagrams of cross-sectioned chambers and vasculature. AHA and CIBA slides AHA charts: 3 views of heart	
	6. To identify the function of the moderator band	Lecture, discussion	Slides	Multiple-choice item
	7. To characterize each cardiac chamber in terms of its pressure generation requirement and the resistance to its ejection	Class discussion Clinical reinforcement	Chalkboard	Written testing Clinical conference
	8. To compare and contrast the functional anatomy of atrioventricular valves and semilunar valves	Class discussion Lecture	Slides Chalkboard	Multiple-choice item
	9. To state the name, location, and function of each cardiac valve	Lecture, discussion Clinical reinforcement	Slides	Diagram labels
	10. To specify the anatomy, location, and functional significance of the sinuses of Valsalva	Lecture Class discussion	Handouts Coronary arterial circulation system: areas of distribution. Dominance or preponderance.	Multiple-choice item
	11. To identify the coronary arterial blood supply to any given area of the myocardium	Review of handout Clinical reinforcement with MI patients		Multiple-choice item Clinical conference

296

	Objective	Teaching activity	Resources	Evaluation
	12. To explain the concept of "dominance" ("preponderance") in relation to coronary circulation	Review of handout / Clinical reinforcement	Reading / Andreoli, pp. 3–4.	Short essay item
	13. To recognize the structures involved in draining venous cardiac blood to the right atrium	Lecture, discussion		Multiple-choice item
	14. To compare and contrast the coronary arterial distribution to all major portions of the cardiac conduction system	Review of handout / Class discussion / Clinical reinforcement	Handouts / Coronary arterial distribution to conduction system.	Multiple-choice item / Clinical conference review
	15. To identify the structure and course of all divisions and subdivisions of the cardiac conduction system	Review of handout / Class discussion	Basic anatomy of cardiac conduction.	Completion item
	16. To specify how pacemaking control, rate, and rhythm are determined	Lecture, discussion / Clinical reinforcement		Clinical conference. / Multiple-choice item / Written testing
	17. To recognize the type of tissue composing the conduction system structure	Lecture		
	18. To explain the anatomical basis of conduction delay in the A-V junction	Lecture, discussion / Clinical reinforcement	Slides / Chalkboard	Multiple-choice item
	19. To differentiate between the two segments of the Bundle of His	Review of handout		Multiple-choice item
	20. To compare and contrast the pathological vulnerability of the three ventricular fasicles	Class discussion		Clinical conference
	21. To compare and contrast the major structural and functional characteristics of systemic arteries, capillaries, and veins	Lecture, discussion		Matching item
	22. To label all arterial branches of the ascending aorta and aortic arch	Lecture	Chalkboard / Slides / AHA diagrams / Videocassette / Cardiac A and P.	Labelling of blank / AHA diagrams
■ Cardiovascular physiology	To correlate and apply principles of cardiovascular physiology to nursing management of patients with or without cardiovascular dysfunction			
	1. To describe the events involved in the three sequential steps of excitation–contraction coupling in cardiac muscle fibers	Lecture, discussion	Reading / Warner p. 1.	Essay item
	2. To specify the most important ions involved in muscle contraction and their primary function in this process	Class discussion / Lecture / Clinical reinforcement	Handout / Excitation–contraction.	Multiple-choice item / Clinical conference
	3. To trace the pathway of impulse conduction necessary for muscle contraction	Lecture, discussion	Readings / Katz, AM, and Brady, AJ: Mechanical and biochemical correlates of cardiac contraction. I and II.	
	4. To identify the clinical significance of Starling's law of the heart	Lecture, discussion / Clinical reinforcement		Clinical conference / Written testing
	5. To define the functional significance of the All or None principle in relation to cardiac muscle contraction	Class discussion		Multiple-choice item
	6. To recognize the factors that influence myocardial contractility	Lecture, discussion	Warner.	Clinical conference / Written testing
	7. To define and give examples of positive and negative inotropism, chronotropism, and dromotropism	Lecture, discussion	Chalkboard / Cardiac drug game	

Continued.

III. CARDIOVASCULAR COMPONENT—cont'd

Topic	Participant objectives	Teaching method	Instructional media	Method of evaluation
Physiological effects of stress— cont'd	8. To define the functional properties of cardiac muscle: a. Automaticity b. Conductivity c. Contractility d. Irritability e. Refractoriness	Lecture, discussion Clinical instruction (arrhythmia mechanisms)	Readings Andreoli, pp. 131-133. Fisch. Slides	Multiple-choice item Clinical conference
	9. To identify the clinical significance of the following in relation to venous return: a. Skeletal muscle pump b. Thoracoabdominal pump c. Respiratory cycle d. Venous valves e. Gravity f. IPPB, PEEP, and CPAP g. Cardiac systole	Class discussion Bedside rounds	Slides Chalkboard	Clinical conference Multiple-choice item
	10. To delineate the various mechanisms by which cardiac output may be augmented	Class discussion Clinical reinforcement	Slides Chalkboard	Essay item
	11. To describe the clinical significance of interfascicular tension	Class discussion	Chalkboard	Written testing
	12. To specify the location and results of stimulation of autonomic nervous system connections to the heart	Lecture, discussion Clinical instruction	Reading Andreoli, pp. 5-7. Slides	Written testing Clinical conference
	13. To explain and illustrate the concept of reciprocal innervation	Class discussion		Essay item
	14. To differentiate sympathetic and parasympathetic neurotransmitters with respect to their origin and resultants of release	Class discussion Lecture	Chalkboard	Completion item
	15. To describe autonomic nervous system innervation to systemic blood vessels	Lecture, discussion Clinical reinforcement		Written testing
	16. To identify the major resistance and capacitance vessels of the systemic circulation	Lecture	Chalkboard	Multiple-choice item
	17. To specify the location, functional significance, and limits of sensitivity of arterial baroreceptors and chemoreceptors	Lecture, discussion Clinical conference	Slides Chalkboard	Written testing Clinical conference
■ **Electrochemical physiology**	To use and apply the principles of electrochemical physiology to nursing management of patient care 1. To define: electrical a. Potential b. Voltage c. Current d. Polarity e. Permeability f. Na+ pump g. Polarized state h. Depolarization	Lecture, discussion	Readings Andreoli, pp. 87-91. Fisch. Surawicz, B: The input of cellular electrophysiology into the practice of clinical cardiography.	Matching item

Content	Objectives	Teaching methods	Resources/media	Evaluation
i. Repolarization j. Membrane potential k. Threshold potential l. Action potential				
	2. To list the major ions involved in creating cellular membrane potential and the extracellular vs intracellular distribution of each	Class discussion Lecture Clinical reinforcement	Slides	Written testing Clinical conference
	3. To identify the role of the Na+ pump in electrophysiology	Class discussion	Chalkboard	Multiple-choice item
	4. To describe the major ionic and electrical events associated with the four phases of an action potential	Lecture, discussion	Handout Action potential phases. Slides	True-false item
	5. To apply the concepts of excitability and automaticity to the generation of action potentials	Lecture, discussion Clinical instruction on application	Reading Fisch, C. Electrophysiologic basis of clinical arrhythmias.	Essay item Clinical conference
	6. To distinguish between the electrochemical characteristics and functional properties of pacemaking and nonpacemaking myocardial cells	Lecture, discussion Clinical reinforcement	Slides	True-false item
■ Clinical assessment of the cardiovascular system	To formulate a valid clinical assessment of the cardiovascular system	Performance checklist	Handout Clinical assessment of the cardiovascular system.	
A. Patient history	A. To obtain and record a pertinent history of a patient's cardiovascular health	Performance checklist	Samples of patient history formats presently used	Return demonstration of ability with written recording by participants
B. Inspection	B. To obtain and record a valid clinical assessment of a patient's cardiovascular status by means of inspection	Lecture, discussion Clinical instruction and demonstration	Assigned and selected patients or peers Readings Andreoli, chapter 3. Delaney, MT: Examining the chest. Winslow, EH: Visual inspection of the patient with cardiopulmonary disease.	Clinical demonstration of ability Performance checklist
	1. To enumerate the general and specific parameters that should be inspected to assess a patient's cardiovascular system	Class discussion Lecture Clinical reinforcement Written recording as assignment	Chalkboard A-V Initial segment of Examination of the thorax and lungs filmstrip.	Review of written recording of assessment Multiple-choice item Individual clinical conferences
	2. To correlate abnormal findings of inspection with their clinical interpretation and implications for care	Lecture, discussion Clinical rounds		

Continued.

299

III. CARDIOVASCULAR COMPONENT—cont'd

Topic	Participant objectives	Teaching method	Instructional media	Method of evaluation
Physiological effects of stress— cont'd	3. To differentiate between central and peripheral cyanosis in terms of clinical significance and areas involved	Class discussion	Readings Winslow, EH: Visual inspection.	Clinical discussion Multiple-choice item
	4. To define clubbing and describe how it is clinically recognized	Class discussion Clinical instruction	Delaney, MT: Examining the chest.	Completion item Clinical return demonstration of how to assess for
	5. To identify the funduscopic evidence of papilledema and its associated vascular findings	Lecture, discussion Clinical instruction Clinical laboratory sessions	CIBA slides Ophthalmoscope	Multiple-choice item
	6. To perform and describe the procedure for evaluating venous pressure by inspection	Lecture, discussion Clinical instruction and reinforcement Clinical laboratory sessions	Reading Winslow, EH: Visual inspection.	Clinical demonstration of ability Essay item
	7. To explain the clinical significance of cannon A waves and how they may be recognized	Class discussion		Written testing
	8. To identify clinically the seven areas of the chest that should be inspected for abnormal pulsations	Lecture, discussion Performance checklist	Assigned or selected patients or peers CIBA and Anderson slides A-V Anderson: An introduction to cardiac auscultation (slides and cassette).	Clinical demonstration of ability Written testing
	9. To specify the clinical significance of abnormal pulsations in each of the seven areas of inspection on the chest	Lecture, discussion Clinical rounds	CIBA and Anderson slides	Clinical discussion Multiple-choice item
	10. To define "precordial heave" and its clinical significance	Class discussion	Selected patients	Written testing Clinical discussion
	11. To locate angle of Louis on a patient's chest	Performance checklist		Clinical demonstration of ability
	12. To state what proportion of the normal population has a visible apical impulse	Class discussion	Readings Winslow, EH: Visual inspection.	Written testing
	13. To specify the anticipated clinical findings associated with inadequate peripheral circulation	Class discussion Clinical rounds	Roberts, B: The acutely ischemic limb.	Written testing Clinical discussion
	14. To identify the clinical significance of various types of facies observed in patients with cardiopulmonary disease	Class discussion Case conference	Winslow, EH: Visual inspection.	Multiple-choice item
	15. To specify the rationale for and techniques of taking PAPs and PAWPs	Clinical demonstration and practice in laboratory and patient areas Preceptor	Andreoli, pp. 79-82, 287-289. Bolognini, V: The Swan-Ganz pulmonary catheter: implications for nursing.	Clinical demonstration of ability Written testing

300

Content	Objectives	Learning experiences	Reading / Equipment for PAWP monitoring	Evaluation
	16. To demonstrate and describe how accurately to take PAP, PAWP, and CVP readings	Performance checklist	Reading Woods, SL: Monitoring pulmonary artery pressures.	Clinical demonstration of ability: checklist / Written testing
	17. To demonstrate and describe how to assemble the equipment necessary for central venous, pulmonary artery, and radial artery blood pressure monitoring	Clinical demonstration in laboratory; practice sessions in small groups	Selected patients / Necessary equipment / Reading Adams, NR: Reducing the perils of intracardiac monitoring.	Clinical demonstration of ability
	18. To specify the advantages of PAP and PAWP measurements over CVP measurements in managing the fluid balance of patients in left ventricular failure	Bedside rounds		Multiple-choice item
C. Palpation and percussion	To obtain and record a valid clinical assessment of a patient's cardiovascular status by means of palpation and percussion			
	1. To identify the seven chest and abdominal areas that should be palpated for abnormal pulsations and the lifts and normal findings at each area	Lecture, discussion / Clinical instruction and demonstration	Slides / Assigned or selected patients / A-V Anderson: An introduction to cardiac auscultation.	Clinical demonstration of ability: checklist / Written testing / Clinical conference
	2. To define: a. Thrills b. Lifts or heaves c. PMI	Class discussion / Clinical reinforcement		Written testing / Clinical discussion
	3. To specify the sites and methods of evaluating peripheral pulses	Clinical instruction and demonstration	Reading Sparks, C: Peripheral pulses.	Clinical demonstration of ability: rating scale
	4. To identify the normal findings of each peripheral arterial pulse site by means of a four-point rating scale	Class discussion / Clinical reinforcement		Clinical discussion
	5. To delineate the technique for eliciting a Homans' sign and state the clinical implications of a positive finding	Clinical demonstration	Selected or assigned patients	Clinical demonstration of ability / Multiple-choice item
	6. To describe how peripheral venous pressures may be evaluated and estimated	Clinical demonstration / Lecture, discussion	Assigned patients	Clinical demonstration of ability / Completion item
	7. To identify the normal characteristics of the PMI: size, location, timing, forcefulness	Class discussion / Clinical reinforcement	Assigned patients	Clinical demonstration of ability / True-false item
	8. To specify the clinical significance of abnormal findings related to the PMI	Bedside rounds	Chalkboard	Clinical conference / Multiple-choice item
D. Auscultation	To obtain and record a valid clinical assessment of a patient's cardiovascular status by means of auscultation			
	1. To relate the anatomical location of the heart valves to their respective areas of auscultation	Lecture, discussion / Preceptor	Readings Andreoli, pp. 34-45. / Lehman, J: Auscultation of heart sounds. / Littman, D: Stethoscopes and auscultation.	Clinical discussion / Matching item

Continued.

III. CARDIOVASCULAR COMPONENT—cont'd

Topic	Participant objectives	Teaching method	Instructional media	Method of evaluation
Physiological effects of stress— cont'd	2. To differentiate between the two major mechanisms producing heart sounds and the nature of the sounds they produce, citing examples of each	Lecture, discussion Clinical reinforcement	A-V Anderson: An introduction to cardiac auscultation.	Essay item
	3. To describe the four major aspects of heart sounds	Lecture	Slides	Written testing
	4. To relate appropriate use of stethoscopic headpieces with the mechanisms for producing heart sounds	Clinical instruction Class discussion	Videotape	Clinical conference Written testing
	5. To identify the features of a good quality stethoscope	Class discussion	Videotape Stethoscope	True-false item
	6. To differentiate between heart sounds proper and extra heart sounds, murmurs, and rubs	Lecture, discussion Clinical discussion	Selected patients	Clinical demonstration of ability Multiple-choice item
	7. To relate heart sounds to hemodynamic events in the cardiac cycle	Lecture, discussion Clinical reinforcement	CIBA slides	Clinical conference True-false item
	8. To demonstrate and describe a systematic approach to auscultating and evaluating heart sounds	Clinical demonstration Class discussion	Videotape Assigned patients	Clinical demonstration of ability: checklist
	9. To distinguish between normal and abnormal heart sounds	Performance checklist	Assigned or selected patients	Clinical demonstration of ability: rating scale Written testing
	10. To describe each heart sound (S$_{1-4}$) in terms of the following:	Lecture, discussion Clinical instruction and reinforcement	Reading Lehman, J: Auscultation.	Multiple-choice item Clinical demonstration of ability
	a. Hemodynamic events involved in its production	Bedside rounds	Anderson and CIBA slides	
	b. Its relationship to the cardiac cycle (systolic or diastolic)		Chalkboard	
	c. Its components			
	d. Where it may be best heard			
	e. Which head of stethoscope to use (bell or diaphragm)			
	f. Variations, clinical implications of abnormalities, or presence			
	11. To differentiate among the clinical significance of physiological, fixed, and paradoxical splitting of the second heart sound	Class discussion	Chalkboard Anderson slides	Matching item
	12. To define:	Lecture, discussion Clinical reinforcement	Chalkboard Videotape	Completion item Clinical conference
	a. Gallop sounds			
	b. Atrial gallop			
	c. Ventricular gallop			
	d. Summation gallop			
	13. To recognize and distinguish systolic and diastolic murmurs, citing examples of each	Class discussion Lecture Clinical reinforcement	Slides	Written testing Audiotapes
	14. To compare and delineate how pericardial friction rubs may be distinguished from pleural friction rubs	Clinical rounds	Chalkboard	Multiple-choice item
E. Diagnostic procedures	E. To identify the purpose, technique, potential complications, and nursing responsibilities related to the following diagnostic procedures:		CIBA slides Chalkboard Readings Andreoli, pp. 53-59. Kory, RC: Cardiac catheterization and related procedures.	

	Objectives	Teaching methods	Resources	Evaluation

1. Invasive
  a. Cardiac catheterization
  b. Coronary arteriography
2. Noninvasive
  a. Echocardiography
  b. Phonocardiography
  c. Stress testing
  d. Vectorcardiography
		Lecture
		Case study
			Coats, K. Non-invasive cardiac diagnostic procedures.	Simulated patients
				Role-playing

■ Electrocardiography A. General information	A. To demonstrate a satisfactory working knowledge of electrocardiographic monitoring and recording	Lecture Clinical instruction and demonstration		
	1. To specify the purpose of ECG monitoring	Preceptor	Andreoli, pp. 280-286.	Clinical conference
	2. To identify the major functions and appropriate use of each of the components of an ECG monitor	Clinical instruction	Andreoli, EK: The cardiac monitor. Meltzer, LE: Coronary care, electrocardiography and the nurse.	Clinical demonstration of ability: checklist Written testing
	3. To demonstrate how to set and adjust ECG monitor settings to varying patients' situations.	Class discussion Performance checklist	ECG monitor	Clinical demonstration of ability: checklist
1. ECG paper	a. To delineate the four major methods by which ECG recordings are standardized	Lecture, discussion Clinical reinforcement	Chalkboard AHA slides Handouts	Completion item Clinical discussions Multiple-choice item
	b. To identify the specific ECG standardizations for each method	Lecture, discussion	ECG paper, and P-Q-R-S-T Cycle.	
	c. From conventional standards of time and amplitude, to determine accurately a patient's heart rate and duration and amplitude of various ECG waves and intervals	Classroom practice Clinical instruction and demonstration	Heart rate. Practice rhythm strips for determining heart rate and rhythm.	Clinical and written demonstration of ability: checklist
	d. To compare and contrast how heart rates may be accurately determined from ECG recording based on regularity of heart rhythm	Class discussion Lecture Clinical demonstration	Rhythm strips of assigned and selected patients	Clinical demonstration of ability: checklist Written testing Clinical discussion
	e. To identify accurately how 12-lead ECG recordings are lead-coded in this hospital	Clinical instruction and demonstration	Handout Lead identification. 12-Lead ECG	Demonstrated ability to recognize specific leads
	f. To explain how an electrocardiograph transposes the electrical activity of the heart into a scalar ECG	Class discussion Lecture	Chalkboard Readings Andreoli readings under Cardiac monitor.	Clinical conference Multiple-choice item
	g. To demonstrate how to record correctly a 12-lead ECG	Performance checklist	Electrocardiograph Reading. Andreoli, pp. 297-298.	Clinical demonstration of ability: checklist

Continued.

III. CARDIOVASCULAR COMPONENT—cont'd

Topic	Participant objectives	Teaching method	Instructional media	Method of evaluation
Physiological effects of stress—cont'd				
2. Electrocardiographic deflections	h. To describe and differentiate the electrophysiological phenomena responsible for producing the following types of ECG deflections: (1) Isoelectric (2) Positive (3) Negative (4) Di- or biphasic (5) Equiphasic	Lecture ECG games	Handouts Basic definitions and laws of electrocardiography. Some definitions pertaining to electrocardiography. Chalkboard Slides Readings See Andreoli readings above.	Multiple-choice item Clinical discussion
B. Cardiac cycle	B. To correlate the electrophysiological and hemodynamic events occurring throughout the entire cardiac cycle with the various ECG waves, segments, and intervals	Lecture, discussion Clinical reinforcement	Handout P-Q-R-S-T cycle. Reading Andreoli, pp. 91-95, 101-103, 128-131.	Multiple-choice item Individual clinical conferences
	1. To demonstrate how to measure accurately the duration and amplitude of each ECG wave, interval, and segment.	Lecture, discussion Classroom practice Performance checklist	Handout Rhythm strips: practice. Slides	Clinical demonstration of ability: checklist Written testing Review of charting record
	2. To identify how each ECG wave, interval, and segment is defined in terms of its general characteristics, normal contour, amplitude, duration, and variations	Lecture, discussion Clinical reinforcement	Handout ECG: normal limits. Slides	Written testing Clinical conference
	3. To specify how correctly to identify, describe, and record normal and abnormal variations of ECG waves, intervals, segments	Lecture Clinical instruction	Slides	Clinical demonstration of ability: rating scale Written testing Review of nursing notes
C. ECG lead systems	C. To demonstrate a satisfactory working knowledge of various ECG lead systems	Performance checklist	Reading Andreoli, pp. 95-100.	Clinical demonstration of ability: rating scale
	1. To define: a. Electrode b. Lead c. Lead axis d. Artifact e. Einthoven's triangle f. Hexaxial reference system g. Vector h. Bipolar lead i. Unipolar lead j. Augmented lead k. Limb lead l. Precordial lead m. Frontal plane n. Horizontal plane	Lecture Class discussion	Handouts Some basic definitions and laws of electrocardiography. Definitions pertaining to electrocardiography. Lead identification. Standard positions for C or V leads.	True-false item Clinical conference
	2. To specify the causal relationship between cardiac vectors and ECG deflections	Lecture		True-false item

Objective	Methods	Resources	Evaluation
3. To differentiate between standard limb leads and augmented limb leads	Class discussion	Slides	Multiple-choice item
4. To differentiate between bipolar and unipolar leads	Class discussion	Slides	Clinical demonstration of ability
5. To identify the location of the negative and positive (or exploring) electrodes of the 12 ECG leads and the normal appearance of the P-Q-R-S-T cycle in each lead	Lecture / Performance checklist	Readings Andreoli articles in this section above.	Matching item
6. To relate the cardiac surfaces or areas represented by the standard ECG leads	Lecture, discussion	Handouts Normal 12 lead ECG. Areas/surfaces of the heart leads reflect.	Written testing / Clinical demonstration of ability
7. To compare and contrast ECG telemetry and hardwire monitoring		Readings Alspach, J: Electrical axis: how to recognize deviations on the ECG and interpret them. Beaumont, E: ECG telemetry.	
8. To describe the advantages of using leads MCL$_1$ and an esophageal lead for monitoring purposes	Lecture, discussion	Chalkboard Readings Marriott, HJL, and Fogg, E: Constant monitoring for cardiac dysrhythmias and blocks.	Clinical discussion / Multiple-choice item
D. Electrical axis			
To describe the clinical significance and method of determining electrical axis	Lecture, discussion / Clinical reinforcement	Alspach, J. Electrical axis.	Essay item / Clinical demonstration of ability
1. To delineate the three major references implied in determining electrical axis	Lecture	Andreoli, pp. 101-108. Schamroth, L: The electrical axis.	Written testing
2. To specify how the hexaxial reference system is demarcated for determining electrical axis	Lecture	Chalkboard CIBA slides	Diagram completion
3. To identify the normal sequence of ventricular depolarization in terms of the major vectoral shifts and directions	Lecture, discussion / Clinical reinforcement / Multiple-choice item	Chalkboard CIBA slides	Clinical discussion / Multiple-choice item
4. To describe a systematic method for clinically determining mean electrical axis	Homework practice	Handouts Determining electrical axis practice strips. Lead identification.	Clinical demonstration of ability: checklist / Review of practice sheets / Written testing / Clinical demonstration of ability with ECGs
5. To accurately plot and determine a patient's mean (QRS) electrical axis in degrees	Lecture, discussion / Classroom practice / Performance checklist		
6. To specify the parameters of normal electrical axis, right axis deviation, and left axis deviation	Lecture	ECG: normal limits.	Multiple-choice item
7. To identify clinical examples when axis deviations would be anticipated	Class discussion / Clinical rounds	Chalkboard Selected patients	Clinical conference / Case study
8. To identify the clinical significance of axis deviations	Class discussions	Chalkboard	Multiple-choice item / Clinical conference

Continued.

III. CARDIOVASCULAR COMPONENT—cont'd

Topic	Participant objectives	Teaching method	Instructional media	Method of evaluation
Physiological effects of stress—cont'd ■ Cardiac dysrhythmias A. Mechanisms	A. 1. To differentiate among the primary mechanisms responsible for producing cardiac dysrhythmias	Lecture, discussion Clinical instruction	Readings Andreoli, pp. 120-121. Fisch, C: Electrophysiologic basis of clinical arrhythmias.	Matching item
	2. To specify the electrophysiological basis of each mechanism producing cardiac dysrhythmias			Multiple-choice item
B. General considerations in approaching dysrhythmias	B. To enumerate the general considerations the nurse should make before interpreting any cardiac dysrhythmia	Lecture Clinical reinforcement Class discussion Written simualtions	Andreoli, pp. 131-134.	Clinical discussion rating scale
C. Approach to analysis and interpretation of cardiac dysrhythmias	C. To use a systematic approach to the analysis and interpretation of cardiac dysrhythmias	Lecture, discussion Clinical checklist	Handout How to read an electrocardiogram. Readings Andreoli, p. 134. Chung, EK: How to approach cardiac arrhythmias. Homework sheets	Clinical demonstration of ability: rating scale
D. Normal sinus rhythm	D. To recognize the ECG parameters of normal sinus rhythm	Lecture, discussion Performance checklist	Handout ECG: normal limits. Reading Andreoli, p. 141. Slides	Clinical demonstration of ability Rating scale
E. Analysis, interpretation, and clinical management of cardiac dysrhythmias (dysrhythmias are disturbances of automaticity or conductivity)	E. For the following cardiac dysrhythmias, the participant will be able to differentiate and: —Analyze the: a. Atrial rate and rhythm b. P wave: (1) Configuration (2) Duration c. P-R interval duration d. Ventricular rate and rhythm e. QRS complex: (1) Configuration (2) Duration f. S-T segment: contour g. Mean electrical axis	Lecture Discussion Classroom practice on ECG analysis and interpretation Performance checklist	Handouts Cardiac rhythms (site of origin). Cardiac rhythms (regular vs irregular). Slides CIBA. Tampa tracings. Schreiner, D. Introduction to cardiac arrhythmia interpretation (American Heart Association). Mountain Press: ECG workbook Series. (practice strips)	Checklist Review of practice slides in class Review of homework assignments (ECG workbook sheets) Clinical demonstration of ability: checklist
	—Interpret the specific dysrhythmia based on previous analysis	Lecture Discussion ECG workshop		

Content	Objectives	Teaching strategies	Resources	Evaluation
	—Classify the mechanisms responsible for producing the dysrhythmia —Delineate the dysrhythmia's clinical significance —Specify the major therapeutic objectives —Identify the clinical implications for a. Nursing management of the patient, and b. Appropriate drug therapy	Class and clinical discussion Simulated patient ECGs Class and clinical practice Group discussion Bedside rounds Class and clinical instruction Homework assignments on interpreting dysrhythmias	Chalkboard Slides Chalkboard Chalkboard Patient care plans (kardex) Mountain Press: ECG workbook sheets, pp. 60-120.	Checklist Review of practice slides in class Review of homework assignments (ECG workbook sheets) Clinical demonstration of ability: checklist Multiple-choice item Static ECG exams
1. Dysrhythmias originating in the sinoatrial node	1. To describe sinus dysrhythmias: a. Sinus bradycardia b. Sinus tachycardia c. Sinus arrhythmia d. Sinus arrest e. Sinus exit block f. Sick sinus syndrome	Didactic instruction and practice Clinical instruction and reinforcement Performance checklist	Readings Andreoli, pp. 142-150. Van Meter, M. and Lavine, PG: What every nurse should know about EKG's. Part 1. Slides Chalkboard	Checklist Review of practice slides in class Review of homework assignments (ECG workbook sheets) Clinical demonstration of ability: checklist
2. Dysrhythmias originating in the atria	2. To describe atrial dysrhythmias: a. Wandering atrial pacemaker b. Atrial ectopic beats c. Multifocal atrial tachycardia d. Paroxysmal atrial tachycardia (with and without block) e. Atrial flutter f. Atrial fibrillation	Didactic instruction and practice Clinical instruction and reinforcement Performance checklist	Readings Andreoli, pp. 152-173. Van Meter, M. and Lavine, PG: What every nurse should know about EKG's. Part 2. Slides Chalkboard	
3. Dysrhythmias originating in the atrioventricular junction	3. To describe junctional dysrhythmias: a. Junctional ectopic beats b. Junctional rhythm c. Nonparoxysmal junctional tachycardia d. Paroxysmal junctional tachycardia	Didactic instruction and practice Clinical instruction and reinforcement Performance checklist	Readings Andreoli, pp. 174-179. Van Meter, M. and Lavine, PG: What every nurse should know about EKG's. Part 3. Slides Chalkboard	
4. Ventricular dysrhythmias	4. a. To describe ventricular dysrhythmias: (1) Ventricular ectopic beats (2) Idioventricular rhythm (3) Accelerated idioventricular rhythm (slow ventricular tachycardia) (4) Ventricular tachycardia (5) Ventricular flutter (6) Ventricular fibrillation	Didactic instruction and practice Clinical instruction and reinforcement Performance checklist	Readings Andreoli, pp. 180-197. Van Meter, M. and Lavine, PG: What every nurse should know about EKG's. Part 4. Slides Chalkboard	Checklist Review of practice slides in class Review of homework assignments (ECG workbook sheets) Clinical demonstration of ability: checklist

Continued.

III. CARDIOVASCULAR COMPONENT—cont'd

Topic	Participant objectives	Teaching method	Instructional media	Method of evaluation
Physiological effects of stress—cont'd	b. To identify the "rule of bigeminy" and its application to precipitating ventricular dysrhythmias	Group discussion	Reading Schamroth, L., and Perlman, MM: The rule of bigeminy.	Multiple-choice item
	c. To specify the ECG parameters of the four types of "lethal PVCs"	Didactic instruction and practice Clinical instruction and reinforcement Performance checklist	Slides Reading Van Meter and Lavine: Part 4, p. 32. Slides	Checklist Review of practice slides in class Review of homework assignments (ECG workbook sheets) Clinical demonstration of ability: checklist
5. Atrioventricular conduction defects	5. a. To describe atrioventricular blocks: (1) 1st degree A-V block (2) 2nd degree A-V block (a) Mobitz Type I (Wenchebach) (b) Mobitz Type II b. To describe His bundle electrograms: (3) 3rd degree (complete) A-V block	Didactic instruction and practice Clinical instruction and reinforcement Performance checklist	Readings Andreoli, pp. 198-207. Van Meter and Lavine, Part 3, pp. 21-25. Slides Reading Andreoli, p. 230. Chalkboard	Checklist Review of practice slides in class Review of homework assignments (ECG workbook sheets) Clinical demonstration of ability: checklist
6. Intraventricular conduction defects	6. To describe: a. Bundle branch blocks: (1) Incomplete vs complete (2) RBBB (3) LBBB	Didactic instruction and practice Clinical instruction and reinforcement Performance checlist	Readings Andreoli, pp. 208-211. Castellanos, A, Spence, MI, and Chapell, DE: Hemiblock and bundle branch block: a nursing approach. Lichstein, E: Pitfalls in interpretation of electrocardiograms.	
	b. Hemiblocks and fascicular blocks: (1) LAH: left anterior hemiblock (2) LPH: left posterior hemiblock		Andreoli, pp. 212-214. Castellanos. Lichstein.	Checklist Review of practice slides in class Review of homework assignments (ECG workbook sheets) Clinical demonstration of ability: checklist
	c. Bifascicular blocks d. Trifascicular blocks		Slides Chalkboard	

Content	Objectives	Methods	Resources	Evaluation
7. ECG phenomena of mixed origin	7. To describe other ECG phenomena a. Reentry phenomena: (1) Circus reentry (2) Focal reentry (3) Reciprocal rhythms	Didactic instruction and practice Clinical instruction and reinforcement Performance checklist	Reading Segal, I, and Schamroth, L: The basic forms of reciprocal rhythm. Chalkboard	Checklist Review of practice slides in class Review of homework assignments (ECG workbook sheets) Clinical demonstration of ability: checklist
	b. Pre-excitation syndromes: (1) Wolff-Parkinson-White (2) Lown-Ganong-Levine		Reading Andreoli, pp. 216-221. Chalkboard	
	c. Parasystole		Readings Andreoli, pp. 214-215.	
	d. A-V dissociation		Andreoli, p. 222.	
	e. Fusion beats		Andreoli, p. 181.	
	f. Escape beats		Andreoli, p. 132.	
	g. Aberration vs ectopy		Andreoli, pp. 223-226. Handouts Action potential correlated with ECG. Features favoring aberration. Features favoring ectopy. Pauses. Slides	
	h. Pauses in rhythm		Chalkboard	
8. ECG changes in electrolyte imbalance	8. To identify the ECG changes characteristically produced by the following electrolyte imbalances and specify the clinical implications of each: a. Hypokalemia b. Hyperkalemia c. Hypocalcemia d. Hypercalcemia	Didactic instruction and practice Clinical instruction and reinforcement Performance checklist	Reading Andreoli, pp. 227-230. Handouts Hypokalemia. Hyperkalemia. Hypocalcemia. Hypercalcemia. Slides	Checklist Review of practice slides in class Review of homework assignments (ECG workbook sheets) Clinical demonstration of ability: checklist Matching item
■ Management of care	To demonstrate the knowledge and ability required for managing nursing care of patients with cardiovascular system dysfunction based on a valid data base and rationale for care	Lecture, discussion Written simulations Clinical instruction and reinforcement	Chalkboard	Written testing Clinical demonstration of ability Direct observation Performance checklists
A. Patients with acute myocardial infarction	A. To describe the rationale and provide for nursing management of the patient with acute myocardial infarction as determined by the:	Lecture, discussion Team conference	Chalkboard AHA slides	Multiple-choice item
1. Pathogenesis	1. Various pathophysiological processes involved in the pathogenesis of acute myocardial infarction a. To identify the triad of risk factors most predisposing to coronary heart disease and MI			

Continued.

III. CARDIOVASCULAR COMPONENT—cont'd

Topic	Participant objectives	Teaching method	Instructional media	Method of evaluation
Physiological effects of stress—cont'd	b. To specify the major constitutional metabolic, non-metabolic, and environmental factors identified as contributory influences in the pathogenesis of coronary artery disease	Class discussion	Readings Andreoli, pp. 8-13. Kannel, WB, and Dawber, TR: Contributors to coronary risk implications for pre- and public health: the Framingham Study.	Clinical conferences in reference to specific patients Written testing
	c. To relate the mechanism by which each identified risk factor predisposes to coronary artery disease	Lecture, discussion	Transparencies Risk factors.	Multiple-choice item
	d. To identify the psychosocial and cultural risk factors associated with the pathogenesis of coronary artery disease and the postulated mechanisms of their association	Lecture, discussion Written simulations	Reading Syme, SL: Social and psychological risk factors in coronary heart disease.	Clinical conference on selected patients Multiple-choice item
	e. To differentiate the proposed relationships of coronary thrombosis to myocardial infarction	Lecture, discussion	Chalkboard	True-false item
	f. To specify the potential role of the subendocardium in the pathogenesis of myocardial infarction	Lecture	Reading Eliot, RS, and Holsinger, JW, Jr: A unified concept of the pathophysiology of myocardial infarction and sudden death.	Multiple-choice item
	g. To enumerate three mechanisms by which an MI may be produced in the presence of patent coronary arteries	Class discussion Lecture	Chalkboard Slides	Completion item Clinical conference
	h. To differentiate between major and minor risk factors of coronary artery disease	Class discussion Lecture	Chalkboard	Multiple-choice item
2. Pathophysiology	2. Major pathophysiological features involved in the various types of myocardial infarction			
	a. To describe the coronary metabolic and hormonal alterations that are produced with myocardial infarction	Lecture, discussion Care conference	Readings Andreoli, pp. 8-13. Eliot. Kennedy, JW: Myocardial function in coronary artery disease.	Essay item Clinical discussion Multiple-choice item
	b. To identify the primary hemodynamic changes produced in myocardial infarction	Class discussion Lecture Clinical reinforcement		Multiple-choice item
	c. To specify the deleterious effects of acidosis on cardiac performance	Lecture Case study	Oliver, MF: The metabolic response to a heart attack.	Clinical discussion
	d. To define and relate the following terms to myocardial performance with acute infarction: (1) Hypokinesis (2) Akinesis (3) Dyskinesis	Lecture, discussion Clinical instruction	Videocassette Impaired contractility. Chalkboard	Multiple-choice item Clinical conference

Content	Objective	Methods	Resources	Evaluation
	e. To delineate the primary systemic metabolic responses to myocardial damage	Lecture, discussion; Clinical reinforcement	Chalkboard; Slides; Flipchart	Multiple-choice item; Clinical conference; Case study
	f. To identify the major determinants of prognosis and clinical course following an acute myocardial infarction	Lecture, discussion; Case study		
3. Clinical assessment	3. Clinical and laboratory evaluation of the patient with an acute MI			
	a. To list the most pertinent parameters to be evaluated in determining whether the patient has sustained an MI	Class discussion; Bedside rounds	Readings: Andreoli, pp. 69-71. Houser, D: What to do first when a patient complains of chest pain.	Clinical conference; Case study
	b. To state the relative value of each parameter in the diagnosis of an MI	Class discussion; Bedside rounds; Class discussion	Chalkboard	Written testing
	c. To describe the major facets of a typical patient history in MI	Class discussion; Case study		Clinical conference
	d. To compare and contrast the enzyme changes characteristically produced with an MI in terms of the onset, peak, and duration of elevation of each	Lecture, discussion; Case study	Handout: Typical enzyme changes following myocardial infarction.	Written testing; Clinical discussion
	e. To differentiate among nonspecific and more cardiospecific enzyme changes in MI, citing examples of each	Lecture, discussion; Case study	Readings: Andreoli, pp. 51-53. Smith, AM, Theiner, JA, and Huang, SH: Serum enzymes in myocardial infarction.	Completion item
	f. To differentiate the ECG changes produced with: (1) Myocardial ischemia (2) Myocardial injury (3) Myocardial infarction	Lecture, discussion; Classroom practice; Performance checklist	Readings: Andreoli, pp. 115-116. Slides; ECG homework sheets; Patient charts	Clinical demonstration of ability: checklist; Multiple-choice item
	g. To compare and contrast ECG evidence of acute: (1) Transmural MI (2) Intramural MI (3) Subendocardial MI	Lecture, discussion; Classroom practice; Performance checklist	Slides; Patient charts	Clinical demonstration of ability; Multiple-choice item
	h. To contrast the ECG changes characteristically observed during evolution of an acute MI with those observed during its resolution and healing	Lecture, discussion; Classroom practice; Clinical instruction and reinforcement	Readings: Andreoli, pp. 109-115. Van Meter and Lavine: Part 4, p. 32. Slides	Multiple-choice item; Clinical discussion and conference; Clinical demonstration of ability
	i. To determine the age, location, and quality of resolution of an acute MI from ECG and laboratory evidence	Lecture, discussion; Classroom practice; Clinical instruction and reinforcement	Readings: Andreoli, pp. 118-127 (review pp. 45-46). Van Meter and Lavine: Part 4, p. 35. ECG homework sheets; Slides	Clinical demonstration of ability: checklist; Written testing; Review of homework sheets

Continued.

311

III. CARDIOVASCULAR COMPONENT—cont'd

Topic	Participant objectives	Teaching method	Instructional media	Method of evaluation
Physiological effects of stress—cont'd	j. To identify the anticipated clinical presentation of an MI patient (inclusive of both signs and symptoms) relating the pathophysiological basis for this characteristic presentation	Lecture, discussion Nursing care conference	Readings Andreoli: pp. 69-71.	Case study Clinical conference
	k. To differentiate between the characteristics of chest pain associated with an MI and with various types of angina	Lecture, discussion Nursing care conference	Houser.	Written testing Clinical conference
	l. To interpret the findings of clinical assessment in terms of their implications for patient care	Simulated patients Bedside rounds	Selected patients	Clinical conference Case study
4. Clinical problems	4. Priority of clinical problems associated with acute myocardial infarction			
	a. From the pathophysiology and clinical evaluation of the patient with an acute MI, to delineate the anticipated clinical problems according to their life-threatening potential	Class discussion Bedside rounds Written simulations	Readings Bunke, B: Respiratory function after acute myocardial infarction. Col, JJ, and Weinberg, SE: Factors affecting prognosis in acute myocardial infarction.	Clinical conference on selected patients Simulated patient
	b. To identify the most common complications of acute MI in order of their prevalence, indicating at least two means to recognize the development of each	Lecture, discussion Bedside rounds	Andreoli: pp. 70-71. Romhilt and Fowler.	Essay item Clinical discussion
	c. To identify the basic pathophysiology and clinical presentation observed in patients with Dressler's syndrome	Lecture, discussion Nursing care conference	Andreoli: p. 73. Programmed instruction	Multiple-choice item
	d. To specify the objectives of care for nursing management of the patient with acute myocardial infarction	Class discussion Nursing care conference	Selected patients	Clinical discussion Written testing
5. Modes of therapy	5. Currently available modes of therapy for patient with an acute MI			
	a. To describe the rationale for and techniques of alternative modes of care for the MI patient	Class discussion Team conference	Readings Andreoli: chapter 8. Braunwald, E, and Maroko, R: The reduction of infarct size.	Written testing Clinical conference
	b. To determine the priority of care needs of the MI patient during the initial 48 hours following admission to the hospital	Discussion, lecture Multiple assignment	Romhilt and Fowler.	Clinical conference Multiple-choice item
	c. To specify at least two measures to take to prevent or minimize complications in the MI patient	Lecture, discussion Bedside rounds	Chalkboard	Written testing Clinical discussion

Objectives	Teaching/Learning methods	Resources	Evaluation
d. In relation to Cassem and Hackett's "stages of recovery" following an MI, identify the nursing interventions appropriate to each stage of psychological recovery	Lecture, discussion / Team conference	Readings Andreoli: pp. 311-317. Cassem, NH, and Hackett, TP: Psychological rehabilitation of MI patients in the acute phase.	Clinical demonstration of ability / Written testing: role-play
e. To identify the most prevalent long-term physical and psychosocial complications of MI, indicating nursing interventions that can minimize these barriers to rehabilitation	Lecture / Team conference	Scalzi, C: Nursing management of behavioral responses, following an acute myocardial infarction.	Clinical discussion / Multiple-choice item
f. To specify areas in which the recovering patient with an MI should receive instructions before discharge	Class discussion / Team conference		Clinical conference
g. To design an appropriate discharge plan of care for the post-MI patient	Homework assignment on specific patient / Performance checklist	Andreoli: pp. 319-332. Kardex care plan	Review of homework assignment (discharge planning)
h. To demonstrate satisfactory performance and knowledge of CPR techniques according to American Heart Association standards for CPR certification	Laboratory and classroom demonstration and practice / Simulated situations / Performance checklist	Reading Andreoli: pp. 303-306. Manikins	Return satisfactory demonstrations of proper techniques / Written tests on CPR (Heart Association)
i. To demonstrate the knowledge and technical proficiency required to become certified in cardiac defibrillation according to the standards and policies established	Lectures and classes as outlined in hospital policies / Clinical instruction / Simulated situations / Performance checklist	Defibrillator / Crash cart / Manikins	Clinical demonstration of ability together with examination as outlined / Checklists
j. To differentiate between the rationale, techniques, and nursing implications of cardioversion and those of defibrillation	Lecture, discussion	Reading Andreoli: pp. 300-303. Slides	Essay item
k. To describe the most commonly used cardiac drugs in terms of their therapeutic effect and dosages, routes of administration, and side and toxic effects	Lecture, discussion / Clinical instruction and reinforcement	Reading Andreoli: Appendix A. ACLS slides	Clinical discussion / Multiple-choice item
B. Patients with acute or chronic cardiac conduction system dysfunction — B. To describe the rationale and provide for nursing management of patients needing artificial cardiac pacemaking systems	Lecture, discussion / Bedside rounds	Readings Andreoli: pp. 258-261. Jenkins, AC: Patients with pacers.	Multiple-choice item / Clinical conference
1. Indications for pacing — 1. To specify the clinical indications for both temporary and permanent artificial cardiac pacing			

Continued.

III. CARDIOVASCULAR COMPONENT—cont'd

Topic	Participant objectives	Teaching method	Instructional media	Method of evaluation
Physiological effects of stress—cont'd				
a. Temporary	a. Temporary			
	(1) To identify the clinical (therapeutic and diagnostic) indications for temporary cardiac pacing, indicating the rationale for each	Lecture, discussion Case presentations	Spence, MI, and Lemberg, L: Cardiac pacemakers. II. Indications for pacing.	Multiple-choice item Clinical discussion
	(2) To differentiate the rationale for temporary cardiac pacing based on the location of an acute MI	Class discussion Case study	Warkentin slides Chalkboard	Completion item
	(3) To identify the situations when prophylactic temporary pacing may be indicated	Lecture, discussion Bedside rounds		Multiple-choice item
b. Permanent	b. Permanent			
	(1) To identify the clinical indications for permanent cardiac pacing	Lecture, discussion Case study	Reading Andreoli: pp. 258-261.	Clinical conference Multiple-choice item
	(2) To delineate the clinical situations that may lead to heart block	Lecture, discussion Nursing team conference	Chalkboard	Written testing Clinical discussion
	(3) To specify the pathophysiological features of the two primary causes of complete heart block	Lecture	Chalkboard	True-false item
	(4) To define the clinical features of Stokes-Adams syndrome	Class discussion Case presentation	Chalkboard	Multiple-choice item
	(5) To identify the types of intraventricular conduction defects that would most likely require permanent cardiac pacing	Class discussion Lecture	Warkentin slides	Multiple-choice item Clinical conference
2. Pacemaker components a. Temporary pacemakers	2. a. Temporary pacemakers			
	(1) To describe the general components of a temporary (transvenous) pacemaking system	Lecture, discussion Demonstration of various pacemaker systems	Readings Andreoli: p. 258. Barold, SS: Modern concepts of cardiac pacing.	Clinical discussion Written testing
	(2) To specify the function of each component of a temporary pacemaker unit	Class discussion Lecture Laboratory session	Samples of various types of pacemakers systems	Clinical demonstration of ability: rating scale Written testing
	(3) To explain what each setting and indicator on an external pacing unit represents and how settings may be adjusted	Class discussion Lecture Laboratory session	Pictures of various types of pacemakers	Clinical demonstration of ability: laboratory Written testing
b. Permanent pacemakers	b. Permanent pacemakers			
	(1) To describe the general components of a permanent (implantable) pacemaking system	Laboratory session with pacemakers Class discussion	Readings Andreoli, p. 263-265. Barold. Equipment used with pacemakers	Written testing Clinical discussion

314

Content	Objectives	Learning activities	Resources	Evaluation
3. Methods of pacemaker electrode insertion a. Temporary	3. a. Temporary (1) To differentiate transvenous from transthoracic pacemaker insertion techniques	Class discussion Lab demonstration	Readings Andreoli: pp. 261-265. Jenkins.	Clinical conference True-false item
	(2) To describe the technique for inserting a temporary transvenous pacemaker	Class discussion Lab demonstration	Warkentin and CIBA slides	Essay item
	(3) To identify where each component of a transvenous pacing system is placed for temporary pacing and indicate how it is secured in place	Class demonstration Laboratory session Clinical reinforcement and instruction	Chalkboard Warkentin slides Temporary pacemaker system and ancillary equipment necessary	Clinical demonstration of ability to secure equipment in place
	(4) To specify the nursing responsibilities in assisting with insertion of a temporary (transvenous) pacemaker	Lecture, discussion Multiple assignment	Reading Friedberg, HD: Crucial measurements during pacemaker implantation.	Clinical demonstration of ability to assist: rating scale
	(5) To identify the characteristic ECG waves associated with advancement and placement of a transvenous pacing catheter	Lecture, discussion Participation at pacemaker insertion	Pacemaker insertion slides	Written testing Demonstration of ability to recognize
	(6) To describe the criteria used initially to evaluate the adequacy of transvenous pacemaker insertion	Class discussion Nursing care conference	Chalkboard	Multiple-choice item
	(7) To delineate the nursing responsibilities for the patient immediately following the insertion of a temporary pacemaker	Lecture, discussion Nursing care conference	Flipchart	Written testing Clinical conference
b. Permanent	b. Permanent (1) To describe the various approaches that may be used for inserting a permanent pacemaker	Class discussion Nursing care conference	Readings Andreoli: pp. 263-265. Friedberg. Kardex care plan	Multiple-choice item
	(2) To delineate the preoperative and postoperative nursing care for a patient having a permanent pacemaker insertion	Class discussion Nursing care conference		Essay item Clinical demonstration of ability
4. Pacemaker lead systems	4. To differentiate and distinguish between unipolar and bipolar pacemaker lead systems	Lecture, discussion	Readings Andreoli: p. 263. Barold: p. 238. Chalkboard	Multiple-choice item
5. General features and concepts related to pacemakers	5. To relate the general features and concepts of cardiac pacing to specific modalities and functioning of pacemakers			
	a. To distinguish between atrial and ventricular stimulating electrodes in the ECG response produced	Slide presentation Lecture, discussion Clinical preceptor	Readings Andreoli: p. 265. Barold. Warkentin slides	Clinical demonstration of ability to distinguish: rating scale
	b. To differentiate between a pacemaker's automatic interval and its escape interval	Lecture, discussion	Chalkboard Slides	True-false item
	c. To list the advantages and disadvantages of the pacemaker hysteresis feature of some pacemakers	Class discussion Lecture	Chalkboard	Written testing Clinical conference

Continued.

III. CARDIOVASCULAR COMPONENT—cont'd

Physiological effects of stress—cont'd

Topic	Participant objectives	Teaching method	Instructional media	Method of evaluation
6. Modalities of pacing	6. To describe each of the modalities of pacing in terms of the: —Location of stimulating and sensing electrodes —Intervals or waves sensed —Response to sensing of intervals and waves —Response produced by stimulating electrode —Potential problems associated with its use —Clinical indications for its use —ECG it produces when functioning properly and improperly	Lecture, discussion Slide presentation Clinical instruction and reinforcement	Readings Andreoli: pp. 266-271. Barold. Jenkins: pp. 608-609. Spence, MI, and Lemberg, L. Cardiac pacemakers. I. Modalities of pacing. Homework ECG sheets	Multiple-choice item Slide review Homework sheets review Clinical discussion
a. Ventricular pacing modes	a. To describe ventricular pacing modalities in terms of the above characteristics (1) Continuous asynchronous (2) QRS: inhibited (3) QRS: triggered (4) P wave: triggered	Lecture, discussion Slide presentation Clinical instruction and reinforcement	Readings Andreoli: pp. 266-271. Barold. Jenkins: pp. 608-609. Spence and Lemberg.	Multiple-choice item Slide review Homework sheets review Clinical discussion
b. Atrial pacing modes	b. To describe atrial pacing modalities in terms of the above characteristics (1) Continuous atrial (2) P wave: triggered (3) P wave: inhibited (4) QRS: inhibited	Lecture, discussion Slide presentation Clinical instruction and reinforcement	Andreoli: pp. 266-271. Barold. Jenkins: pp. 608-609. Spence and Lemberg.	Multiple-choice item Slide review Homework sheets review Clinical discussion
c. Atrial and ventricular pacing modes	c. To describe atrial and ventricular pacing modalities in terms of the above characteristics (1) Continuous sequential (2) QRS: inhibited sequential	Lecture, discussion Slide presentation Clinical instruction and reinforcement	Andreoli: pp. 266-271. Barold. Jenkins: pp. 608-609. Spence and Lemberg.	Multiple-choice item Slide review Homework sheets review Clinical discussion
7. Complications of pacemakers	7. To describe and demonstrate how to deal effectively with the potential complications associated with pacemakers	Lecture, discussion Laboratory and clinical instruction, demonstration, checklist		Written testing Clinical demonstration of ability
	a. To explain what is implied by the following terms: (1) Failure to sense adequately (2) Failure to stimulate adequately	Lecture, discussion Bedside rounds	Andreoli: pp. 271-272. Barold: pp. 245-249.	Completion item

316

(3) Failure to capture adequately

Objective	Teaching method	Resources	Evaluation
		Spence, MI, and Lemberg, L: Cardiac pacemakers. IV. Complications of pacing.	
b. To list at least three potential causes of failure to sense, stimulate, and capture adequately	Class discussion Nursing care conference	Chalkboard Slides	True-false item Clinical conference
c. To describe the appropriate nursing interventions for each failure situation	Lecture, discussion Clinical instruction Laboratory practice session	Pacemaker equipment	Multiple-choice item Laboratory practice of interventions
d. To enumerate factors that increase or decrease a pacemaker's threshold level	Lecture Clinical preceptor	Chalkboard	Multiple-choice item
e. To identify the additional hazards of surgical implantation of a pacemaker	Class discussion Case study	Chalkboard	Clinical discussion Multiple choice item
f. To describe the ECG problems created by pacemakers	Lecture, discussion Case study	Readings Marriott, HJL, and Gozensky, C: Electrocardiogram problems created by pacemakers.	Slide review Written testing ECG sheet review
g. To recognize the complications of pacemakers as evidenced on the ECG	Slide presentation Lecture, discussion	Homework ECG sheets	
h. To describe and perform appropriate nursing interventions aimed at preventing the electrical hazards posed in pacemakers	Class discussion Laboratory session Performance checklist Simulated situations	Readings Andreoli: p. 273. Merkel, R, and Savie, M: Electrocution hazards with transvenous pacemaker electrodes. Equipment used to reduce electrical hazard potential	Clinical demonstration of ability: rating scale Written testing Return demonstration
8. Nursing management of patients with pacemakers			
a. Patients with temporary pacemakers			
8. a. To specify the objectives of nursing management of the patient with a temporary pacemaker and how these may be achieved	Lecture, discussion Nursing team conference	Readings Andreoli: pp. 272-274. Jenkins. Chalkboard Selected patients	Multiple-choice item Clinical demonstration of ability

Continued.

317

III. CARDIOVASCULAR COMPONENT—cont'd

Topic	Participant objectives	Teaching method	Instructional media	Method of evaluation
Physiological effects of stress—cont'd a. Patients with permanent pacemakers—cont'd	b. To specify the objectives of nursing management of the patient with a permanent pacemaker and describe how these may be achieved	Lecture, discussion Multiple assignment	Readings Andreoli: pp. 274-275. Cortes, TS: Pacemakers today. Jenkins. Selected patients	Written testing Clinical demonstration of ability
	(1) To identify areas needing patient and family teaching before discharge of the pacemaker patient from the hospital	Case study	Readings Andreoli: pp. 276-278. Kos, BA, and Culbert, P: Teaching the patient with a pacemaker. Sweetwood, H: Patients with pacemakers.	Clinical conference
	(2) To formulate a discharge plan of care for patients having permanent cardiac pacemakers	Class discussion Class assignment Class presentation	Andreoli: pp. 276-278.	Essay item Review of assignment Case review
C. Patients with acute congestive heart failure	C. To describe the rationale for nursing management of patients with acute congestive heart failure as determined by the:			
1. Pathogenesis	1. Pathogenesis of congestive heart failure	Lecture Discussion	Andreoli: pp. 73-78.	Clinical conference
	a. To define the term "congestive heart failure"			
	b. To identify the three principal causes of CHF	Lecture	Filmstrip CHF. Handout Upjohn: Cardiac failure, pp. 4-7.	Multiple-choice item
	c. To cite at least two clinical disorders that exemplify each of the principal causes of CHF	Class discussion	CIBA slides	Written testing Clinical conference Multiple-choice item
	d. To distinguish low-output failure from high-output failure	Lecture, discussion Case study	Chalkboard	
	e. To specify two clinical situations in which CHF exists in the presence of a normal cardiac output	Class discussion	Chalkboard	Clinical discussion
	f. To identify the common underlying causes of CHF	Care conference Lecture, discussion Clinical rounds	Slides Chalkboard	Multiple-choice item Completion item
	g. To list four factors that may precipitate or aggravate CHF			
2. Pathophysiology	2. To describe the pathophysiology of CHF			
	a. To describe the acute, subacute, and chronic compensatory mechanisms that are activated in severe CHF, their physiological limits, and their clinical effects:	Lecture Clinical instruction and reinforcement Nursing team conference	Filmstrip CHF. Reading Andreoli: pp. 73-78. Handout Upjohn: Cardiac failure, pp. 7-10.	Multiple-choice item Clinical conference
	(1) Acute (a) Circulatory reflexes (Starling's law of the heart)		Slides	

Content / Objectives	Teaching methods	Resources	Evaluation

(b) Sympathetic nervous system
(2) Subacute
  (a) Renal retention of NaCl and H_2O (Aldosterone, ADH, reninangiotensin)
(3) Chronic
  (a) Ventricular hypertrophy and dilatation
		Chalkboard	

b. To relate the clinical effects of compensatory mechanisms in CHF to Starling's law of the heart c. To differentiate between compensated and decompensated CHF	Lecture, discussion Case study Class discussion	Filmstrip CHF.	Multiple-choice item Clinical discussion Clinical conference
d. To identify the biochemical abnormalities that seem to be associated with CHF and their pathophysiological effects	Lecture, discussion	Slides	Multiple-choice item
e. To differentiate between the primary pathophysiological features of left heart failure and right heart failure	Class discussion Case study	Slides Chalkboard	Clinical discussion True-false item
f. To specify at least three causes (each) of left and right heart failure	Class discussion		Written testing
g. To describe the physiological effects of CHF in each of the following organs: (1) Heart (2) Lungs (3) Kidneys (4) Splanchnic organs (5) Endocrine organs	Lecture, discussion Case study	Handout Upjohn: Cardiac failure.	Multiple-choice item Clinical conference
h. To define clinically "acute pulmonary edema" and describe its relationship to left ventricular failure	Lecture, discussion Written simulations	Reading Larsen, EL. The patient with acute pulmonary edema. Handout Pathophysiology of pulmonary edema due to heart disease.	Multiple-choice item Clinical discussion
i. To define clinically "cor pulmonale" and describe its relationship to right ventricular failure	Lecture, discussion	Slides	Multiple-choice item Clinical discussion
j. To define "preload," "afterload," and LVEDV and relate each to the pathophysiology of CHF	Lecture, discussion		
3. Clinical assessment 3. To perform clinical and laboratory evaluation of the patient with acute CHF	Written simulations	Readings Andreoli: pp. 74-75. Hanchett, ES. and Johnson, R: Early signs of congestive heart failure.	
a. To differentiate between the early and late signs and symptoms of left ventricular failure and those of right ventricular failure	Lecture, discussion	Handout Upjohn: Cardiac failure, pp. 11-14. Selected patients	Clinical conference True-false item
b. To relate the signs and symptoms of CHF to their pathophysiological bases	Class discussion Clinical reinforcement		Multiple-choice item Clinical conference
c. To recognize the ECG findings characteristic of left and right ventricular hypertrophy and strain	Lecture, discussion	Slides Patient charts	Demonstrated ability to recognize: rating scale Written testing

Continued.

III. CARDIOVASCULAR COMPONENT—cont'd

Topic	Participant objectives	Teaching method	Instructional media	Method of evaluation
Physiological effects of stress—cont'd	d. To identify the early radiological findings associated with acute and chronic CHF; to state the clinical significance of Kerley's lines for the patient suspected of having CHF	Lecture, discussion Clinical instruction and correlation	Representative chest roentgenograms	Multiple-choice item
	e. To specify the clinical findings to anticipate finding in a patient with acute CHF when the patient's CVP, PAP, PAWP, circulation time, and ABGs are measured	Class discussion Lecture Bedside rounds	Chalkboard Slides	Clinical discussion Multiple-choice item
	f. To describe the cardiac auscultatory findings to anticipate hearing in a patient with acute CHF	Lecture, discussion Clinical rounds	Chalkboard Audiotape CHF.	Clinical discussion Case study
	g. To classify functionally a CHF patient according to the NY Heart Association's "Functional Classification of Cardiac Patients"	Lecture Clinical rounds	Copies of NY Heart Association: Functional classification of cardiac patients	Multiple-choice item Clinical conference
	h. To explain the clinical significance of paroxysmal nocturnal dyspnea (PND)	Bedside rounds		Multiple-choice item
4. Clinical problems	To set the priority of clinical problems associated with acute CHF		Reading Andreoli: pp. 60-62.	
	a. To list the primary clinical problems associated with LVF and with RVF in order of their immediacy.	Nursing care conference		Clinical conference
	b. To compare and contrast the priority of clinical problems of LVF and those of RVF	Clinical instruction and reinforcement Lecture	Handout Upjohn: Cardiac failure, pp. 14-19.	Written testing Clinical conference
	c. To state the objectives of care for management of the patient with acute CHF	Class discussion	Chalkboard Nursing care plan Homework: nursing care plan (kardex)	Review of written plan of nursing care
5. Modes of therapy	To describe currently available modes of therapy for the patient in acute CHF		Reading Andreoli: pp. 75-76.	
	a. To identify the primary modes of therapy used to: (1) Improve pulmonary ventilation and gas exchange (2) Reduce cardiac workload (3) Improve myocardial contractility (4) Reduce venous return (5) Decrease intravascular volume (6) Relieve anxiety (7) Correct dysrhythmias	Lecture, discussion Nursing care conference	Handout Upjohn: Cardiac failure, pp. 14-19.	Clinical discussion Multiple-choice item
	b. To delineate the nursing responsibilities inherent in providing these modes of therapy	Lecture, discussion Clinical conference	Reading Smith, BC: Congestive heart failure.	Clinical return demonstration Written testing

Content	Teaching methods	Resources (Chalkboard)	Completion item
c. To enumerate the additional interventions that may be necessitated in a patient with acute pulmonary edema	Nursing care conference	Chalkboard	Completion item
d. To describe the rationale for and demonstrate the technique of applying both automatic and manual rotating tourniquets	Laboratory instruction on technique of using automatic rotating tourniquets / Class discussion	Automatic rotating tourniquets	Laboratory demonstration of ability to use tourniquets: checklist
D. Patients with cardiogenic shock / 1. Pathogenesis / To describe the rationale for nursing management of patients with cardiogenic shock as determined by the: / 1. Pathogenesis of cardiogenic shock	Nursing care conference		
a. To define "cardiogenic shock"	Lecture, discussion	Handout / Cardiogenic shock. / Readings / Andreoli: pp. 78-79. / Evans, RW: Cardiogenic shock: can the prognosis be improved?	Multiple-choice item
b. To identify the clinical criteria of cardiogenic shock as defined by the National Heart and Lung Institute MIRU	Lecture, discussion	O'Rourke, MF: Cardiogenic shock following myocardial infarction.	
c. To recognize the spectrum of clinical problems that may lead to cardiogenic shock	Lecture, discussion / Clinical reinforcement		Clinical conference / Multiple-choice item
d. To describe the characteristics of patients most likely to develop cardiogenic shock	Nursing care conference	Chalkboard	Clinical conference / Written testing
e. To identify the incidence, mortality, and descriptive statistics related to post-MI cardiogenic shock	Lecture, discussion / Clinical conference	Videocassette / Cardiogenic shock.	Multiple-choice item
2. Pathophysiological features of cardiogenic shock		Handout / Cardiogenic shock.	
2. Pathophysiology / a. To describe the major hemodynamic consequences of cardiogenic shock at both the central and peripheral levels	Lecture, discussion / Case study	Readings / Andreoli: pp. 78-79. / O'Rourke. / Stude, C: Cardiogenic shock.	Clinical discussion / Multiple-choice item
b. To describe the major systemic effects of reduced tissue perfusion caused by cardiogenic shock	Lecture, discussion / Case study	Chalkboard / Slides	Clinical discussion / Written testing
c. To specify the neuroendocrine responses to cardiogenic shock	Class discussion	Chalkboard	Clinical discussion / Multiple-choice item
d. To identify the postulated role of a myocardial depressant factor in shock states	Lecture	Chalkboard	Written testing
e. To delineate the primary mechanisms by which the heart may compensate for a diminished cardiac output and describe their efficiency in cardiogenic shock	Lecture, discussion / Case study	Handout / Cardiogenic shock. / Chalkboard / Slides	Written testing / Clinical conference

Continued.

III. CARDIOVASCULAR COMPONENT—cont'd

Topic	Participant objectives	Teaching method	Instructional media	Method of evaluation

Physiological effects of stress—cont'd	f. To relate the following terms and abbreviations to the pathophysiology of cardiogenic shock:
	(1) Preload
	(2) Afterload
	(3) MVO_2
	(4) MAP
	(5) SVR
	(6) Starling's law of the heart
	(7) Contractility
	(8) LVEDV
	(9) LVEDP
	(10) PAP and PAWP
	(11) $CO = HR \times SV$
		Lecture, discussion
		Bedside rounds
			Slides
			Handout
			  Cardiogenic shock.
			Chalkboard.
			Videocassette
			  Cardiogenic shock.
				Matching item
				Clinical conference

	g. To differentiate the three progressive stages of cardiogenic shock	Lecture	Readings Stude.	Completion item
3. Clinical assessment	3. To perform clinical and laboratory evaluation of the patient with cardiogenic shock			
	a. To identify the early clinical evidence of cardiogenic shock	Lecture Case study	Adams, CW: Recognition and evaluation of cardiogenic shock.	Multiple-choice item
	b. To specify the clinical findings to anticipate when a patient develops cardiogenic shock (signs, symptoms, clinical presentation)	Clinical instruction Lecture Class discussion Case study	Evans: pp. 82-83. Stude: pp. 1636-1638. Selected patients	Clinical demonstration of ability to relate Written testing Review of case illustration
	c. To describe the laboratory results that would support the diagnosis of cardiogenic shock	Lecture, discussion Case study	Chalkboard	Clinical conference Multiple-choice item
	d. To describe the laboratory results that would support the diagnosis of cardiogenic shock	Lecture, discussion Clinical rounds	Chalkboard	Clinical conference Multiple-choice item
	e. To relate the clinical and laboratory findings in cardiogenic shock with their pathophysiological correlates	Case study	Chalkboard	Demonstration of ability to relate Written testing
	f. To compare and contrast the usefulness and reliability of CVP and PAP and PAWP monitoring in a patient suspected of having cardiogenic shock	Lecture Bedside rounds	Slides	Multiple-choice item Clinical discussion

	g. To identify the clinical advantages of intro-arterial measurement of BP in patients with cardiogenic shock	Class discussion	Readings
			  Evans.
			  Scheidt and Killip.
				Clinical discussion: case study

	h. To describe the prognostic factors in cardiogenic shock	Lecture, discussion	Evans. Scheidt and Killip.	Clinical conference
4. Clinical problems	4. To set the priority of clinical problems associated with cardiogenic shock			
	a. To identify the clinical problems of patients in cardiogenic shock	Case study		Clinical conference: multiple assignment
	b. To rank the clinical problems of patients in cardiogenic shock according to their immediacy	Case study	Chalkboard	Written testing Clinical conference

Content	Objectives	Teaching method	Readings / Resources	Evaluation
	c. From the priority listing of clinical problems, to state the objectives of care for nursing management of the patient in cardiogenic shock	Homework: written plan	Nursing care plans (kardex)	Review of kardexes
5. Modes of therapy	5. To describe currently available modes of therapy for patients in cardiogenic shock		Readings Andreoli: pp. 79-86.	
	a. To describe the rationale and currently available means by which myocardial infarct size may be reduced	Lecture, discussion		Completion item
	b. To identify the rationale for using diastolic augmentation devices in a patient with cardiogenic shock	Lecture, discussion Case study	Amsterdam, EA, et al: Evaluation and management of cardiogenic shock. Amsterdam, EA, et al: Roles of cardiac surgery and mechanical assist.	Multiple-choice item
	c. To explain how various circulatory assist devices function in management of patients with cardiogenic shock	Class discussion Case study		Essay item
	d. To distinguish and differentiate among the various pharmacological agents used to treat patients in cardiogenic shock: (1) Vasopressors (2) Vasodilators (3) Steroids (4) Inotropic agents (5) Anticoagulants (6) Glucagon (7) Oxygen	Lecture, discussion Clinical instruction and reinforcement	Amsterdam, EA, et al: II. Drug therapy. Evans. O'Rourke. Shinn, AF: Corticosteroids and their use in shock.	Demonstration of ability to distinguish in selected patients Matching item
	e. To describe the rationale for surgical interventions used in treating cardiogenic shock	Class discussion	Amsterdam, et al: III.	Clinical conference: case study
	f. To identify the nursing responsibilities associated with managing the care of a patient in cardiogenic shock	Lecture, discussion Case study	Selected patients	Multiple-choice item Clinical demonstration of ability in selected patients
E. Patients with pericarditis 1. Pathogenesis	F. To describe the rationale for nursing management of patients with acute pericarditis as determined by the: 1. Pathogenesis of pericarditis			
	a. To delineate the clinical characteristics of the patient population most likely to develop acute pericarditis or pericardial tamponade	Lecture, discussion	Readings Kuhn, L. Clinical problems of pericardial disease. In: S.E. Moolten (Ed.)	Written testing Clinical conference
	b. To describe the clinical history of patients who may present an auto-immune or acute idiopathic pericarditis	Lecture, discussion Simulated patient	Yan, V: Pericarditis in acute myocardial infarction. Slide-tape program Pericarditis	Clinical discussion Written testing: simulated situations
	c. To distinguish acute infectious pericarditis from its autoimmune and acute idiopathic forms	Lecture, discussion	Pericarditis	Written testing

Continued.

III. CARDIOVASCULAR COMPONENT—cont'd

Physiological effects of stress—cont'd

Topic	Participant objectives	Teaching method	Instructional media	Method of evaluation
2. Pathophysiology	2. To describe the pathophysiology of various forms of pericarditis		Slide-tape program Pericarditis.	
	a. To identify the primary determinant of the hemodynamic effects of acute pericarditis	Lecture, discussion Bedside rounds	Readings Andreoli: p. 376. Kuhn. Yan.	Multiple-choice item
	b. To compare and contrast the hemodynamic alterations produced by acute pericarditis as they are reflected in the systemic venous and arterial systems	Lecture, discussion Bedside rounds	CIBA slides Chalkboard	Clinical discussion Written testing
	c. To identify the limiting factor of pericardial anatomy that determines intrapericardial pressure	Class discussion	CIBA slides	Multiple-choice item
	d. To describe the cardiac events that accompany acute pericarditis as compensatory mechanisms	Lecture Bedside rounds	Chalkboard	Clinical conference Completion item
	e. To specify the major pathophysiologic events leading to pericardial tamponade	Lecture, discussion	Chalkboard	Multiple-choice item
3. Clinical assessment	3. To perform clinical and laboratory evaluation of the patient with acute pericarditis			
	a. To differentiate between the pain syndrome of pericarditis and of myocardial infarction	Simulated patient Class discussion	Readings Andreoli: pp. 375-378. Kuhn: pp. 211-213. Yan.	Clinical conference True-false item
	b. To identify the primary characteristics of a pericardial friction rub caused by pericarditis	Lecture Clinical rounds	Kuhn: p. 211. Anderson and CIBA slides Audiotapes	Clinical discussion Written testing with audiotapes
	c. To compare and contrast the physical ECG, and laboratory findings of patients with pericarditis and those of the MI patient	Class discussion Written simulation	Reading Andreoli: pp. 375-378. Chalkboard	Written testing Clinical conference
	d. To explain the clinical significance of pulsus paradoxus and electrical alternans in patients with pericarditis	Lecture Class discussion	Reading Kuhn: pp. 216-217.	Multiple-choice item
	e. To identify the signs of pericardial effusion and the clinical situations when it is most likely to occur	Class discussion Simulated patient	Slide-tape program Pericarditis.	Written testing Clinical discussion
	f. To enumerate the physical signs of pericardial tamponade and the clinical situations when it is likely to be observed	Bedside rounds	Reading Kuhn: pp. 216-218. CIBA slides	True-false item Clinical discussion
	g. To distinguish between pulsus alternans and electrical alternans	Class discussion	Slides	True-false item
4. Clinical problems	4. To set the priority of clinical problems associated with pericarditis			
	a. To enumerate the major clinical problems of a patient with acute pericarditis	Class discussion Multiple assignment	Chalkboard	Clinical conference

Objective	Teaching/Learning activities	Resources	Evaluation
b. To compare and contrast the priority of clinical problems faced by patients with acute pericarditis and those with pericardial effusion and tamponade	Homework: written listing of clinical problems in order of priority	Chalkboard, Nursing care plans (kardex)	Review of care plans and problem lists, Multiple-choice item
c. To list the objectives of care for nursing management of the patient with acute pericarditis	Homework: written set of objectives of care	Kardex	Review of objectives
5. Modes of therapy			
a. To specify the usual modes of treatment for the pain and fever of pericarditis	Multiple assignment	Readings Kuhn: pp. 214-215, 218-219, 221-222. Yan.	Multiple-choice item, Clinical conference
b. To explain the rationale for steroid therapy in patients with acute pericarditis	Class discussion		Completion item, Clinical conference
c. To identify the contraindications of anticoagulant therapy in patients with acute pericarditis	Class discussion, Clinical reinforcement	Chalkboard	Multiple-choice item
d. To describe how the nurse may determine if a pulsus paradoxus, pulsus alternans, or electrical alternans is present	Clinical rounds, Lecture	Clinical laboratory with selected patients	Clinical demonstration of ability to determine, Written testing, Rating scale
e. To describe the nursing responsibilities in assisting with a pericardiocentesis	Lecture, discussion, Simulated patient	Reading Kuhn: pp. 218-219. Equipment for pericardiocentesis	Clinical demonstration of ability to assist, Essay item
F. Patients with hypertensive crisis 1. Pathogenesis			
E. To describe the rationale for nursing management of the patient with hypertensive crisis as determined by the: 1. Pathogenesis of hypertensive crisis a. To define the following terms: (1) Hypertensive crisis (2) Accelerated hypertension (3) Hypertensive encephalopathy (4) Malignant hypertension	Lecture, discussion, Incident process	Transparencies, Readings Finnerty, FA: Aggressive drug therapy in accelerated hypertension. Finnerty, FA: Hypertensive crisis. Shank, LF, and Ludewig, J: Hypertension.	Clinical conference, Matching item
b. To describe the known risk factors and epidemiological data on patients with hypertension	Class discussion	Transparencies	Clinical conference
c. To identify the clinical factors implicated in the etiology of hypertension and the approximate incidence of each factor	Lecture, discussion	Transparencies	Clinical conference
d. To specify the characteristics of patient population at greatest risk for developing hypertensive crisis	Class discussion	Transparencies	Multiple-choice item, Clinical discussion
e. To identify common areas of patient ignorance or misunderstanding that may predispose a patient to developing hypertensive crisis	Incident process	Transparencies	Clinical conference

Continued.

III. CARDIOVASCULAR COMPONENT—cont'd

Physiological effects of stress—cont'd

Topic	Participant objectives	Teaching method	Instructional media	Method of evaluation
2. Pathophysiology	2. Pathophysiology of hypertensive crises			
	a. To identify the primary physiological mechanisms responsible for control of mean arterial blood pressure	Lecture, discussion Incident process	Readings Campbell, WB: Axioms on malignant hypertension.	Multiple-choice item Clinical discussion
	b. To explain the essential pathological defect of hypertension in terms of Starling's law of the heart	Lecture, discussion	Finnerty: Hypertensive crisis, pp. 32, 34. Finnerty: Aggressive drug therapy, pp. 2178-2179. Shank and Ludewig: pp. 679-680.	Completion item
	c. To describe how the five mechanisms that regulate arterial blood pressure normally function as blood pressure levels vary	Lecture, discussion	Transparencies	Essay item Clinical discussion
	d. To specify the interrelation of renin, angiotensin I and II, and aldosterone in control of blood pressure	Lecture Incident process	Slides	Written testing
	e. To identify the progressive vascular changes associated with sustained hypertension	Lecture, discussion	Transparencies	True-false item
	f. To recognize the major end organs usually affected by progressive hypertensive disease	Incident process	Chalkboard Netter illustrations	True-false item
	g. To describe the pathological sequelae of severe hypertension observed in each of the affected end organs	Lecture, discussion Incident process	Chalkboard Netter illustrations	Clinical discussion Multiple-choice item
	h. To specify the cardiac compensatory mechanisms observed in patients with severe hypertension	Class discussion	Chalkboard	Written testing Clinical conference
	i. To explain the pathophysiology of hypertensive encephalopathy	Lecture, discussion Incident process	Slides Chalkboard	Multiple-choice item Clinical discussion
3. Clinical assessment	3. To perform clinical and laboratory evaluation of the patient in hypertensive crisis			
	a. To identify the clinical complications that may be anticipated in each of the end organs affected by severe hypertension	Lecture Class discussion Incident process	Readings Campbell: pp. 10-12. Finnerty: Hypertensive crisis, p. 34.	Multiple-choice item Clinical conference

	Objective	Learning experiences	Resources	Evaluation
	b. To classify a patient's degree of hypertension according to the development of complications	Lecture, discussion	Finnerty: Aggressive drug therapy, p. 2179.	True-false item
	c. To differentiate between the early and late clinical signs of hypertensive vascular disease	Lecture / Incident process	Transparencies	Multiple-choice item
	d. To demonstrate the proper technique of funduscopic examination	Laboratory session / Clinical instruction / Preceptor	Transparencies / Ophthalmascope / Assigned patients	Return demonstration of ability in lab and clinical settings / Written testing
	e. To recognize the varying findings of normal and pathological funduscopic architecture	Lecture / Clinical instruction / Preceptor	CIBA slides	Clinical demonstration of ability
	f. To describe the clinical significance and appearance of papilledema	Lecture, discussion / Bedside rounds	Slides	Multiple-choice item
	g. To explain how to assess a patient for development of the end-organ complications of hypertension	Incident process	Readings / Campbell. / Finnerty: Aggressive drug therapy, p. 2179.	Clinical demonstration of ability: rating scale / Written testing
	h. To delineate the clinical features of a patient in hypertensive crisis	Lecture, discussion / Incident process / Clinical instruction	Slides	Multiple-choice item / Clinical discussion / Demonstration of ability
	i. To demonstrate how to measure correctly a patient's arterial blood pressure	Return demonstration with preceptor	Videotape / Measuring arterial blood pressure.	Videotape
4. Clinical problems	4. To set the priority of clinical problems associated with hypertensive crisis			
	a. To identify the clinical problems of a patient in hypertensive crisis according to the end-organ involved	Lecture, discussion	Readings / Campbell. / Finnerty. / Shank and Ludewig.	Multiple-choice item / Clinical discussion
	b. To rank the clinical problems of patients in hypertensive crisis according to their immediacy	Class discussion	Chalkboard	Completion item / Clinical conference
	c. From the priority of clinical problems identified, to state the objectives of care for nursing management of patients with hypertensive crisis	Homework: written record of nursing care objectives / Incident process	Nursing care plans (kardex)	Review of written objectives (kardex)

Continued.

III. CARDIOVASCULAR COMPONENT—cont'd

Physiological effects of stress—cont'd

Topic	Participant objectives	Teaching method	Instructional media	Method of evaluation
5. Modes of therapy	5. To describe currently available modes of therapy for patients with hypertensive crisis			
	a. To identify the drugs of choice for hypertensive crisis, the rationale for their use, and their side effects	Lecture, discussion Bedside rounds	Transparencies	Multiple-choice item Clinical discussion
	b. To state the clinical precautions and disadvantages of selected antihypertensive agents	Bedside rounds	Handout Drugs used to control accelerated hypertension.	Completion item
	c. To specify the modes of therapy currently favored for treating the renal, cardiac, cerebral, and other end-organ dysfunctions of severe hypertension	Class discussion Incident process	Chalkboard	Clinical discussion Multiple-choice item
	d. To recognize the clinical criteria used for judging the effectiveness of therapy in patients with hypertensive crisis	Lecture, discussion Bedside rounds	Chalkboard	Multiple-choice item Clinical conference
	e. To describe areas in need of predischarge instruction for patients (and their families) who are hypertensive	Class discussion Team conference	Handouts National Institutes of Health: Patient education in high blood pressure. National Institutes of Health: The 120/80 notebook.	Review of written care plans (kardex)
	f. To identify nursing interventions that may reduce the noncompliance problem observed in hypertensive patients	Team conference	Reading Shank and Ludewig.	Clinical conference Case study
	g. To formulate a written discharge plan of care for a hypertensive patient.	Homework: incorporate into kardex plan of care	Nursing care plan (kardex)	Review of written plan
G. Patients requiring surgery for peripheral arterial insufficiency 1. Pathogenesis	G. To describe the rationale for nursing management of patients with peripheral arterial insufficiency as determined by the: 1. Pathogenesis of various forms and locations of peripheral arterial disease		Slides Readings Roberts, B: The acutely ischemic limb.	
	a. To identify the peripheral arteries most commonly affected by occlusive arterial processes	Lecture, discussion	Spittell, JA, and Schirger, A: Occlusive arterial disease.	Multiple-choice item Clinical conference
	b. To enumerate the anatomical and physiological characteristics of these arterial occlusion sites that predispose them to occlusive episodes	Class discussion Lecture	Wheeler, HB: Management of acute arterial insufficiency.	Multiple-choice item
	c. To specify the most common clinical causes of acute arterial insufficiency relative to its location	Lecture, discussion	Chalkboard	Clinical discussion Matching item
	d. To recognize the risk factors associated with arterial occlusive disease	Case study	Slides	Clinical conference Multiple-choice item

328

Objective	Teaching method	Resources	Evaluation
e. To specify the cardiac conditions most frequently associated with arterial emboli	Lecture, discussion	Reading Roberts: p. 274. Chalkboard	Clinical conference Multiple-choice item
f. To identify the patient population at greatest risk for the development of acute peripheral arterial occlusive disease	Class discussion Case study	Slides	Clinical conference Written testing
2. Pathophysiology Pathophysiology of the various forms of arterial insufficiency			
a. To distinguish and differentiate the pathophysiology of large vessel arterial disease and that of small vessel arterial disease	Lecture Class discussion	Reading Cobey and Cobey. Chalkboard	Essay item
b. To compare and contrast the pathophysiology of peripheral arterial occlusive disease caused by arterial embolization and that caused by arterial thrombosis	Class discussion	Readings Robert: p. 273, 275. Spittell: pp. 31-33.	
c. To describe the mechanisms by which local trauma may produce arterial insufficiency	Lecture Class discussion	Spittell: p. 31. Wheeler: p. 852. Chalkboard	Clinical conference Completion item
d. To identify the major factors involved in the pathophysiology of aortic aneurysms	Written simulation	Chalkboard Slides	Multiple-choice item
3. Clinical assessment To perform clinical and laboratory evaluation of the patient with peripheral arterial insufficiency.			
a. To demonstrate how to evaluate major peripheral arterial pulses: (1) Temporal (2) Carotid (3) Subclavian (4) Brachial (5) Radial (6) Ulnar (7) Abdominal aortic (8) Femoral (9) Popliteal (10) Dorsalis pedis (11) Posterior tibialis	Clinical instruction and reinforcement with preceptor	Reading Sparks. Slides	Clinical demonstration of ability to evaluate Videotape
b. To recognize the usual order of signs and symptoms that develop following peripheral artery occlusion	Case study	Reading Roberts: pp. 273-274. Chalkboard	Multiple-choice item Clinical discussion
c. To identify the clinical picture presented with embolization at an arterial bifurcation	Class discussion	Slides	Clinical conference Written testing: video-trainer
d. To specify the clinical significance of claudication and the presence of arterial bruits in a patient with peripheral arterial disease	Case study Class discussion	Readings Spittell: p. 21.	Multiple-choice item Clinical conference
e. To identify the clinical findings to anticipate observing in a patient with arterial insufficiency to an extremity	Class discussion Case study	Wheeler: p. 852. Slides	Clinical discussion Multiple-choice item
f. To specify the most reliable index of tissue viability in peripheral arterial insufficiency and cerebrovascular insufficiency	Class discussion	Slides	Completion item
g. To describe the clinical significance of unequal arterial blood pressure readings in the arms	Written simulation	Slides	Multiple-choice item Clinical conference
h. To describe how to assess the effect of postural changes in evaluating the degree of arterial insufficiency	Clinical instruction with preceptor	Readings Spittell: pp. 21-22.	Clinical demonstration of ability to assess Essay item

Continued.

III. CARDIOVASCULAR COMPONENT—cont'd

Topic	Participant objectives	Teaching method	Instructional media	Method of evaluation
Physiological effects of stress—cont'd	i. To identify the cardinal and associated signs and symptoms of acute arterial occlusion in an extremity	Lecture, discussion	Slides	Clinical conference
	j. To recognize the signs and symptoms of a dissecting thoracic or abdominal aortic aneurysm	Written simulation Written simulation	Chalkboard	Multiple-choice item Multiple-choice item
	k. To describe how the following diagnostic procedures may assist in evaluating the extent of peripheral arterial insufficiency: (1) Ultrasonic flow detector (2) Plethysmography (3) Radioisotopic tracers (4) Ophthalmodynamometry	Class discussion Case study	Videotape Detection of peripheral arterial disease.	Matching item Clinical discussion
4. Clinical problems	4. To set the priority of clinical problems associated with peripheral arterial insufficiency			
	a. To identify the common clinical problems posed by acute arterial insufficiency in the peripheral arteries and the aorta	Class discussion Case study	Markerboard	Clinical conference Completion item
	b. To differentiate between the priority of clinical problems associated with arterial insufficiency in an extremity and that occurring in cerebral, mesenteric, and aortic vasculature	Lecture, discussion	Markerboard	Multiple-choice item Clinical discussion
	c. To recognize how surgery for peripheral arterial occlusion or insufficiency affects the priority of clinical problems	Class discussion Case study	Markerboard	Clinical conference Written testing; case study
	d. To identify the primary indications and contraindications for surgery for arterial insufficiency	Lecture, discussion	Reading Spittell and Schirger: pp. 23, 27, 35.	Clinical conference Multiple-choice item
	e. To state the objectives of care for nursing management of patients with acute arterial insufficiency	Case study	Markerboard	Written testing Review of written objectives
5. Modes of therapy a. Nonoperative	5. a. To describe currently available modes of therapy for the patient having acute arterial insufficiency	Class discussion	Readings Breslau, RC: Intensive care following vascular surgery. Roberts: pp. 275-276. Spittell and Schirger: p. 23, 27, 34-35. Wheeler: pp. 858-861.	Clinical conference
	(1) To describe the nonoperative measures to use in caring for a patient with arterial insufficiency, together with the rationale for each measure	Clinical instruction and reinforcement with preceptor		Essay item

	(2) To specify the rationale, advantages and disadvantages for each of the following in the care of a patient with arterial insufficiency: (a) Heparin therapy (b) Sympathectomy (c) Fogarty catheter embolectomy (d) LMW Dextran	Lecture, discussion Case study	Markerboard Transparencies	Multiple-choice item Clinical conference
b. Operative	b. To delineate the postoperative nursing responsibilities in caring for a patient with each of the following types of vascular surgery: (1) Carotid endarterectomy (2) Thoracic and abdominal aortic aneurysm resection and graft (3) Aorto-iliac endarterectomy (4) Aorto-iliac resection and graft (5) Aorto-femoral resection and graft (6) Femoral-popliteal graft	Lecture, discussion Case study	Markerboard Slides	Clinical conference Essay item
H. Patients with disseminated intravascular coagulation (DIC) 1. Pathogenesis	H. To describe the rationale for nursing management of patients with disseminated intravascular coagulation as determined by the: 1. Pathogenesis of DIC a. To recognize the various clinical references used to describe DIC	Lecture, discussion	Slides Readings Colman, R, Mihna, J, and Robboy, S: Disseminated intravascular coagulation: a problem in critical care medicine.	Multiple-choice item
	b. To characterize the primary clinical factors of DIC	Lecture, discussion Clinical rounds		Clinical conference Multiple-choice item
	c. To identify DIC as a secondary vs primary clinical disorder	Class discussion	Mayer, GG: Disseminated intravascular coagulation.	Clinical discussion
	d. To specify the primary clinical conditions or mechanisms associated with DIC and the clinical factor common to all	Class discussion Bedside rounds	Witmer, SE: Disseminated intravascular coagulation.	Multiple-choice item
	e. To characterize the patient population most at risk for developing DIC	Class discussion Clinical rounds		Clinical conference Completion item

Continued.

III. CARDIOVASCULAR COMPONENT—cont'd

Topic	Participant objectives	Teaching method	Instructional media	Method of evaluation
Physiological effects of stress— cont'd				
2. Pathophysiology	2. Pathophysiology of DIC			
	a. To describe DIC in terms of its relationship to normal hemostatic mechanisms	Lecture, discussion Clinical rounds	DIC slide-tape	True-false item Clinical conference
	b. To differentiate between the primary features of intrinsic coagulation and those of extrinsic coagulation	Lecture	Chalkboard	True-false item
	c. To describe the major role and mechanisms involved in fibrinolysis	Lecture, discussion	DIC slide-tape	Essay item
	d. To delineate the primary phases involved in the normal hemostatic mechanism	Lecture, discussion	Readings Byrne, J: Coagulation studies. Part I. Witmer: pp. 5-6.	Completion item
	e. To identify the basic pathophysiological defect associated with DIC	Class discussion Clinical reinforcement		Clinical conference Multiple-choice item
	f. To identify the possible mechanisms that may precipitate DIC	Bedside rounds	Colman: p. 792. Witmer: p. 7.	Multiple-choice item
	g. To describe the three major pathophysiological processes involved in DIC and the clinical effects of each	Lecture, discussion Clinical reinforcement	DIC slide-tape	Clinical discussion Written testing
	h. To recognize the three clinical forms of DIC based on the rapidity of clotting	Class discussion	DIC slide-tape	Clinical conference
	i. To identify the variables that determine the clinical severity of DIC	Class discussion	Readings Colman: pp. 792-793. Mayer: p. 2068.	Clinical conference Written testing Case study
3. Clinical assessment	3. To perform clinical and laboratory evaluation of the patient suspected of having DIC			
	a. To identify the signs and symptoms to anticipate finding in a patient with DIC	Lecture, discussion Game: DICE	Selected patients Game materials Dice Cards Markerboard	Multiple-choice item
	b. To relate the clinical picture of DIC to its pathophysiological causes	Game: DICE	Chalkboard	Clinical ability to relate Multiple-choice item
	c. To recognize a variety of subtle clinical clues to the presence of DIC	Lecture Game: DICE	Selected patients	Clinical ability to recognize: rating scale Written testing
	d. To define, recognize, and relate the following to the pathophysiology of DIC: (1) Petechiae (2) Purpura	Lecture, discussion Clinical rounds Game: DICE	Reading Witmer: p. 10.	Clinical ability to recognize and relate Matching item

Topic	Objective	Teaching method	Resources / Readings	Evaluation
	(3) Hemorrhagic bullae (4) Acrocyanosis			
	e. To specify the hematologic and coagulation studies most pertinent to verifying the diagnosis of DIC	Lecture Clinical rounds	DIC slide-tape	Clinical discussions Multiple-choice item
	f. To relate the normal and abnormal findings of coagulation studies used to support the diagnosis of DIC, specifying the reasons for the observed abnormalities	Clinical rounds Lecture Game: DICE	Readings Bryne: Part I. Bryne, J: Coagulation studies. Part II. Tests of plasma clotting factors. Mayer: pp. 2068-2069. Witmer: pp. 10-12. DIC slide-tape Readings	Clinical ability to relate Written testing
4. Clinical problems	To set the priority of clinical problems associated with DIC	Game: DICE		Written testing Clinical conference
	a. To enumerate the spectrum of clinical problems posed by DIC	Class discussion Clinical rounds	Mayer: pp. 2068-2069. Witmer: pp. 10-11. DIC slide-tape	Clinical conference Multiple-choice item
	b. To rank the clinical problems associated with DIC in their relative order of immediacy	Class discussion		Review of written objectives
	c. To list the objectives of care for nursing management of the patient with DIC according to the priority of clinical problems identified	Class discussion Clinical rounds Homework: written objectives of care for patient with DIC	Nursing care plans (kardex)	
5. Modes of therapy	To describe currently available modes of therapy for the patient with DIC	Game: DICE	Readings Colman: pp. 793-796.	Multiple-choice item Clinical conference
	a. To identify the therapeutic agent of choice for treatment of DIC, and the rationale and regime for its use	Lecture, discussion Clinical rounds	Mayer: pp. 2068-2069. Witmer: pp. 11-12; 14-15.	Clinical discussion Completion item
	b. To specify the blood component therapy that may be used in the management of patients with DIC and the potential hazards associated with its administration	Lecture, discussion Clinical instruction and reinforcement	DIC slide-tape	Clinical conference Multiple-choice item
	c. To describe appropriate nursing interventions for each of the clinical problems faced by patients with DIC	Class discussion Lecture Game: DICE	DIC slide-tape	Multiple-choice item
	d. To identify appropriate therapy in managing the primary disorders associated with DIC	Class discussion Clinical rounds		Multiple-choice item

Continued.

IV. NEUROLOGICAL COMPONENT

Topic	Participant objectives	Teaching method	Instructional media	Method of evaluation
Physiological effects of stress—cont'd ■ Functional neurological anatomy	To describe the functional anatomy of the neurological system in terms of its correlation and application to nursing management of patients with neurological dysfunctions			
	1. To specify the functional significance of the major divisions and subdivisions of the central nervous system	Lecture, discussion	Physical simulations CNS Peripheral system	Matching item
	2. To identify the functional divisions of the peripheral nervous system and the respective physiological features of each	Lecture, discussion	CIBA slides CNS model	Matching item
	3. To describe the anatomical location of the eight cranial bones	Lecture, discussion	CIBA slides CNS model	Written testing: diagram

	4. To define each of the following according to its clinical significance:
	  a. Galea aponeurotica
	  b. Diploic space
	  c. Cranial fossae
		Lecture	Chalkboard	Multiple-choice item

	5. To differentiate between the anatomical features of cervical vertebrae and those of thoracic and lumbar vertebrae	Lecture Class discussion	CIBA slides CNS model	Multiple-choice item
	6. To describe the anatomy of a representative vertebra	Lecture, discussion	CIBA slides Chalkboard Vertebra model	Written testing: slide illustration
	7. To compare and contrast the structural, physiological and vulnerability characteristics of the three meningeal layers and three meningeal spaces	Lecture, discussion Case study	Slides CNS model	Clinical conference Multiple-choice item
	8. To identify the major functions of each component of a neuron	Lecture, discussion	Slides	Matching item
	9. To describe the synthesis and functional significance of the myelin sheath	Lecture, discussion	Slides	Multiple-choice item Clinical discussion
	10. To identify the primary functions of each division and major subdivision of cerebral structure	Lecture, discussion Case study	CIBA slides CNS model	Matching item Clinical conference
	11. To differentiate between the composition of gray matter and white matter	Lecture	Chalkboard	Multiple-choice item
	12. To describe the synthesis and circulation of cerebrospinal fluid	Lecture, discussion	CIBA slides CNS model	Clinical discussion Essay item
	13. To compare and contrast the functional anatomy of the carotid arterial system with that of the vertebrobasilar arterial system in providing for perfusion to specific cerebral areas	Lecture, discussion Case study	CIBA slides CNS model	Written testing Clinical conference
	14. To specify the blood vessels that comprise the circle of Willis	Class discussion	CIBA slides CNS model	Completion item

Neurological physiology	To describe neurological physiology in terms of its correlation and application to nursing management of the patient with neurological system dysfunction		Videocassette Neurophysiology.	
	1. To delineate the major structures and events involved in transmission of nerve impulses	Lecture, discussion	Reading Hewitt, W: Functional neuroanatomy for nurses. Slides	Essay item
	2. To identify the factors that alter the speed of impulse transmission	Class discussion	Slides	Multiple-choice item
	3. To compare and contrast impulse conduction along an unmyelinated nerve fiber and that along a myelinated nerve fiber	Lecture, discussion	Chalkboard Videocassette Neurophysiology.	Multiple-choice item
	4. To specify the functional significance of the following: a. Nodes of Ranvier b. Saltatory conduction c. Nissl granules d. Schwann cells e. Oligodendrocytes	Lecture, discussion	Slides Videocassette Neurophysiology.	Multiple-choice item
	5. To relate the primary functions controlled by the various spinal cord tracts	Lecture Clinical rounds	CNS Model Videocassette Neurophysiology.	Clinical discussion Matching item
	6. To enumerate the anatomical structures responsible for control of: a. Level of consciousness b. Pupillary responses c. Motor function d. Cardiovascular responses e. Respiratory responses f. Vital signs g. Sensory ability	Lecture, discussion Clinical rounds	CIBA slides Videocassette Neurophysiology.	Clinical conference Multiple-choice item
	7. To identify the primary functions served by cerebrospinal fluid	Class discussion	Chalkboard Videocassette Neurophysiology.	True-false item
	8. To specify the role of pacchionian granules in CSF physiology	Lecture	Chalkboard Videocassette Neurophysiology.	Multiple-choice item
	9. To distinguish the substrates normally used in cerebral metabolism from those used in compromised states of perfusion	Lecture, discussion Case study	Chalkboard Videocassette Neurophysiology.	Multiple-choice item Clinical conference
	10. To define cerebral "autoregulation" and to describe the cerebral responses to altered circulatory requirements	Lecture, discussion Case study	Chalkboard Neurophysiology.	Multiple-choice item Clinical conference
	11. To explain the components and physiology of a reflex arc	Lecture, discussion	CIBA slides Videocassette Neurophysiology.	Essay item

Continued.

Topic	Participant objectives	Teaching method	Instructional media	Method of evaluation
Physiological effects of stress— cont'd	12. To characterize CSF fluid in terms of its: a. Variable pressures b. Limits of normal pressure c. Pressure correlation with overt signs and symptoms d. Acid-base physiology	Lecture, discussion Clinical preceptor with reinforcement	Reading Mitchell, PH, and Mauss, N: Intracranial pressure: fact and fancy. Videocassette Neurophysiology.	True-false item Clinical discussion
	13. To specify the function of the major neurotransmitters	Class discussion Lecture		Multiple-choice item
■ Clinical assessment of the neurological system	To perform clinical and laboratory evaluation of the patient with suspected or actual neurological system dysfunction		Handout Nursing neurological assessment.	
	1. To identify five parameters of generalized cerebral function to use in initiating a neurological assessment and describe how these may be evaluated and described	Class discussion Clinical preceptor Simulated patients	Reading Alexander, MM, and Brown, MS: Neurological examination. Part 17. Selected patients	Essay item Clinical demonstration of ability to identify and describe
	2. To specify how to determine validly and describe appropriately a patient's: a. Level of consciousness b. Pupillary size and responses	Role model Clinical instruction and reinforcement Simulated patients	Readings Alexander and Brown: Part 17. Alexander, MM, and Brown, MS: Neurological examination. Part 18.	Written testing with videotape and performance checklist
	c. Eye movements d. Respiratory pattern e. Sensory responses and reflexes f. Motor responses g. Cranial nerve integrity h. Posturing	Simulated patients Demonstration with preceptor	Bordeaux, MP: The intensive-care unit and observation of the patient acutely ill with neurologic disease. Gifford, RRM, and Plant, MR: Abnormal respiratory patterns in the comatose patient caused by intracranial dysfunction. Gifford, RRM, and Plant, MR: On describing altered state of consciousness.	Clinical demonstration of ability to determine and describe Performance checklist

3. To interpret normal and abnormal CNS functioning in relation to its clinical significance, implications for nursing care, and prognostic indications	Lecture, discussion Clinical rounds	Handout Cranial nerves. Handout Neurological and neurosurgical nursing assessment: a glossary of pertinent terms and observations.	Written testing Clinical demonstration of ability to interpret Bedside rounds with rating scale
4. To perform satisfactorily and record appropriately a neurological assessment	Performance checklist	Selected patients Form Neurological assessment.	Clinical demonstration of ability to perform and record Performance checklist Videotape Review of recordings
5. To correlate abnormal CSF lab values with their pathophysiological significance and clinical implications for care	Lecture, discussion Clinical rounds	Selected patient charts Chalkboard	Written testing Clinical conference Simulated situations
6. To assist and describe how to assist with a lumbar puncture and perform the attendant nursing responsibilities	Clinical instruction Role model demonstration Simulated situation	Readings McGuckin, M: Tips for assisting with cultures of CSF and other body fluids.	Clinical demonstration of ability to assist Essay item
7. To identify the purpose and nursing responsibilities involved in various radiological examinations of the neurological system: a. Cerebral angiography b. Cerebral echoencephalogram c. EEG d. CAT scan e. Pneumoencephalogram f. Myelogram	Lecture, discussion Bedside rounds Chart review	Blackwell, CA: PEG and angiography: a patient's sensations. Pohutsky, LC, and Pohutsky, KR: Computerized axial tomography of the brain: a new diagnostic tool. Selected patient charts	Multiple-choice item Clinical discussion
8. To describe the principles and nursing responsibilities involved with intracranial pressure monitoring	Lecture, discussion Clinical rounds with preceptor	Readings Bell, M, Lorig, RJ, and Weiss, MH: Nursing involvement with monitoring of ICP. Hanlon, K: Description and uses of intracranial pressure monitoring. See readings in acute head trauma section.	Multiple-choice item Clinical conference Workshop on ICPM

Continued.

IV. NEUROLOGICAL COMPONENT—cont'd

Topic	Participant objectives	Teaching method	Instructional media	Method of evaluation
Physiological effects of stress— cont'd				
■ Patients with neurological system dysfunction	To describe the rationale for and provide for nursing management of patients with neurological system dysfunction			
A. Patients with an acute cerebrovascular accident (CVA)	A. To describe the rationale for and provide for nursing management of patients with an acute cerebrovascular accident (CVA) as determined by the:			
1. Pathogenesis	1. Pathogenesis of CVA			
	a. To define the term "stroke"	Lecture, discussion	Programmed instruction Stroke.	Clinical conference True-false item
			Reading Feldman, JL, and Schultz, ME: Rehabilitation after stroke.	
	b. To recognize the major epidemiological characteristics of stroke in the US population.	Lecture	Programmed instruction Stroke.	Clinical discussion
	c. To enumerate the precipitating factors in stroke categorized by the American Heart Association's listing of the "stroke-prone profile"	Class discussion	Chalkboard	True-false item Clinical conference
	d. To identify the clinical problems that usually accompany stroke	Multiple assignment	Programmed instruction Stroke.	Completion item
	e. To characterize the patient population at greatest risk for developing stroke	Lecture, discussion Clinical rounds	Programmed instruction Stroke.	True-false item Clinical conference
	f. From a listing of the various etiological causes of stroke, to identify the three primary causes of stroke.	Class discussion	Programmed instruction Stroke.	Completion item
	g. To specify the evolutionary stages (temporal profile) of a CVA	Lecture, discussion Multiple assignment	Chalkboard	Multiple-choice item Clinical conference Completion item
	h. To define a transient ischemic attack (TIA) and state its relationship to the pathogenesis of stroke	Lecture, discussion	Reading Keller, MR, and Truscott, BL. Transient ischemic attacks.	
	i. To differentiate between the predisposing factors of cerebral thrombosis, embolism, and hemorrhage	Class discussion	Programmed instruction Stroke.	Multiple-choice item
2. Pathophysiology	2. Pathophysiology of acute CVA		Programmed instruction Stroke.	

Objective	Teaching Method	Resource	Evaluation
a. To compare and contrast the pathophysiology of cerebral thrombosis, embolism, and hemorrhage	Lecture, discussion; Clinical rounds	Readings Elwood, E: Nursing the patient with a cerebrovascular accident.	Multiple-choice item
b. To describe the pathophysiological features of a TIA	Lecture, discussion	Feldman and Schultz: pp. 29-30. Keller and Truscott.	Multiple-choice item
c. To describe the major pathophysiological features of a cerebral aneurysm in relation to the development of subarachnoid hemorrhage	Lecture, discussion; Case study	Breunig, KA: After the blowup. . . . how to care for the patient with a ruptured aneurysm.	Clinical discussion; Multiple-choice item
d. To specify the pathophysiological significance of cerebral A-V malformation in the pathogenesis of CVAs	Lecture, discussion; Case study	Toole: pp. 13-14. Programmed instruction Stroke.	True-false item
e. To compare and contrast the overall prognosis of patients incurring cerebral thrombosis and those incurring cerebral embolism and hemorrhage	Lecture, discussion; Clinical reinforcement	Programmed instruction Stroke.	True-false item; Clinical conference
f. To identify the effects of an acute CVA on cerebral autoregulation	Lecture; Clinical rounds	Chalkboard	Essay item
3. Clinical assessment To perform clinical and laboratory evaluation of the patient with an acute CVA		Readings Bruenig: pp. 37-39; 42-43. Elwood: pp. 48-50.	
a. To distinguish the clinical history characteristic of patients with cerebral thrombosis from that of patients with cerebral embolism and hemorrhage	Bedside rounds	Programmed instruction Stroke.	Matching item
b. To compare and contrast the clinical presentation of patients having cerebral thrombosis and that of patients having cerebral embolism and hemorrhage	Lecture; Clinical rounds	Selected patients	Matching item; Clinical conference
c. To distinguish between decerebrate and decorticate posturing	Performance checklist	Selected patients	Demonstrated ability to distinguish: checklist
d. To correlate the laboratory values of CSF in acute stroke with their pathophysiological causes	Lecture, discussion; Clinical rounds	Chalkboard; Selected patients	Matching item; Demonstrated ability to correlate
e. To differentiate between the clinical picture of middle cerebral artery CVAs and that of vertebrobasilar CVAs	Clinical instruction; Written simulation	Chalkboard; Programmed instruction Stroke.	Multiple-choice item
f. To explain how to determine the temporal profile of an acute CVA	Class discussion; Clinical preceptor	Selected patients	Written testing; Demonstrated ability to determine
g. To differentiate between the clinical presentation of TIA and that of acute CVA	Lecture, discussion	Programmed instruction Stroke.	Matching item

Continued.

IV. NEUROLOGICAL COMPONENT—cont'd

Physiological effects of stress—cont'd

Topic	Participant objectives	Teaching method	Instructional media	Method of evaluation
4. Clinical problems	4. To set the priority of clinical problems associated with the various types of acute CVA			
	a. To specify the general clinical problems to anticipate in patients with acute CVA	Class discussion / Nursing care conference	Readings / Feldman and Schultz: pp. 30-34. / Guidelines to stroke-patient care	Multiple-choice item / Clinical conference
	b. To distinguish between the anticipated clinical problems of patients having cerebral thrombosis and those having embolism and hemorrhage	Lecture / Class discussion	Chalkboard	Matching item / Clinical conference
	c. To enumerate an appropriate priority of anticipated clinical problems in patients with acute CVA according to their life-threatening potential	Multiple assignment	Chalkboard	Multiple-choice item
	d. To contrast the objectives of care for the patient with an acute CVA during the acute phase with those applicable during the rehabilitative phase of care	Multiple assignment / Homework: written objectives of care	Selected patients / Nursing care plans (kardex)	Essay item / Review of written objectives
5. Modes of therapy	5. To describe currently available modes of therapy for the patient with acute CVA			
	a. To explain the rationale for various modes of therapy used for the patient with acute CVA during the acute phase of care	Lecture, discussion / Nursing care conference	Readings / Bruenig: pp. 39-40; 44-45. / Elwood. / Schultz, LCM: Nursing care of the stroke patient—rehabilitative aspects.	Essay item / Clinical conference
	b. To identify the complications of acute CVA the nurse must take measures to prevent during the acute phase of care, and the interventions appropriate for each	Class discussion / Nursing care conference	Chalkboard / Programmed instruction. Stroke.	Multiple-choice item / Clinical conference
	c. To specify the indications and contraindications of anticoagulant therapy in patients with acute CVA	Bedside rounds	Selected patients	True-false item
	d. To recognize the indications and contraindications of surgical therapy in patients with acute CVA	Class discussion	Programmed instruction. Stroke.	True-false item
	e. To delineate the primary modes of care appropriate to each stage of recovery following acute CVA	Lecture, discussion / Clinical conference	Chalkboard	Completion item / Clinical conference
B. Patients with acute head trauma	B. To describe the rationale for nursing management of patients with acute head trauma as determined by the:			

Content	Objectives	Methods	Resources	Evaluation
1. Pathogenesis	1. Various types and classifications involved in the pathogenesis of acute head trauma		Readings Berkovsky, D: Physiological effects of closed head injury. Hinkhouse, A: Craniocerebral trauma. Swift, N: Head injury: essentials of excellent care.	
	a. To identify the anatomical characteristics that make certain cranial vault areas more vulnerable to traumatic insult	Lecture, discussion		Multiple-choice item
	b. To differentiate the structural alterations produced by the following types of acute head trauma: (1) Cerebral concussion (2) Cerebral contusion (3) Simple skull fracture (4) Comminuted skull fracture (5) Depressed skull fracture (6) Compound skull fracture (7) Hematomas: (a) Epidural (b) Subdural (c) Intracerebral (8) Gunshot wound	Lecture, discussion Written simulations Written simulations	CIBA slides Chalkboard CIBA slides	Clinical conference Multiple-choice item Multiple-choice item
2. Pathophysiology	2. Pathophysiology of various types of acute head trauma		Readings Berkovsky.	
	a. To compare and contrast the primary pathophysiological features associated with the various types of acute head trauma	Lecture, discussion Nursing team conference	Glass, SJ: Nursing care of the neurosurgical patient: head injuries. Hinkhouse. Swift: pp. 27-30.	Multiple-choice item Clinical discussion
	b. To distinguish between the clinical courses and clinical significances of subdural and epidural hematomas	Case studies	Written case histories	Clinical conference Matching item
	c. To explain why diabetes insipidus and stress ulcers may be observed in the patient who has sustained head trauma	Lecture Clinical rounds	Selected patients	Essay item Clinical discussion
3. Clinical assessment	3. To perform clinical and laboratory evaluation of the patient with acute head trauma		Readings Berkovsky. Glass: pp. 50-52. Hinkhouse. Swift: pp. 30-32.	
	a. To specify the advantages of computerized axial tomography over arteriography and burr holes in evaluating the patient with acute head trauma	Lecture, discussion		Multiple-choice item
	b. To rank the relative importance of neurological parameters to be assessed in the patient with acute head trauma	Class discussion Clinical rounds	Slides	Clinical conference True-false item

Continued.

IV. NEUROLOGICAL COMPONENT—cont'd

Topic	Participant objectives	Teaching method	Instructional media	Method of evaluation
Physiological effects of stress—cont'd	c. To identify the signs and symptoms of herniation of the brainstem and of increased intracranial pressure	Lecture, discussion Clinical preceptor	Readings Bell. Hanlon. Jimm, LR: Nursing management of patients for increased intracranial pressure.	Multiple-choice item Clinical discussion
	d. To identify the clinical significance of otorrhea and rhinorrhea in a patient who has sustained head injury	Class discussion Clinical reinforcement		Multiple-choice item Clinical conference
4. Clinical problems	4. To set the priority of clinical problems associated with various types of acute head trauma			
	a. To specify the priority of the three most important clinical problems associated with various types of head trauma	Nursing team conference	Chalkboard	Multiple-choice item
	b. To correlate alterations in vital signs with their associated clinical significance in patients who have sustained cerebral trauma	Clinical rounds Lecture, discussion Case presentation	Chalkboard Selected patients	Matching item Review of case presentation
	c. To list the objectives of care for nursing management of the patient with head trauma	Class discussion Homework: written objectives of care	Chalkboard Nursing care plans (kardex)	Review of written objectives
5. Modes of therapy	5. To describe currently available modes of therapy for the patient having acute head trauma		Readings Glass: pp. 52-55. Hinkhouse: pp. 1720-1722. Swift: pp. 31-33. Wound suction	
	a. To correlate alterations in vital signs with their associated clinical significance in patients who have sustained cerebral trauma	Class discussion Clinical preceptor		Clinical discussion Matching item
	b. To indicate the rationale for using the following modes of therapy in management of the patient with head trauma: (1) Dexamethasone (Decadron)	Clinical instruction and reinforcement with preceptor Nursing team conference	CIBA slides	Multiple-choice item Clinical conference
	(2) Mannitol, urea (3) Steroids	Case presentation	Chalkboard Selected patients	Review of case presentation
	(4) Phenobarbital (5) Diphenylhydantoin (Dilantin) (6) Primidone (Mysoline) (7) Antibiotics (8) Restricted fluid intake (9) Hyperventilation (10) Antacids (11) Hypothermia, hyperthermia			

Content	Teaching methods	Resources	Evaluation
C. Patients with acute spinal cord trauma			
1. Pathogenesis			
c. To indicate the nursing responsibilities associated with these modes of therapy for the patient with acute head trauma	Class discussion / Team conference	Selected patients	Written testing / Clinical conference
C. To describe the rationale and provide for nursing management of the patient with acute spinal cord trauma as determined by the:			
1. Various types and classifications of injury associated with the pathogenesis of acute spinal cord trauma		Reading / Mack, EW, and Dawson, WN: Injury to the spine and spinal cord.	
a. To compare and contrast the arterial blood supplies of the three major spinal cord areas in relation to the relative adequacy of each for recovering from traumatic insult	Lecture, discussion / Clinical rounds	CIBA slides / Chalkboard	True-false item
b. To differentiate the potential structural damage produced by the following types of trauma at various levels of the spinal cord: (1) Simple fracture (2) Fracture dislocation (3) Hyperflexion (4) Hyperextension	Lecture, discussion / Clinical instruction and reinforcement with preceptor	CIBA slides / Chalkboard	Multiple-choice item / Clinical conference
2. Pathophysiology			
Pathophysiology of various types and levels of acute spinal cord trauma			
a. To describe the following types of traumatic spinal cord lesions and differentiate between their major pathophysiological features:	Lecture, discussion / Team conference	Readings / Culp, P: Nursing care of the patient with spinal cord injury. / Mack and Dawson: pp. 25-34. / Selected patients	Clinical discussion / Essay item
(1) Complete transsection	Case presentation		Clinical conference / Simulated situations
(2) Incomplete transsection (3) Contusion (4) Laceration (5) Herniated nucleus pulposus		CIBA slides	
b. To relate specific motor and sensory dysfunctions to their appropriate anatomical level of spinal cord injury	Lecture / Performance checklist	Selected patients	Clinical conference / Matching item
c. To describe the following clinical conditions in terms of their etiology, course, and clinical significance: (1) Spinal shock (2) Autonomic dysreflexia	Class discussion / Lecture / Clinical preceptor	Readings / Feustal, D: Autonomic dysreflexia. / Lindh and Rickerson: p. 41. / Talbot, HS: Adjunctive care of spinal cord injury.	Multiple-choice item

Continued.

343

IV. NEUROLOGICAL COMPONENT—cont'd

Physiological effects of stress—cont'd

Topic	Participant objectives	Teaching method	Instructional media	Method of evaluation
3. Clinical assessment	3. To perform clinical and laboratory evaluation of patients with acute spinal cord trauma			
	a. To identify the most relevant parameters that should be evaluated in a patient who has sustained various levels of spinal cord trauma	Class discussion Clinical reinforcement with preceptor	Culp. Feustel: pp. 228-229. Mack and Dawson: pp. 24-28, 33-34.	Written testing Clinical conference
	b. To specify the signs and symptoms characteristic of: (1) Spinal shock (2) Autonomic dysreflexia (3) Brown-Séquard syndrome	Lecture, discussion	Slides	Multiple-choice item Clinical conference
	c. To perform and indicate the nursing responsibilities in assisting with and appropriate location for performance of a lumbar puncture.	Class discussion Lecture Clinical instruction by preceptor	Filmstrip Assisting with lumbar puncture.	Clinical discussion and demonstration of ability to assist with an LP Rating scale
	d. To identify the clinical significance of Queckenstedt's test.	Lecture, discussion	CIBA slides	Multiple-choice item
4. Clinical problems	4. To set the priority and types of acute spinal trauma			
	a. To compare and contrast the priority of anticipated clinical problems following high cervical spine fracture and those of thoracic and sacral fractures	Class discussion Team conference	Readings Lindh and Rickerson: pp. 41-42. See next section readings.	Multiple-choice item Clinical conference
	b. To identify factors that predispose patients with spinal cord trauma to decubiti	Class discussion	Chalkboard	Clinical conference Multiple assignment
	c. To specify the priority of clinical problems resulting from spinal shock and autonomic dysreflexia	Lecture, discussion Team conference	Chalkboard	Multiple-choice item
	d. To enumerate the objectives of care for nursing management of patients with various levels and types of spinal cord trauma	Homework: written objectives of care	Nursing care plan (kardex)	Review of written objectives Case study
5. Modes of therapy	5. To describe currently available modes of therapy for the patient who has sustained acute spinal cord trauma			
	a. To specify the major modes of therapy used for meeting each objective of care	Team conference		Clinical conference
	b. To explain why tracheostomy may be preferred to endotracheal intubation in a patient with acute spinal cord trauma	Bedside rounds	Selected patients	Multiple-choice item
	c. To identify the appropriate nursing interventions necessitated by the development of autonomic dysreflexia	Lecture, discussion	Slides	

Content	Objectives	Teaching/learning activities	Resources	Evaluation
	d. To demonstrate how to use a Stryker frame and a Circoelectric bed in caring for a patient with acute spinal cord trauma	Laboratory practice session with student patients / Clinical instruction by preceptor / Performance checklist	Stryker frame / Circoelectric bed / Student patients / Selected patients as available	Clinical demonstration of ability to operate equipment safely / Performance checklist
	e. To demonstrate how to care for patients with various forms of cervical traction appliances (e.g., Crutchfield tongs)	Clinical instruction / Performance checklist	Various cervical traction appliances (Halo system, tongs)	Demonstration of ability to care for patients requiring these appliances / Clinical conference / Written testing
	f. To determine the general prognosis and rehabilitation potential of patients with various levels and types of spinal cord trauma	Lecture, discussion / Team conference	Chalkboard	Clinical conference / Case study
	g. To describe the patient teaching necessary before discharge for the quadriplegic patient and the family	Class discussion / Case study	Chalkboard	
D. Patients with acute meningitis	D. To describe the rationale and provide for nursing management of patients with acute meningitis as determined by the:			
1. Pathogenesis	1. Pathogenesis of the various types and classifications of acute meningitis	Lecture	Handout / Meningitis.	
	a. To describe the epidemiological and clinical situations that may predispose a patient to develop acute meningitis	Lecture, discussion / Clinical reinforcement / Review of charts	Readings / Hyslop, NE, and Swartz, MN: Bacterial meningitis.	Multiple-choice item / Clinical discussion
	b. To identify the most common organisms implicated in a bacterial meningitis	Chart review / Lecture	Meade, RH, Ross, S, and Wehrle, PF: Relearning to cope with meningitis.	
2. Pathophysiology	2. Pathophysiology of various types and classifications of acute meningitis		Smith, DH: The challenge of bacterial meningitis.	
	a. To identify the routes of infection in acute meningitis in terms of their viral or bacterial vs posttraumatic etiology	Class discussion	Selected patient charts	Clinical conference / Written testing
	b. To differentiate between the pathophysiology of meningitis and that of encephalitis.	Lecture, discussion		True-false item
	c. To describe the major pathophysiological features of acute meningitis	Case study		Multiple-choice item
	d. To specify the pathological features of the Waterhouse-Friderichsen syndrome	Lecture, discussion	Slides	Multiple-choice item
3. Clinical assessment	3. To perform psychophysical and laboratory evaluation of the patient with aute meningitis		Readings / See readings above.	
	a. To distinguish and differentiate the typical clinical course of a patient with bacterial vs viral meningitis in terms of their history and anticipated clinical presentation	Lecture, discussion	Chalkboard	Clinical conference / Matching item

Continued.

IV. NEUROLOGICAL COMPONENT—cont'd

Topic	Participant objectives	Teaching method	Instructional media	Method of evaluation
Physiological effects of stress—cont'd				
	b. To compare and contrast the CSF findings of bacterial and viral meningitis	Class discussion Clinical reinforcement	Overhead projector	Matching item
	c. To identify and state the clinical significance of a positive Brudzinski's sign	Lecture, discussion	Slides	Multiple-choice item
	d. To rank the most important clinical parameters to assess in a patient with acute meningitis	Class discussion Bedside rounds		Clinical conference
4. Clinical problems	4. To set the priority of clinical problems associated with various types and etiologies of acute meningitis		Readings See readings above.	
	a. To compare and contrast the priority of clinical problems associated with bacterial meningitis and viral (aseptic) meningitis	Lecture, discussion Clinical rounds	Chalkboard	Clinical discussion Matching item
	b. To differentiate how development of the Waterhouse-Friderichsen syndrome alters the priority of clinical problems associated with bacterial and viral meningitis	Lecture, discussion	Slides	Multiple-choice item
	c. To identify the potential clinical complications of meningitis and how to recognize the appearance of each	Clinical instruction and reinforcement by preceptor Bedside rounds	Selected patients	Clinical discussion Completion item
5. Modes of therapy	5. To describe currently available modes of therapy for the patient with acute meningitis		Readings See readings above.	
	a. To specify the objectives of care for nursing management of patients with acute meningitis	Case study	Chalkboard	Clinical conference Case study
	b. To identify the most likely antibiotics to be administered to a patient with bacterial meningitis	Lecture, discussion		Multiple-choice item
	c. To specify the currently suggested modes of therapy for meeting the objectives of care	Lecture, discussion		Multiple-choice item
	d. To describe the recommended therapy for managing each of the potential complications of meningitis, including epidemiological aspects	Lecture, discussion Case study	Slides	Clinical conference Essay item
E. Patients with acute seizure disorders	E. To describe the rationale for nursing management of patients with acute seizure disorders as determined by the:		Readings Bruya, MA, and Bolin, RH: Epilepsy: a controllable disease. Part I. Classification and diagnosis of seizures. Zwang, HJ: Epilepsy.	
1. Pathogenesis	1. Pathogenesis of various types of seizure disorders			
	a. To identify the acute and traumatic situations that may precipitate seizures	Lecture, discussion		Multiple-choice item
	b. To list the chronic clinical problems that may be manifested by seizure activity	Lecture, discussion Clinical reinforcement		Completion item

	Objectives	Teaching method	Media/Resources	Evaluation
2. Pathophysiology	2. Pathophysiology of various causes of seizure activity			
	a. To describe the major pathophysiological features of tetanus in relaton to the three degrees of tetanus	Lecture, discussion	Weinstein, L: Current concepts: tetanus. See above readings.	Essay item
	b. To describe the general pathophysiology of seizures based on the properties of epileptogenic neurons	Lecture, discussion	Slides	Multiple-choice item
	c. To relate the pathophysiology of seizure activity to the precipatory factors or events	Class discussion	Chalkboard	Clinical conference / Written testing
	d. To compare and contrast the pathophysiology of status epilepticus and less severe forms of seizure activity	Simulated patient / Class discussion		Written testing
3. Clinical assessment	3. To perform psycholphysical and laboratory evaluation or patients with seizure disorders			
	a. To specify the most important diagnostic study in evaluating the patient with seizures	Class discussion	Handout / Outline for describing and recording a convulsion.	True-false item
	b. To compare and contrast the clinical presentations and findings of patients in each stage of severity of tetantus	Lecture, discussion	Slides	Matching item
	c. To recognize the differentiating clinical findings observed in grand mal and petit mal seizures	Lecture, discussion / Clinical reinforcement by preceptor / Simulated patient	Slides / Chalkboard	Matching item / Clinical conference
	d. To identify a clinical description of the following types of seizure activity: (1) Psychomotor (2) Myoclonic (3) Trismus (4) Akinetic (5) Jacksonian epilepsy (6) Status epilepticus	Lecture, discussion / Written simulations	Slides	Matching item
	e. To identify the purpose and nature of information that can be obtained by each of the following in evaluating patients' seizure activity: (1) EEG (2) Brain scan (3) Echoencephalogram (4) CAT scan	Class discussion / Clinical reinforcement by preceptor	Chalkboard	Clinical conference / Multiple-choice item
	f. To distinguish among the three stages of progression in a grand mal seizure	Lecture, discussion	Slides	Multiple-choice item
	g. To list the clinically significant characteristics of seizure activity necessary to observe and record	Class discussion / Clinical instruction and reinforcement by preceptor	Handout / Outline for describing and recording a convulsion.	Demonstration of ability to note and record / Completion item

Continued.

IV. NEUROLOGICAL COMPONENT—cont'd

Topic	Participant objectives	Teaching method	Instructional media	Method of evaluation
Physiological effects of stress—cont'd				
4. Clinical problems	4. To set the priority of clinical problems associated with seizure disorders		Readings See readings above.	
	a. To enumerate the priority of potential clinical problems of a patient with a seizure disorder	Class discussion Clinical rounds	Chalkboard Selected patients	Clinical conference Completion item
	b. To compare and contrast the clinical problems of a patient having a single grand mal seizure and one having status epilepticus	Bedside rounds		
5. Modes of therapy	5. To describe currently available modes of therapy for the patient with a seizure disorder		Readings Bruya, MA, and Bolin, RH: Epilepsy: a controllable disease. Part II. Drug therapy and nursing care.	
	a. To enumerate the priority of care objectives for nursing management of the patient with a seizure disorder	Class discussion Clinical conference	Zwang,	Clinical conference Demonstration of ability to intervene appropriately
	b. To recognize appropriate and inappropriate nursing interventions for maintaining the airway of a patient having grand mal seizures or status epilepticus	Lecture, discussion Simulated situations	Intubation manikin Artificial airways	Written testing Rating scale
	c. To identify appropriate nursing interventions for maintaining patient safety during seizure activity	Simulated situations	Models Manikin Padding	Written testing Rating scale
	d. To specify the recommended pharmacological therapy for various seizure disorders and the rationale and side effects of these in acute and maintenance situations	Lecture, discussion Clinical conference	Chalkboard	Multiple-choice item
	e. To describe content areas of teaching required for patients who have seizure disorders	Class discussion Clinical conference		Clinical conference

348

	Objectives	Teaching method	Resources	Evaluation
F. Patients with Guillain-Barré syndrome	F. To describe the rationale and provide for nursing management of patients with Guillain-Barré syndrome as determined by the:			Because of little likelihood of having patients with GBS in unit, nearly all evaluation probably be via written testing
1. Pathogenesis	1. Pathogenesis of GBS			
	a. To identify the various clinical terms used to characterize GBS, indicating the reasons for the appropriateness of these synonyms	Lecture Class discussion	Readings Polk, BV: Cardiopulmonary complications of Guillain-Barré syndrome.	Multiple-choice item
	b. To specify the general incidence characteristics of GBS according to patient's sex, age, health status, and seasonal variation	Class discussion	Sodaro, E, and Perlick, N: Guillain-Barré; the syndrome, patient care and some case findings.	Multiple-choice item
	c. To identify the postulated etiologic factors in GBS and the basis for their probable role in the pathogenesis of GBS	Lecture, discussion	Vonk, H: Guillain-Barré syndrome.	True-false item
	d. To describe the patient population most at risk for developing GBS	Class discussion	Chalkboard	True-false item
2. Pathophysiology	2. Pathophysiology of GBS			
	a. To identify the pathophysiological features responsible for cardiovascular complications of GBS	Lecture, discussion	Readings Polk: p. 968. Sodaro: pp. 97-100.	Multiple-choice item
	b. To specify the pathophysiological basis of respiratory complications in GBS	Class discussion	Polk: pp. 968-969.	Multiple-choice item
	c. To describe the pathophysiology of GBS as a disease of: (1) Viral or infectious origin	Lecture, discussion	Sodaro and Perlick: p. 99.	Essay item
	(2) Hypersensitivity or autoimmunity d. To delineate the neurological lesions produced by GBS in the: (1) Reflex arc (motor and sensory nerve roots) (2) Brain (3) Spinal cord (4) Peripheral nerve (5) Cranial nerves (6) Other major body organs	Lecture, discussion	Sodaro and Perlick: p. 100. Slides Readings Sodaro and Perlick: p. 100.	Completion item

Continued.

IV. NEUROLOGICAL COMPONENT—cont'd

Topic	Participant objectives	Teaching method	Instructional media	Method of evaluation
Physiological effects of stress— cont'd	e. To describe the pathophysiological basis of nerve conduction deficits in GBS	Class discussion		Multiple-choice item
	f. To specify the postulated causes of CSF composition changes in patients with GBS	Lecture, discussion		Essay item
3. Clinical assessment	3. To perform clinical and laboratory evaluation of patients with GBS			
	a. To delineate the typical clinical history related by patients with GBS	Class discussion Written simulation	Polk: pp. 967-968. Sodaro and Perlick: pp. 97-98, 100-102. Vonk	Multiple-choice item
	b. To identify the clinical presentation of patients with GBS with respect to: (1) Characteristics of paralysis (2) Sensory dysfunctions (3) Order of cranial nerve involvement (4) Respiratory manifestations (5) Cardiovascular manifestations (6) Pain	Lecture, discussion Simulated patient	Polk: pp. 967-968. Sodaro and Perlick: pp. 98. 100-102. Vonk.	Essay item
	c. To describe the clinical manifestations of autonomic dysfunction seen in patients with GBS	Lecture, discussion Simulated patient	Polk: p. 968. Sodaro and Perlick: p. 101. Vonk.	Essay item
	d. To explain why patients with GBS must be evaluated for evidence of nephritis and papilledema	Lecture, discussion		Multiple-choice item
	e. To identify the earliest clinical signs and cardinal features of GBS	Simulated patient	Sodaro and Perlick: pp. 98-99. Vonk.	Multiple-choice item
	f. To specify the CSF findings characteristic of patients with GBS	Lecture	Chalkboard	Multiple-choice item
	g. To recognize the potential cardiovascular, GI, respiratory, renal, and fluid balance complications of GBS	Lecture, discussion Simulated patient		Written testing: simulated patients
4. Clinical problems	4. To set the priority of clinical problems associated with GBS			

a. To delineate the clinical problems anticipated in a patient with a severe case of GBS	Class discussion	Readings Polk: pp. 967-969. Sodaro and Perlick: pp. 100-106 Vonk.	Clinical conference
b. To rank the clinical problems associated with GBS according to their clinical immediacy	Class discussion	Chalkboard	Clinical conference
c. To describe the usual clinical course of patients with GBS	Simulated patient	Readings Polk: pp. 967-969. Sodaro and Perlick: p. 102. Vonk.	Multiple-choice item
d. To specify the psychosocial problems the GBS patient may face	Class discussion	Chalkboard	Clinical conference
e. To delineate the general prognosis and factors affecting prognosis in patients with GBS	Class discussion Lecture	Readings Polk: p. 968. Sodaro and Perlick: p. 102.	Multiple-choice item
f. To identify the usual causes of death in patients with GBS	Class discussion	Slides	Multiple-choice item
g. To list the objectives of nursing management of patients with GBS	Class discussion Homework: written objectives of care		Review of written objectives
5. Modes of therapy	5. To describe currently available modes of therapy for patients with severe GBS		
	a. To summarize the primary approach to therapy in patients with GBS	Class discussion	Readings Polk: p. 969.	Clinical conference
	b. To enumerate the most important clinical situations to be prevented in patients with GBS	Lecture, discussion	Sodaro and Perlick: p. 102.	Multiple-choice item
	c. To identify the means to assess a GBS patient's respiratory muscle adequacy	Clinical demonstration and reinforcement by preceptor	Wright respirometer Student patients	Demonstration of ability to assess: checklist
	d. To discuss the rationale for using the following in caring for patients with GBS: (1) Steroids (2) Tracheostomy vs E-T tube (3) Alpha-adrenergic blocking agents (4) Vasopressors (5) Anticoagulants	Lecture, discussion Written simulations	Readings Polk: pp. 968-969. Sodaro and Perlick: pp. 102-104.	Multiple-choice item Written testing Clinical conference: written simulation

Continued.

IV. NEUROLOGICAL COMPONENT—cont'd

Topic	Participant objectives	Teaching method	Instructional media	Method of evaluation
Physiological effects of stress—cont'd	e. To describe nursing interventions appropriate to caring for an alert, young, quadriplegic patient's possible psychosocial reactions in GBS	Class discussion	Sodaro and Perlick: p. 104.	Clinical conference: written simulation
	d. To specify nursing management techniques designed to deal with each clinical problem identified in patients with GBS	Lecture, discussion	Polk: pp. 968-969. Sodaro and Perlick: pp. 102-107.	Essay item
G. Patients with myasthenia gravis 1. Pathogenesis	G. To describe and provide for nursing management of patients with acute myasthenia gravis as determined by the: 1. Pathogenesis of myasthenia gravis			
	a. To describe clinical evidence supporting the pathogenesis of myasthenia gravis as an autoimmune disorder	Lecture, discussion	Stackhouse, J: Myasthenia gravis.	Essay item
	b. To differentiate between the factors that may precipitate a myasthenic crisis and a cholinergic crisis	Lecture, discussion	Chalkboard Slides	Matching item
2. Pathophysiology	2. Pathophysiology of myasthenia gravis			
	a. To identify the primary pathophysiological defect in myasthenia gravis	Class discussion	Reading Stackhouse: p. 1544. Slides	Multiple-choice item
	b. To specify the possible causes of the primary pathophysiological defect in myasthenia gravis	Class discussion	Chalkboard	Multiple-choice item
3. Clinical assessment	3. To perform clinical and laboratory evaluation of the patient with severe, acute myasthenia gravis	Written simulation: case history		
	a. To enumerate the earliest clinical signs of myasthenia gravis	Lecture, discussion	Reading Stackhouse, pp: 1544, 1546.	True-false item
	b. To describe the clinical presentation of patients with severe, fulminating myasthenia gravis	Class discussion Written simulation	Stackhouse: p. 1546.	Multiple-choice item
	c. To differentiate between the clinical picture of myasthic crisis and cholinergic crisis	Lecture, discussion	Slides	True-false item
	d. To recognize the symptoms of cholinergic drug overdose and underdosage	Lecture, discussion	Reading Stackhouse: p. 1545.	True-false item

	Learning experience	Resource	Evaluation
e. To describe the use of IV Tensilon in evaluating myasthenic patients	Lecture, discussion	Stackhouse: p. 1545.	Multiple-choice item
f. To demonstrate how strength of various muscle groups may be evaluated	Clinical instruction and demonstration in clinic	Stackhouse: p. 1546.	Clinical demonstration of ability to test: checklist
4. Clinical problems To set the priority of clinical problems associated with acute, severe myasthenia gravis	Written simulation		
a. To identify the most life-threatening problems associated with acute, severe myasthenia gravis and its associated forms of crisis	Class discussion	Slides Chalkboard	True-false item
b. To recognize the concomitant psychological problems that the myasthenic patient faces	Role-playing		Clinical conference
c. To differentiate between the clinical problems of cholinergic crisis and myasthenic crisis	Lecture, discussion	Reading Stackhouse: p. 1545.	True-false item
d. To explain the severe myasthenic patient's management problems in relation to taking medications	Role-playing		Clinical conference
5. Modes of therapy To describe currently available modes of therapy for myasthenia gravis	Lecture, discussion	Slides	Multiple-choice item
a. To explain the rationale for using cholinergic drugs in the management of myasthenic patients	Written simulation	Reading Stackhouse: p. 1545.	Multiple-choice item
b. To identify the rationale and potential side effects of the following drugs used for myasthenic patients: (1) Neostigmine (Prostigmine) (2) Atropine sulfate (3) Ephedrine (4) ACTH (5) Prednisone			Multiple-choice item
c. To describe the rationale and indications for thymectomy in myasthenic patients who are likely to benefit by this procedure	Class discussion	Stackhouse: pp. 1545-1546.	Clinical conference
d. To describe postoperative nursing care measures for a thymectomy patient	Simulated situation	Stackhouse: p. 1547.	Clinical conference
e. To list means to communicate effectively with an acutely ill myasthenic patient	Role-playing		Clinical conference
f. To identify areas requiring instruction for the myasthenic patient and the family	Written simulation		Clinical conference: written simulation

Continued.

V. RENAL COMPONENT

Topic	Participant objectives	Teaching method	Instructional media	Method of evaluation
Physiological effects of stress— cont'd				
■ Functional renal anatomy	To describe functional renal anatomy as it related to nursing management of patients with renal system dysfunction		Slides Handouts Renal anatomy. Renal physiology.	
	1. To describe the kidneys in terms of their size, location, and gross anatomy	Lecture, discussion	Reading Schramm, MA: Anatomy and physiology of the kidney.	Completion item
	2. To specify the functional unit of the kidney and its components	Class discussion		Multiple-choice item
	3. To identify the components of the renal tubular system and their medullary and cortical location within the kidney	Lecture, discussion	CIBA slides	Multiple-choice item
	4. To identify the location of structures comprising the renal vascular system	Lecture, discussion	CIBA slides Videotape Renal physiology.	Multiple-choice item
■ Renal physiology	To describe renal physiology as it relates to nursing management of patients with renal system dysfunction		Handout Renal physiology.	
	1. To specify the physiological processes involved in urine formation	Lecture, discussion	Reading Schramm.	True-false item
	2. To identify the major functions of each portion of the nephron	Class discussion	Handouts Renal anatomy. Renal physiology.	Matching item
	3. To differentiate the physiological processes involved in urine formation according to the structures involved and their effects	Lecture, discussion Clinical reinforcement	Reading Schramm: pp. 40-42. CIBA slides	Multiple-choice item Clinical discussion
	4. To describe the principles of renal clearance with illustrative examples of each	Lecture, discussion	Chalkboard	Essay item
	5. To explain how the renal system regulates specific electrolytes:	Lecture, discussion Clinical instruction and reinforcement at rounds	Handout Abbott Labs: Fluid and electrolytes.	Multiple-choice item
	a. Sodium			
	b. Chloride		Videotape Renal physiology.	
	c. Potassium			
	d. Calcium		CIBA slides	
	e. Magnesium			
	f. Phosphorus			
	6. To describe renal regulation of fluid balance as it occurs by:	Lecture, discussion	Handout Abbott Labs: Fluid and electrolytes. Videotape Renal physiology.	Essay item
	a. Hormonal mechanisms	Clinical reinforcement by preceptor	Readings Schramm: pp. 42-43.	Clinical discussion

Content	Objectives	Instructional methods	Resources	Evaluation
	b. Counter-current mechanism			
	c. Autoregulation			
	7. To describe the processes involved in renal regulation of blood pressure	Lecture, discussion Clinical reinforcement	Federspiel. CIBA slides	Essay item Clinical conference
	8. To specify the processes involved in renal regulation of acid-base balance	Lecture Clinical rounds	Reading Schramm: pp. 43–46. Videotape Renal physiology.	Multiple-choice item
	9. To differentiate between the terms "osmolality" and "osmolarity" in relation to renal physiology	Class discussion	Reading Renal physiology	True-false item
	10. To recognize the substances actively reabsorbed by the kidneys	Class discussion Clinical instruction	Reading Schramm: pp. 41–42.	True-false item Clinical discussion
	11. To distinguish between active and passive renal reabsorption	Lecture, discussion	Schramm, pp. 41–42.	True-false item
	12. To identify the roles of the following in renal physiology:	Lecture, discussion Clinical conference	CIBA slides Reading	Multiple-choice item Clinical discussion
	a. Renin-angiotensin system		Federspiel. B: Renin and blood pressure.	
	b. Aldosterone			
	c. ADH			
	13. To identify the major physiological functions of each electrolyte listed above	Lecture Clinical reinforcement by preceptor	Handouts Abbott Labs: Fluid and electrolytes. Diagnostic entities of body fluid disturbances.	Matching item
	14. To recognize the causes and primary physiological effects of electrolyte imbalances	Lecture, discussion Clinical instruction and reinforcement by preceptor	Videotape Renal physiology.	Multiple-choice item Clinical conference
■ Clinical assessment of the renal system	To describe the clinical and laboratory assessment of the renal system as it relates to nursing management of the patient with renal system dysfunction			
	1. To specify the normal values for:	Lecture, discussion Clinical instruction and reinforcement at bedside rounds	Reading Pillary, VKG: Clinical testing of renal function. Hospital lab sheets	Completion item Clinical discussion
	a. Urinalysis			
	b. GFR			
	c. Serum electrolytes, BUN, creatinine, uric acid			
	d. Urine electrolytes			
	e. Urinary creatinine clearance	Case presentation	Selected patients	Clinical conference
	f. Serum osmolarity			
	g. Urine osmolarity			
	2. To identify the clinical and laboratory findings characteristic of patients with systemic fluid and electrolyte imbalances	Clinical rounds Lecture	Handout Diagnostic entities of body fluid disturbances.	Demonstrated ability to identify Multiple-choice item
	3. To delineate the general and specific clinical findings characteristic of patients with various renal dysfunctions as determined by:	Clinical rounds Lecture, discussion Performance checklist	CIBA slides Chalkboard	Clinical demonstration of ability to delineate findings; checklist Written testing
	a. Inspection			
	b. Palpation	Bedside rounds	Selected patients	Clinical conference

Continued.

V. RENAL COMPONENT—cont'd

Topic	Participant objectives	Teaching method	Instructional media	Method of evaluation
Physiological effects of stress—cont'd	c. Percussion d. Auscultation e. Vital signs and ABGs	Performance checklist		
	4. To identify laboratory data that signifies renal system dysfunction	Clinical rounds Lecture	Selected charts	Clinical demonstration of ability to identify Multiple-choice item
	5. To rank the three best overall laboratory indexes of renal function indicating the rationale for their clinical significance	Class discussion	Chalkboard	
	6. To define the following terms related to renal assessment: a. Frequency b. Urgency c. Dysuria d. Retention with overflow	Class discussion	Slides	Completion item
	7. To describe the clinical features of the two types of renal pain and their associated causes	Lecture, discussion	Slides	Essay item
	8. To describe appropriate nursing interventions for monitoring the status of a patient's renal system	Class discussion Clinical instruction and reinforcement with preceptor	Chalkboard	Written testing Clinical conference
	9. To explain the rationale for and nursing responsibilities involved in invasive diagnostic tests of renal function	Lecture, discussion Clinical reinforcement	Readings Fennell, SE: Percutaneous renal biopsy.	Essay item
■ Patients with renal system dysfunction A. Patients with acute renal failure (ARF) 1. Pathogenesis	To describe and provide for nursing management of patients with renal system dysfunction A. To describe and provide for nursing management of patients with acute renal failure as determined by the: 1. Pathogenesis of acute renal failure a. To identify the three etiological categories of ARF and the mechanism by which they precipitate ARF	Lecture, discussion Clinical rounds	Freedman, P, and Smith, EC: Acute renal failure.	Multiple-choice item Clinical discussion

Objectives	Teaching Method	Resources	Evaluation
		Papper, S: Renal failure.	
b. To specify at least two examples of each of the three etiological categories of ARF and their specific mechanism of impairment	Class discussion	Thompson, GE: Acute renal failure.	Completion item
c. To recognize the common initiating event in the pathogenesis of ARF	Lecture, discussion	Freedman and Smith: p. 875.	True-false item Clinical conference
d. To describe the patient population at greatest risk for developing ARF	Class discussion Clinical rounds		Clinical conference Multiple-choice item
e. To identify the most common cause of ARF	Class discussion	Papper: p. 335.	True-false item
2. Pathophysiology of acute renal failure			
a. To describe the functional abnormalities that exist in ARF and their pathophysiological results	Lecture, discussion Nursing care conference	Freedman and Smith: p. 875. Papper: pp. 335-338, 341-345. Thompson: pp. 1580-1581.	Essay item Clinical conference
b. To characterize the net effect of renal dysfunctions present in ARF	Lecture, discussion Care conference	Slides	Multiple-choice item
c. To describe the major pathophysiological features of each of the three stages of acute tubular necrosis (acute tubular ischemia)	Lecture	Readings Papper: pp. 337-338, 341-2.	Multiple-choice item
d. To recognize the two general causes of acute tubular necrosis or ischemia	Lecture, discussion Clinical reinforcement	Papper: p. 336.	True-false item Clinical discussion
e. To explain the renal vascular shunting phenomenon that typically occurs in ARF	Lecture, discussion	Thompson: p. 1580.	Essay item
f. To identify the pathophysiological effects of ARF in each of the following body systems: (1) Renal (2) Respiratory (3) Cardiovascular (4) Gastrointestinal (5) Neuromuscular (6) Integumentary	Lecture, discussion Peer participatory conference (PPC)	Papper: pp. 350-352. CIBA slides Chalkboard	Multiple-choice item Clinical demonstration of ability to identify effects Rating scale

2. Pathophysiology

Continued.

V. RENAL COMPONENT—cont'd

Topic	Participant objectives	Teaching method	Instructional media	Method of evaluation
Physiological effects of stress—cont'd				
3. Clinical assessment	3. To perform clinical and laboratory evaluation of the patient in ARF			
	a. To identify the serum levels of electrolytes, BUN, creatinine, and uric acid that would be expected for a patient in ARF together with the reasons for these expected findings	Lecture, discussion Clinical rounds	Readings Freedman and Smith: pp. 875-876. Papper: pp. 337, 343-352. Thompson: pp. 1581-1584. Selected patients	Multiple-choice item Clinical demonstration of ability to identify characteristic findings Clinical conference
	b. To specify the laboratory findings characteristic of varying causes and stages of ARF	Lecture, discussion Clinical conference (PPC)	Chalkboard	Multiple-choice item Clinical conference
	c. To identify the clinical manifestations of uremia and the reasons for their occurrence	Lecture, discussion Clinical conference (PPC)	Reading Papper: pp. 350-352.	Multiple-choice item Clinical discussion
	d. To define the following terms: (1) Azotemia (2) Oliguria (3) Anuria (4) Polyuria	Class discussion Clinical reinforcement by preceptor	Selected patients Slides	Completion item Clinical discussion
	e. To compare and contrast the reliability of BUN and serum creatinine as an index of renal function in the patient with ARF	Lecture, discussion Clinical reinforcement by preceptor	Chalkboard	Written testing Clinical conference
	f. To explain the use of IV Mannitol, saline, and furosemide in assessing the patient with ARF	Lecture, discussion	Reading Thompson: pp. 1582-1583.	Essay item
	g. To identify the clinical features of high-output renal failure	Lecture, discussion	Slides	Multiple-choice item
	h. To describe the usefulness of the ratio of urine to plasma osmolality in evaluating patients with ARF	Lecture Clinical reinforcement by preceptor	Chalkboard	Clinical discussion Multiple-choice item
4. Clinical problems	4. To set the priority of clinical problems associated with ARF			
	a. To identify the spectrum of clinical problems caused by ARF in each of the following systems: (1) Renal	Lecture, discussion Clinical conference (PPC)	Readings Freedman and Smith: pp. 876-878.	Multiple-choice item Clinical conference Case study

Content	Teaching methods	Media	Evaluation
(2) Cardiovascular			
(3) Pulmonary	Papper: pp. 338-341, 345-356.		
(4) Gastrointestinal	CIBA slides		
(5) Neuromuscular	Chalkboard		
(6) Integumentary			
b. To rank the clinical problems of patients with ARF according to their immediacy	Class discussion at PPC	Chalkboard	Completion item
c. To recognize the most frequent ultimate cause of death in patients with ARF	Class discussion / Clinical reinforcement by preceptor	Chalkboard	True-false item / Clinical conference
d. To recognize the two most common immediate causes of death in ARF	Class discussion / Clinical reinforcement	Chalkboard	True-false item / Clinical conference / Multiple-choice item
e. To describe how the following clinical problems may arise as complications of ARF:	Lecture, discussion / Clinical conference (PPC)	Chalkboard	
(1) Pulmonary edema (2) Cardiac dysrhythmias (3) Anemia (4) GI bleeding (5) Pericarditis (6) Infection (7) Hypertension (8) Convulsions (9) Osteodystrophy (10) Acidosis	Case presentations	Selected patients	Clinical conference / Case presentations
f. To list the objectives of care for nursing management of a patient in ARF	Homework: written objectives of care for patient with ARF / PPC	Nursing care plan (Kardex)	Review of written objectives
5. Modes of therapy a. General			
5. To describe currently available modes of therapy for the patient in acute renal failure			
a. General therapeutic measures	Class discussion / Clinical conference (PPC)	Reading / Papper: p. 335.	Completion item / Clinical conference
(1) To enumerate interventions aimed at managing reversible causes of ARF—both prerenal and postrenal	Lecture, discussion / Clinical reinforcement by preceptor		Clinical discussion / Multiple-choice item
(2) To identify the principles of fluid balance management used as guidelines for regulating fluid intake for the patient with ARF			
(3) To indicate nursing measures helpful in evaluating the adequacy of fluid balance in a patient with ARF	Clinical instruction / Class discussion at PPC	Chalkboard	Clinical discussion / Written testing

Continued.

359

V. RENAL COMPONENT—cont'd

Topic	Participant objectives	Teaching method	Instructional media	Method of evaluation
Physiological effects of stress—cont'd	(4) To enumerate measures to initiate in promoting an anabolic state for the patient in ARF	Class discussion at PPC	Chalkboard	Clinical discussion Multiple-choice item Essay item
	(5) To describe at least four means to correct serum potassium levels in the patient with ARF	Lecture, class discussion Bedside rounds	Reading Dolan, PO, and Greene, HL: Renal failure and peritoneal dialysis.	
	(6) To differentiate between the objectives and modes of care during the oliguric phase of ARF and the diuretic phase	Lecture, discussion Clinical reinforcement by preceptor	Selected patients	True-false item Clinical conference
	(7) To indicate the parameters to use in evaluating the effectiveness of therapeutic measures for the patient in ARF	Class discussion at PPC	Markerboard	Clinical rounds Multiple assignment
b. Peritoneal dialysis	(1) To describe and differentiate the principles upon which peritoneal dialysis is based	Lecture, discussion Clinical instruction and reinforcement by preceptor	Readings Dolan and Greene; pp. 44, 46. Mehbod, H, and Lee, CY: Peritoneal dialysis. Smith, EC, and Freedman, P: Dialysis—current status and future trends.	Completion item Clinical discussion
	(2) To specify the clinical indications and contraindications for peritoneal dialysis	Lecture, discussion Clinical reinforcement	Dolan and Greene: pp. 46-47. Freedman and Smith: pp. 877-878. Mehbod, H. and Lee: pp. 99-100. Thompson: p. 1587.	Multiple-choice item Clinical conference
	(3) To identify the clinical advantages of peritoneal dialysis	Class discussion	Dolan and Greene: p. 47. Freedman and Smith: p. 877. Smith and Freedman: p. 879.	Multiple-choice item Clinical conference

	Behavioral objectives	Teaching methods/activities	Teaching aids/resources	Evaluation methods
	(4) To describe and perform the nursing responsibilities in caring for a patient who requires peritoneal dialysis	Clinical instruction Lecture Laboratory instruction Performance checklist	Equipment for peritoneal dialysis	Clinical demonstration of ability to perform: checklist Multiple-choice item True-false item Clinical conference
	(5) To cite the complications of peritoneal dialysis and measures to prevent their occurrence	Lecture, discussion Clinical instruction and reinforcement by preceptor	Readings Dolan and Greene: pp. 47, 49. Mehbod and Lee: pp. 100-102. Smith and Freedman: pp. 880-881.	
c. Hemodialysis	c. Hemodialysis (1) To describe the principles upon which hemodialysis is based	Lecture, discussion Clinical reinforcement at bedside	Jennrich, JA: Some aspects of the nursing care for patients on hemodialysis. McMahon, MR: Hemodialysis: definitions, techniques and complications. Smith and Freeman: pp. 881-882.	Completion item Clinical discussion
	(2) To specify the clinical indications and contraindications for hemodialysis.	Class discussion Lecture	Jennrich: p. 886. Smith and Freeman: p. 883.	True-false item Clinical conference
	(3) To identify the clinical advantages and disadvantages of hemodialysis.	Class discussion	Jennrich: p. 886. Smith and Freeman, p. 883.	Multiple-choice item Clinical conference
	(4) To describe and perform the nursing responsibilities in caring for a patient who requires hemodialysis.	Clinical instruction Lecture, discussion Laboratory instruction Performance checklist	Jennrich: pp. 886-889. McMahon: p. 7.	Clinical demonstration of ability to perform: checklist Multiple-choice item
	(5) To describe and perform all pertinent nursing responsibilities related to shunt care	Clinical instruction Laboratory instruction Lecture, discussion Performance checklist	Jennrich: p. 887. McMahon: pp. 15-21 Read, M, and Mallison, M: External arteriovenous shunts.	Clinical demonstration of ability to perform: checklist Multiple-choice item
	(6) To recognize the potential complications of hemodialysis and to identify measures to minimize or prevent their occurrence	Lecture, discussion Clinical reinforcement at bedside	Chalkboard Selected patients	Clinical conference True-false item

Continued.

VI. GASTROINTESTINAL COMPONENT

Topic	Participant objectives	Teaching method	Instructional media	Method of evaluation
Physiological effects of stress—cont'd				
■ Functional gastrointestinal anatomy	To relate functional gastrointestinal anatomy to nursing management of patients with gastrointestinal system dysfunction			
	1. To recognize the major anatomical components of the GI tract	Class discussion	Readings Dolan, PO, and Greene, HL: Conquering cirrhosis of the liver and a dangerous complication.	Written testing: diagram matching
				Multiple-choice item
	2. To describe the anatomical connections between the GI tract and the liver	Slide lecture Discussion		
	3. To identify the primary arterial and venous blood supplies to the major portions of the GI tract	Discussion Lecture	Brunner, LS: What to do (and what to teach your patient) about peptic ulcer.	True-false item
	4. To specify the anatomical point of separation between the upper and lower GI tract	Class discussion	CIBA slides	Clinical conference
	5. To describe hepatic arterial and venous blood supplies and relate them to GI tract vasculature	Lecture, discussion Clinical reinforcement by preceptor	Readings Dolan.	Clinical discussion Essay item
■ Gastrointestinal physiology	To describe the physiology of the GI tract in relation to nursing management of patients with gastrointestinal system dysfunction		Consult any appropriate reference on GI anatomy and physiology.	
	1. To specify the primary functions of all major components of the GI system	Lecture, discussion Clinical reinforcement at bedside	Chalkboard CIBA slides	Matching item Clinical discussion
■ Clinical assessment of the gastrointestinal system	To relate clinical and laboratory evaluation of the GI system to nursing management of the patient with GI system dysfunction		Readings Alexander, MM, and Brown, MS: Physical examination, part 13, examining the abdomen.	
	1. To relate the appearance of a normal adult abdomen to the underlying anatomy	Performance checklist	Willacker, J: Bowel sounds.	Clinical demonstration Rating scale
	2. To specify how the abdomen may be divided into four quadrants and nine areas for physical assessment	Clinical instruction by preceptor	CIBA and Anderson slides Videocassette Examination of the abdomen.	Demonstration of ability to specify divisions: rating scale
	3. To identify the abdominal contents underlying each quadrant and area	Clinical instruction and return demonstration	Readings Alexander. Willacker.	Clinical demonstration of ability to identify: checklist
A. Inspection	A. 1. To describe the normal findings in inspection of the abdomen for:	Clinical instruction and reinforcement Performance checklist	Selected patients Videocassette Examination of the abdomen.	Demonstration of ability to describe Completion item Direct observation Checklist

362

Content	Teaching method	Resources	Evaluation
a. Size			
b. Shape (contour)			
c. Symmetry			
d. Visible peristalsis			
e. Visible pulsations			
f. Skin condition			
g. Hair distribution			
2. To explain the clinical significance of selected abnormal findings of abdominal inspection	Lecture, discussion; Clinical instruction and reinforcement	Chalkboard; CIBA slides; Selected patients	Multiple-choice item; Clinical conference
B. Auscultation			
B. To describe and perform the procedure for auscultation of the abdomen	Clinical instruction; Performance checklist	Readings; Willacker.; Alexander & Brown.	Demonstration of ability to perform: checklist
1. To identify the nature of normal bowel sounds	Class discussion; Performance checklist		Demonstration of ability to identify
2. To contrast the nature of hyperactive bowel sounds and normal bowel sounds	Clinical instruction by preceptor	Selected patients	Demonstration of ability to differentiate; Multiple-choice item
3. To specify the clinical significance of selected abnormal auscultatory findings in the abdomen	Bedside rounds	Chalkboard; Videocassette; Examination of the abdomen.	Multiple-choice item; Clinical discussion
4. To state the clinical significance of arterial bruits and venous hums heard over the abdomen	Lecture, discussion		True-false item
C. Percussion			
C. To identify the normal percussion notes present over each area of the abdomen	Lecture, discussion; Performance checklist	Reading; Alexander & Brown.; Assigned patients	Multiple-choice item; Demonstration of ability to identify
1. To recognize how intra-abdominal pathological conditions may alter the findings of an abdominal assessment	Lecture, discussion; Clinical reinforcement by preceptor	Videocassette; Examination of the abdomen.	Multiple-choice item; Clinical discussion
2. To differentiate between the purposes of and procedures for performing superficial palpation and deep palpation of the abdomen	Clinical instruction; Performance checklist	Reading; Alexander & Brown.	Demonstration of ability to perform procedures: checklist; Written testing
■ Patients with gastrointestinal system dysfunction: acute GI bleeding			
A. Pathogenesis			
To describe the rationale and provide for nursing management of patients with acute GI bleeding as determined by the:			
A. Pathogenesis of acute GI bleeding			
1. To identify the most common clinical entities in the pathogenesis of GI bleeding	Lecture, discussion		Multiple-choice item
2. To describe the Mallory-Weiss syndrome and its relationship to GI bleeding	Lecture, discussion	CIBA slides	Multiple-choice item
3. To compare the incidence of upper GI bleeding to lower GI bleeding	Class discussion	Chalkboard	True-false item
4. To recognize the most frequent causes of lower GI bleeding	Class discussion		True-false item
B. Pathophysiology			
B. Pathophysiology of various etiologies of acute GI bleeding			
1. To state the general mechanisms involved in the pathophysiology of acute GI bleeding associated with peptic ulcer and esophageal varices	Lecture, discussion; Clinical reinforcement by preceptor	Readings; Brunner, p: 29.; Dolan and Greene: pp. 44-45.	Multiple-choice item; Clinical discussion
2. To relate the major pathophysiological features of Laennec's cirrhosis to the pathophysiology of acute GI bleeding	Lecture, discussion; Case study	Bielski, MT, and Molander, DW: Laennec's cirrhosis.	Multiple-choice item; Clinical discussion; Case study

Continued.

VI. GASTROINTESTINAL COMPONENT—cont'd

Physiological effects of stress—cont'd

Topic	Participant objectives	Teaching method	Instructional media	Method of evaluation
C. Clinical assessment	C. To perform clinical and laboratory evaluation of the patient with acute GI bleeding associated with Laennec's cirrhosis			
	1. To enumerate the clinical features presented by patients with acute upper GI bleeding	Class discussion Case study		Clinical conference Written testing: simulation
	2. To define and identify the clinical significance of:	Lecture, discussion Clinical reinforcement at bedside rounds	Slides	Matching item Clinical conference
	a. Hematemesis b. Melena c. Grey Turner's sign d. Cullen's sign e. Projectile vomiting f. Vasomotor instability		Readings Alexander and Brown: p. 66. Brunner: p. 28.	
	3. To specify the parameters used to estimate the volume of blood loss in GI bleeding	Lecture, discussion Preceptor instruction	Lamb, C, Apple, S, and Hongok, M: The GI bleeder.	Multiple-choice item Clinical conference
	4. To describe how to determine the site of GI bleeding	Lecture, discussion	Slides	Completion item Clinical discussion Multiple-choice item Clinical conference
	5. To specify the relative value of hemoglobin and hematocrit findings in the course of acute GI bleeding	Class discussion Clinical reinforcement at rounds	Slides Selected patients	
	6. To demonstrate how to test NG drainage and stool for occult blood	Performance checklist	Equipment for occult blood testing	Demonstration of ability to accurately test: checklist Essay item
	7. To identify the diagnostic tests most likely to be performed on a patient with acute UGI bleeding and the nursing responsibilities in each procedure	Lecture, discussion Clinical rounds		
	8. To delineate the clinical characteristics of duodenal ulcer disease	Lecture, discussion		True-false item
	9. To demonstrate how to perform the tilt test and describe its relevance to evaluating the patient with acute UGI bleeding	Clinical instruction Peformance checklist		Demonstration of ability to perform test: checklist Written testing
	10. To identify the clinical findings to anticipate in a patient with Laennec's cirrhosis as they relate to the pathophysiology of cirrhosis	Class discussion Bedside rounds	Reading Bielski and Molander: pp. 83-84.	Clinical conference Written testing: written simulation Clinical demonstration of ability to test for asterixis
	11. To demonstrate how to test for liver flap (asterixis)	Clinical instruction Performance checklist	Selected patients	Performance checklist
D. Clinical problems	D. To set the priority of clinical problems associated with acute GI bleeding	Class discussion Case study	Chalkboard Selected patients	Multiple-choice item
	1. To rank the primary clinical problems of a patient with acute GI bleeding according to their immediacy	Lecture, discussion Case study	Readings Bielski and Molander: pp. 84-86.	Clinical conference Written testing: written simulation
	2. To identify the additional clinical problems posed by Laennec's cirrhosis in a patient with acute GI bleeding—both physiological and behavioral	Lecture, discussion Case study	Dolan and Greene: p. 48.	Clinical conference Multiple-choice item
	3. To describe the clinical problems posed by the various stages of hepatic encephalopathy and delerium tremens			

4. To state the objectives of care for nursing management of the patient with acute upper GI bleeding associated with Laennec's cirrhosis	Case study Homework: written objectives of care	Dolan and Greene: pp. 44, 46. Chalkboard Kardex	Review of written objectives of care Case study
E. Modes of therapy			
To describe currently available modes of therapy for the patient with acute UGI bleeding associated with Laennec's cirrhosis			
1. For each of the identified clinical problems of patients with UGI bleeding and Laennec's cirrhosis, to describe the major modes of therapy currently being employed	Lecture, discussion Case study	Readings Brunner: pp. 28-34. Dolan and Greene. Chalkboard	Clinical discussion Essay item
2. To describe the rationale and procedure for each of the following in nursing management of the patient with acute UGI bleeding	Lecture, discussion Clinical instruction and reinforcement by preceptor Case study	Readings Boyce, HW: Nonsurgical treatment for gastrointestinal hemorrhage. Dolan and Greene. Flipchart	Multiple-choice item Clinical demonstration of ability to lavage Performance checklist
a. Phytonadione b. Iced gastric lavages c. IV crytsalloids and colloids d. Packed RBCs (fresh) e. Vasopression injection (Pitressin) f. Neomycin			
3. To identify the clinical indications and nursing responsibilities inherent in caring for a patient with each of the following types of gastrointestinal tubes:	Lecture, discussion Clinical instruction and reinforcement Performance checklist	Selected patients	Multiple-choice item Demonstration of ability to care for patients requiring these tubes Performance checklist
a. Levine tube b. Salem sump tube c. Cantor tube d. Miller-Abbott tube e. Sengstaken-Blakemore tube	Clinical laboratory on use of tubes	Reading McConnell, EA: All about gastrointestinal intubation. Variety of NG tubes as listed Intubation manikins	
4. To identify the clinical situations to expect a need for surgical intervention in a patient with acute UGI bleeding	Class discussion Case study	Reading Brunner: pp. 32-33. Chalkboard	Clinical conference Case study
5. To describe the more common portal shunting surgical procedures, and their rationale and postoperative nursing care for patients with acute UGI bleeding	Lecture, discussion Case study	Readings Brunner: pp. 32-34. Dolan and Greene: p. 51. CIBA slides	Essay item
6. To specify measures that may be undertaken to avert the hepatorenal syndrome	Lecture, discussion	Readings Dolan and Greene: p. 52.	Clinical conference Multiple-choice item
7. To identify nursing interventions appropriate for managing a patient experiencing alcohol withdrawal and delirium tremens	Class discussion Lecture Clinical reinforcement Role-playing	Lewis, LW: Confronting alcoholism. Lewis, LW: The hidden alcoholic: a nursing dilemma.	Clinical conference Completion item
8. To demonstrate and describe how to insert a nasogastric tube	Clinical instruction and reinforcement Performance checklist	Selected patients	Demonstration of ability to insert NG tube Performance checklist

Continued.

VII. METABOLIC COMPONENT

Physiological effects of stress—cont'd

■ Pituitary gland

Topic	Participant objectives	Teaching method	Instructional media	Method of evaluation
	To describe nursing management of patients with pituitary gland dysfunction			
A. Anatomy and physiology	A. To relate the anatomy and physiology of the pituitary gland to nursing management of patients with pituitary gland dysfunction		Filmstrip-cassette Endocrine physiology.	
1. Adenohypophysis	1. To describe the location of the pituitary gland	Class discussion	CIBA slides	Multiple-choice item
	a. For the following hormones of the adenohypophysis, to identify the secretory control, target cells, physiological effects, and results of hypersecretion and hyposecretion of each:	Lecture, discussion	CIBA slides	Table completion item
	(1) Somatotropic hormone		Chalkboard	
	(2) Adrenocorticotropic hormone			
	(3) Thyroid-stimulating hormone			
	(4) Prolactin hormone			
	(5) Follicle-stimulating hormone			
	(6) Leutinizing hormone			
	(7) Melanocyte-stimulating hormone			
2. Neurohypophysis	2. a. To identify the physiologic significance of the hypothalamo-pituitary portal system	Lecture, discussion	CIBA slides Filmstrip-cassette Endocrine physiology.	Multiple-choice item
	b. To specify the secretory control, target cells, physiological effects, and results of hyper- and hyposecretion of the following posterior pituitary hormones: (1) Oxytocin (Pitocin) (2) ADH (vasopressin)		Chalkboard	Matching item
B. Clinical assessment	B. To describe and perform the appropriate techniques of clinical and laboratory assessment of patients for determining pituitary gland dysfunction		Slides	
	1. To identify appropriate parameters to be assessed in evaluating pituitary gland functioning	Class discussion Clinical reinforcement by preceptor	Chalkboard	Clinical discussion True-false item
	2. To differentiate between the clinical findings characteristic of over-secretion and undersecretion of pituitary gland hormones	Class discussion Lecture	Chalkboard	Multiple-choice item Clinical discussion
C. Patients with pituitary gland dysfunction	C. To describe the rationale and provide for nursing management of patients with selected pituitary gland dysfunctions			
1. Patients with diabetes insipidus	1. To describe the rationale and provide for nursing management of patients with diabetes insipidus as determined by the:		Reading Shucart, WA. and Jackson, I: Management of diabetes insipidus in neurosurgical patients.	

Content	Behavioral objectives	Teaching methods	Teaching aids	Evaluation
a. Pathogenesis	Pathogenesis of diabetes insipidus	Lecture, discussion Clinical reinforcement at bedside rounds	Chalkboard	True-false item
	(1) To describe the basic pathophysiological defect present in diabetes insipidus			
b. Pathophysiology	Pathophysiology of diabetes insipidus			
	(1) To list at least three possible clinical disorders that may precipitate diabetes insipidus	Class discussion Clinical conference	Chalkboard	Completion item
	(2) To explain the mechanisms by which diabetes insipidus could be produced in selected clinical disorders	Clinical instruction Bedside rounds	Chalkboard	Multiple-choice item Clinical conference
c. Clinical assessment	To perform clinical and laboratory evaluation of the patient with diabetes insipidus		Reading Shucart and Jackson.	
	(1) To identify the clinical findings characteristic of a patient with diabetes insipidus	Class discussion Clinical reinforcement at rounds	Handout Laboratory findings in endocrine conditions.	Clinical conference Multiple-choice item
	(2) To explain the laboratory and urinalysis results to anticipate in a patient with diabetes insipidus	Clinical instruction Lecture	Chalkboard	Clinical conference Multiple-choice item
d. Clinical problems	To set the priority of clinical problems associated with diabetes insipidus		Reading Shucart and Jackson.	
	(1) To identify the potential clinical complications of diabetes insipidus	Class discussion Clinical reinforcement	Chalkboard	True-false item Clinical discussion
	(2) To rank the clinical problems of patients with diabetes insipidus in order of their immediacy	Class discussion	Chalkboard	Completion item
e. Modes of therapy	To describe currently available modes of therapy for patients with diabetes insipidus		Reading Shucart and Jackson.	
	(1) From the priority of clinical problems identified, to state the objectives of care for nursing management of patients with diabetes insipidus	Homework: written objectives of care for patient with DI	Nursing care plan (kardex)	Review of written objectives Case study
	(2) To differentiate between the types of IV therapy that would assist in preventing dehydration and those that could aggravate fluid losses in the patient with diabetes insipidus	Lecture, discussion Clinical reinforcement	Chalkboard	Clinical conference Essay item
	(3) To describe the special handling necessary in administering vasopressin therapy to a patient with diabetes insipidus	Class discussion Case study	Necessary equipment	Multiple-choice item Clinical discussion
2. Patients with inappropriate ADH syndrome	To describe and provide for nursing management of patients with inappropriate ADH syndrome as determined by the:			
a. Pathogenesis	Pathogenesis of inappropriate ADH syndrome			
	(1) To identify the clinical situations in which the inappropriate ADH syndrome is most frequently observed	Lecture, discussion Clinical conference Class discussion	Chalkboard	True-false item Clinical discussion
b. Pathophysiology	Pathophysiology of inappropriate ADH syndrome			
	(1) To describe the postulated pathophysiological mechanism working in the inappropriate secretion of ADH	Lecture, discussion	Chalkboard CIBA slides	Essay item

Continued.

VII. METABOLIC COMPONENT—cont'd

Topic	Participant objectives	Teaching method	Instructional media	Method of evaluation
Physiological effects of stress— cont'd				
c. Clinical assessment	c. To perform clinical and laboratory evaluation of the patient with inappropriate ADH syndrome	Lecture, discussion	Chalkboard	Multiple-choice item
	(1) To specify the clinical and laboratory findings to anticipate in a patient with inappropriate ADH syndrome, in addition to the reasons for these findings	Clinical reinforcement by preceptor Written simulation	Selected patient charts	Clinical discussion Rating scale
d. Clinical problems	d. To set the priority of clinical problems in patients with inappropriate ADH secretion	Class discussion Written simulation	Markerboard	Completion item
	(1) To rank the clinical problems of patients with inappropriate ADH secretion in order of their clinical immediacy			
e. Modes of therapy	e. To describe currently available modes of therapy for the patient with inappropriate ADH syndrome	Lecture, discussion	Markerboard	Multiple-choice item
	(1) To identify the rationale for therapy indicated in inappropriate ADH syndrome			
■ Thyroid gland	To describe nursing management of patients with thyroid gland dysfunction			
A. Anatomy and physiology	A. To relate the anatomy and physiology of the thyroid gland to nursing management of patients with thyroid gland dysfunction			
	1. To describe the thyroid gland in terms of its structure, location, and stimuli-controlling secretion of its hormones	Lecture, discussion	CIBA slides Chalkboard	Multiple-choice item
	2. To explain regulation of thyroid gland function by the pituitary and hypothalamus	Lecture, discussion	Filmstrip-cassette Endocrine physiology.	Essay item
	3. To specify how thyroxine (T_4) and triiodothyronine (T_3) are: a. Synthesized b. Stored c. Secreted d. Bound	Lecture, discussion	Filmstrip-cassette Endocrine physiology.	Multiple-choice item Clinical discussion
	4. To identify the primary physiological effects produced by thyroxine and the probable basis for these effects	Lecture, discussion	Chalkboard	True-false item
	5. To describe thyrocalcitonin in terms of its secretion and mechanism of action	Lecture, discussion	Filmstrip-cassette Endocrine physiology.	Multiple-choice item
B. Clinical assessment	B. To relate clinical and laboratory assessment of thyroid function to nursing management of patients with thyroid gland dysfunction			
	1. To specify the rationale and anticipated findings for Achilles tendon reflex time in patients with thyroid dysfunction	Class discussion		Multiple-choice item
	2. To identify the most pertinent laboratory tests of thyroid function, their normal values, and the clinical significance of abnormal values	Lecture Class discussion Bedside rounds	Chalkboard	Clinical discussion Multiple-choice item
C. Patients with thyroid gland dysfunction				

Content	Objectives	Method	Readings	Evaluation
1. Patients with hypothyroidism and myxedema coma	1. To describe and provide for nursing management of patients with hypothyroidism and myxedema coma as determined by:		Readings	
a. Pathogenesis	a. Pathogenesis of hypothyroidism and myxedema coma		McConahey, WM: Hypothyroidism. Menendez, CE, and Rivlin, RS: Thyrotoxic crisis and myxedema coma. Singer, MM: Endocrine emergencies. Winer, N: Endocrine emergencies.	
	(1) To differentiate between primary and secondary causes of hypothyroidism	Class discussion		Multiple-choice item
	(2) To distinguish myxedema from cretinism	Class discussion		True-false item
	(3) To identify the factors that may precipitate myxedema coma.	Class discussion Preceptor reinforcement		Multiple-choice item
b. Pathophysiology	b. Pathophysiology of hypothyroidism and myxedema coma			
	(1) To identify the primary pathophysiological effects of myxedema coma	Lecture, discussion	Slides	Matching item
	(2) To compare and contrast the pathophysiological effects of hypothyroidism (in the adult) and myxedema coma.	Class discussion		Matching item
c. Clinical assessment	c. To perform clinical and laboratory evaluation of patients with hypothyroidism and myxedema coma			
	(1) To indicate the laboratory findings that would support a diagnosis of myxedema	Class discussion	Slides	Multiple-choice item
	(2) To evaluate the reliability of goiter as an indicator of a patient's thyroid function	Class discussion		True-false item
	(3) To identify the clinical findings to anticipate in patients with myxedema coma	Lecture, discussion Written simulation		Multiple-choice item
	(4) To contrast the clinical findings of patients with mild to moderate hypothyroidism with those patients having myxedema coma	Lecture, discussion	Markerboard	Clinical conference Written simulation
	(5) To correlate the clinical and laboratory findings of patients with myxedema with their related pathophysiological causes	Lecture, discussion	Chalkboard Slides	Multiple-choice item
d. Clinical problems	d. To set the priority of clinical problems associated with hypothyroidism and myxedema coma			
	(1) To identify the spectrum of clinical problems associated with myxedema	Class discussion Simulated patient		Completion item
	(2) To compare the priority of clinical problems of patients with hypothyroidism to those with myxedema coma	Class discussion	Markerboard	Essay item
e. Modes of therapy	e. To describe currently available modes of therapy for patients with hypothyroidism and myxedema coma		Readings McConahey. Menendez and Rivlin. Singer. Winer.	
	(1) To specify the most commonly used modes of direct and supportive therapy for each of the clinical problems identified in patients with hypothyroidism and myxedema coma	Lecture Class discussion Clinical conference		Multiple-choice item Clinical conference
	(2) To differentiate the basic composition of various thyroid preparations	Lecture	Chalkboard	Multiple-choice item
	(3) To identify the parameters to use in evaluating the effectiveness of thyroid therapy	Class discussion	Chalkboard	True-false item Clinical discussion

Continued.

VII. METABOLIC COMPONENT—cont'd

Topic	Participant objectives	Teaching method	Instructional media	Method of evaluation
Physiological effects of stress— cont'd				
	(4) To differentiate between the agents of choice in treating patients with hypothyroidism and with myxedema coma, together with the rationale for the differentiation.	Class discussion	Chalkboard	Essay item
2. Patients with hyperthyroidism and thyrotoxic storm	2. To describe and provide for nursing management of patients with hyperthyroidism and thyrotoxic storm as determined by the:			
a. Pathogenesis	a. Pathogenesis of hyperthyroidism and thyrotoxic storm		Readings Menendez and Rivlin: 1463-1470. Singer: 1322-1324. Winer: 93-94.	
	(1) To describe the epidemiological features of hyperthyroidism	Class discussion		True-false item
	(2) To identify the possible mechanisms responsible for hyperthyroidism	Lecture, discussion	Slides	True-false item
	(3) To explain the potential roles of emotion and autoimmunity in the pathogenesis of hyperthyroidism	Class discussion		Multiple-choice item
	(4) To specify the situations that may precipitate thyrotoxic storm	Class discussion	Chalkboard	Completion item
b. Pathophysiology	b. Pathophysiology of hyperthyroidism and thyrotoxic storm			
	(1) To identify the major systemic pathophysiological effects of hyperthyroidism	Lecture, discussion	Slides Markerboard	Multiple-choice item
	(2) To compare and contrast the pathophysiologic effects of hyperthyroidism and thyrotoxic storm	Class discussion		Multiple-choice item
c. Clinical assessment	c. To perform clinical and laboratory evaluation of the patient with hyperthyroidism and thyrotoxic storm		Handouts Clinical picture of thyrotoxic crisis.	
	(1) To specify the laboratory findings that would support a diagnosis of thyrotoxicosis	Lecture, discussion	Slides	True-false item
	(2) To explain the etiology of exophthalmus in hyperthyroidism	Lecture, discussion	Slides	Essay item
	(3) To identify the multiple causes responsible for the clinical presentation typical of patients with hyperthyroidism and thyrotoxic storm	Class discussion Written simulation	Chalkboard	Multiple-choice item
	(4) To identify the clinical findings to anticipate in patients with thyrotoxic storm	Class discussion Written simulation	Flipchart	Multiple-choice item
	(5) To correlate the clinical and laboratory findings of patients with hyperthyroidism and thyrotoxic storm with their related pathophysiological causes	Lecture, discussion Written simulation	Flipchart	Multiple-choice item Written simulation
d. Clinical problems	d. To set the priority of clinical problems associated with hyperthyroidism and thyrotoxic storm		Readings Menendez and Rivlin. Singer. Winer.	

Objective	Learning experience	Resources	Evaluation
(1) To identify the spectrum of clinical problems associated with severe hyperthyroidism	Written simulation		Completion item
(2) To rank the anticipated clinical problems of severe hyperthyroidism in order of their immediacy	Class discussion	Chalkboard	Review of problem priority
(3) To contrast the clinical problems of patients having myxedema coma with those having thyrotoxic storm	Lecture, discussion	Flipchart	True-false item
e. Modes of therapy — To describe currently available modes of therapy for patients with severe hyperthyroidism and thyrotoxic storm		Readings Menendez and Rivlin. Singer. Winer.	
(1) To recognize the anticipated clinical effects of antithyroid drug therapy in hyperthyroidism, illustrating with samples of such drugs	Lecture, discussion		Multiple-choice item
(2) To specify the clinical indications and rationale for iodine therapy in treating patients with hyperthyroidism	Lecture, discussion Clinical reinforcement	Chalkboard	Multiple-choice item Clinical discussion
(3) To identify the agents of choice for immediate therapy of thyrotoxic storm	Class discussion	Chalkboard	True-false item
(4) To specify the indications for surgical intervention as therapy for hyperthyroidism	Class discussion	Chalkboard	Multiple-choice item
(5) To describe nursing interventions appropriate for managing the clinical problems of patients with hyperthyroidism and thyrotoxic storm	Lecture, discussion Clinical reinforcement Homework: written plan of care	Kardex	Essay item Written plan of care
■ Parathyroid gland A. Anatomy and physiology — To relate the anatomy and physiology of the parathyroid gland to nursing management of patients with parathyroid gland dysfunction			
1. To identify the number and location of parathyroid glands.	Class discussion	Filmstrip-cassette Endocrine physiology.	True-false item
2. To describe the feedback mechanism of parathormone	Lecture	CIBA slides	Completion item
3. To specify the physiological effects of parathormone in its three target areas	Lecture, discussion		Multiple-choice item
B. Clinical assessment — To describe and demonstrate the techniques for assessing parathyroid gland functioning	Performance checklist	Selected patients	Performance checklist
1. To state the normal values for serum calcium and serum phosphate	Lecture	Hospital chemistry forms	True-false item
2. To identify the major systems affected in parathyroid gland dysfunction	Lecture, discussion	Filmstrip-cassette Endocrine physiology	True-false item
3. To describe how parathormone levels affect the neuromuscular system	Lecture, discussion	CIBA slides	Multiple-choice item
C. Patients with parathyroid gland dysfunction — To describe the rationale and provide for nursing management of patients with parathyroid gland dysfunction 1. Patients with hypoparathyroidism — To describe the rationale and provide for nursing management of patients with hypoparathyroidism as determined by the:		Reading McGann.	
a. Pathogenesis (1) To recognize the common situations when hypoparathyroidism may occur	Class discussion	Slides	Multiple-choice item

Continued.

Topic	Participant objectives	Teaching method	Instructional media	Method of evaluation
Physiological effects of stress—cont'd				
b. Pathophysiology	b. Pathophysiology of hypoparathyroidism	Lecture, discussion	Chalkboard	Multiple-choice item
	(1) To relate the physiological effects of hypoparathyroidism to calcium and phosphate levels	Clinical reinforcement		Clinical discussion
c. Clinical assessment	c. To perform clinical and laboratory evaluation of the patient with hypoparathyroidism			
	(1) To identify the early neuromuscular signs of tetany	Lecture	Selected patients	True-false item
		Clinical rounds		
	(2) To identify the GI, cardiac, CNS, dermal, and skeletal effects of hypoparathyroidism	Lecture, discussion	Slides	Essay item
	(3) To demonstrate how to assess a patient for Chvostek's sign and Trousseau's phenomenon and relate the clinical significance of each	Clinical instruction	Assigned patients	Demonstration of ability to assess for these signs: checklist
		Performance checklist		
d. Clinical problems	d., e. To identify the priority of clinical problems associated with hypoparathyroidism and to describe nursing interventions appropriate to each	Lecture, discussion	Chalkboard	Multiple-choice item
e. Modes of therapy				Multiple-choice item
2. Patients with hyperparathyroidism	2. To describe the rationale and provide for nursing management of patients with hyperparathyroidism as determined by the:		Readings McGann, M. Function and care of the patient with hyperparathyroidism. Singer: pp. 1326-1327.	
a. Pathogenesis	a. Pathogenesis of hyperparathyroidism	Lecture, discussion	Chalkboard	Multiple-choice item
	(1) To distinguish among the primary, secondary, and tertiary causes of hyperparathyroidism			
b. Pathophysiology	b. Pathophysiology of hyperparathyroidism	Lecture, discussion	Chalkboard	True-false item
	(1) To identify the major pathophysiological effects of hyperparathyroidism			
c. Clinical assessment	c. Clinical and laboratory evaluation of the patient with hyperparathyroidism	Lecture, discussion	Chalkboard	Multiple-choice item
	(1) To describe the most common clinical findings of patients with hyperparathyroidism			
d. Clinical problems	d., e. To identify the priority of clinical problems associated with hyperparathyroidism and to describe the nursing interventions appropriate to each	Class discussion	Chalkboard	Completion item
e. Modes of therapy				
■ **Adrenal gland**				
A. Anatomy and physiology	A. To relate the anatomy and physiology of the adrenal gland to nursing management of patients with adrenal gland dysfunction			
	1. To identify the three zones of the adrenal cortex and the hormones secreted by each zone	Lecture	CIBA slides	Completion item
	2. To differentiate the secretory control and target area effects produced by the:	Lecture, discussion	Filmstrip-cassette Endocrine physiology.	Multiple-choice item
				Clinical conference
	a. Glucocorticoids (cortisol, corticosterone)			
	b. Mineralocorticoids (aldosterone)			
	c. Sex steroids (testosterone, progesterone)			
B. Patients with adrenal gland dysfunction				

Content	Objectives	Teaching method	Teaching aids	Evaluation
1. Patients with Addison's disease or addisonian crisis	B. 1. To describe the rationale and provide for nursing management of patients with addison's disease or addisonian crisis as determined by the:			Filmstrip-cassette Endocrine physiology.
a. Pathogenesis	a. Pathogenesis of Addison's disease and addisonian crisis			Readings McKenna, TJ: Acute adrenal insufficiency. Singer: pp. 1324-1326. Winer: pp. 95-96, 100.
	(1) To recognize the most common causes of Addison's disease and addisonian crisis	Class discussion Lecture		Multiple-choice item
b. Pathophysiology	b. Pathophysiology of Addison's disease and addisonian crisis			
	(1) To identify the major pathological effects of aldosterone and cortisol hormonal deficiencies	Class discussion	Chalkboard	Completion item
c. Clinical assessment	c. To perform clinical and laboratory evaluation of the patient with Addison's disease and addisonian crisis			
	(1) To specify the clinical findings to anticipate in a patient with addisonian crisis	Class discussion Nursing care conference	Chalkboard	True-false item
	(2) To differentiate between the clinical picture of addisonian crisis and Cushing's syndrome	Class discussion Nursing care conference	Chalkboard	Essay item
d. Clinical problems	d. To differentiate between the priority of clinical problems anticipated in a patient having addisonian crisis and a patient having severe effects of Cushing's syndrome	Class discussion	Chalkboard	Essay item
	(1) To enumerate the clinical problems associated with Conn's syndrome (hyperaldosteronism), and pheochromocytoma	Lecture, discussion	Slides	Completion item
e. Modes of therapy	e. To describe currently available modes of therapy for patients with addisonian crisis	Nursing care conference		
	(1) To describe the nursing interventions appropriate to managing each clinical problem associated with an addisonian crisis	Class discussion		Multiple-choice item
■ Pancreas				
A. Anatomy and physiology	A. To relate the anatomy and physiology of the pancreas to nursing management of the patient with pancreatic dysfunction			Filmstrip-cassette Endocrine physiology.
	1. To differentiate the two types of pancreatic tissue according to their hormonal functions	Lecture, discussion	CIBA slides	Matching item
	2. To distinguish the four types of pancreatic cells and their related hormonal functions	Lecture, discussion		Matching item
	3. To describe the two pancreatic hormones according to their respective feedback mechanisms and physiological effects	Lecture, discussion Clinical reinforcement		Multiple-choice item Clinical conference
B. Patients with pancreatic dysfunction or related clinical states	B. To describe and provide for nursing management of patients with pancreatic dysfunction or related clinical states			
1. Patients with diabetic ketoacidosis	1. To describe the rationale and provide for nursing management of patients with diabetic ketoacidosis as determined by the:	Case study		Readings Beigelman, RM, et al: Severe diabetic keotacidosis.

Continued.

373

VII. METABOLIC COMPONENT—cont'd

Physiologic effects of stress—cont'd

Topic	Participant objectives	Teaching method	Instructional media	Method of evaluation
a. Pathogenesis	a. Pathogenesis of diabetic ketoacidosis		Felts, PW: Coma in the diabetic, current concepts.	
	(1) To describe the major pathophysiological effects of hypoinsulinism	Lecture, discussion Clinical reinforcement by preceptor		Completion item Clinical conference
	(2) To recognize the patient population most at risk for developing diabetic ketoacidosis	Class discussion Clinical	Guthrie, DW, and Guthrie, RA: Coping with diabetic ketoacidosis.	True-false item Clinical conference
	(3) To recognize the factors that may precipitate diabetic ketoacidosis	Case study		Multiple-choice item
b. Pathophysiology	b. Pathophysiology of diabetic ketoacidosis			
	(1) To identify the primary pathophysiologic defect of patients who develop diabetic ketoacidosis	Lecture	Slides	True-false item
	(2) To specify the pathophysiologic events responsible for ketogenesis in patients with diabetic ketoacidosis	Lecture, discussion Clinical reinforcement by preceptor	CIBA slides Chalkboard	Multiple-choice item Clinical conference
	(3) To differentiate between the pathophysiology of metabolic acidosis and respiratory alkalosis in patients with diabetic ketoacidosis	Lecture Clinical rounds	Chalkboard	Multiple-choice item Clinical conference
	(4) To identify the major fluid and electrolyte disturbances associated with diabetic ketoacidosis	Lecture, discussion Case study	Flipchart	True-false item Clinical conference
c. Clinical assessment	c. To perform clinical and laboratory evaluation of the patient with diabetic ketoacidosis		Readings Schumann, D: Assessing the diabetic.	
	(1) To identify the triad of salient clinical findings observed in patients with diabetic ketoacidosis	Class discussion Clinical rounds	Schumann, D: Tips for improving urine testing techniques.	Completion item
	(2) To recognize the three ketone bodies and their clinical significance for patients in ketoacidosis	Lecture, discussion Clinical reinforcement by preceptor	Slides	Multiple-choice item Clinical conference
	(3) To relate the clinical findings (signs, symptoms, laboratory) of patients in diabetic ketoacidosis to their pathophysiological correlates	Class discussion Clinical reinforcement Case study	Chalkboard Selected patients	Multiple-choice item Clinical conference Rating scale
	(4) To demonstrate how to test accurately a patient for glucosuria and ketonuria	Clinical instruction Performance checklist	Equipment, supplies, and specimens necessary for testing	Clinical demonstration of ability to test accurately: checklist
	(5) To specify the ABG results expected in diabetic ketoacidosis	Class discussion Clinical rounds	Chalkboard	Multiple-choice item
	(6) To identify the renal threshold for glucose reabsorption	Bedside rounds		True-false item

Content	Objectives	Teaching methods	Resources	Evaluation
d. Clinical problems	d. To set the priority of clinical problems associated with diabetic ketoacidosis			
	(1) To rank the clinical problems of patients with diabetic ketoacidosis according to their clinical immediacy	Class discussion Case study	Chalkboard	Clinical conference Case study
e. Modes of therapy	e. To describe currently available modes of therapy for patients with diabetic ketoacidosis	Case study	Chalkboard	Multiple-choice item Clinical conferences
	(1) To specify the appropriate nursing interventions related to: (a) Insulin therapy (b) IV fluid therapy (c) Electrolyte therapy (d) Alkalinizing therapy in patients with diabetic ketoacidosis	Lecture, discussion Clinical reinforcement		
2. Patients with hyperosmolar hyperglycemic nonketotic coma (HHNK)	2. To describe the rationale and provide for nursing management of patients with hyperosmolar hyperglycemic nonketotic coma as determined by its pathogenesis, pathophysiology, clinical findings, clinical problems, and modes of therapy.		Reading Arieff, AI, and Felts, PW: Hyperosmolar coma, current concepts. McCurdy, DK: Hyperosmolar hyperglycemic nonketotic coma. Witt, K: HHNK. Chalkboard Slides	
	a. To compare and contrast the following characteristics of HHNK with those of diabetic ketoacidosis: (1) Pathogenesis (2) Pathophysiology (3) Clinical assessment (4) Clinical problems (5) Modes of therapy	Clinical conference		Matching item
3. Patients with acute hypoglycemia (insulin shock)	3. To describe the rationale and provide for nursing management of patients with acute hypoglycemia (insulin shock) as determined by its pathogenesis, pathophysiology, clinical findings, clinical problems, and therapy		Readings Conn, JW, and Pek, S: On spontaneous hypoglycemia, current concepts. Schumann, D: Coping with the complex, dangerous, elusive problem of those insulin-induced hypoglycemic reactions. Statement on hypoglycemia, Archives of Internal Medicine. Wolf, BM: Hypoglycemia: some facts about a misunderstood condition.	
	a. To compare and contrast the following characteristics of acute hypoglycemia (insulin shock) with those of HHNK and diabetic ketoacidosis: (1) Pathogenesis (2) Pathophysiology (3) Clinical assessment (4) Clinical problems (5) Modes of therapy	Lecture, discussion Clinical conference		Matching item

Continued.

VIII. BURN COMPONENT

Topic	Participant objectives	Teaching method	Instructional media	Method of evaluation
Physiological effects of stress—cont'd				
■ Anatomy and physiology of the integumentary system: the skin	To describe the major anatomical and physiological features of the skin			
	1. To differentiate between the cellular composition of the epidermis and the dermis.	Lecture, discussion	Reading Consult general references on anatomy and physiology of the skin layers.	True-false item
	2. To identify the five epidermal layers	Lecture	Slides	Completion item
	3. To specify the physiological functions served by the stratum corneum epidermis and stratum germinativum epidermis in relation to the pathophysiology of burns	Lecture, discussion	Chalkboard	Multiple-choice item
	4. To specify the primary functions served by the dermis (corium)	Class discussion	Chalkboard Slides	Completion item
	5. To identify the epidermal appendages and the major functions they provide in intact skin	Lecture, discussion	Chalkboard	Multiple-choice item
	6. To enumerate the general functions of the skin	Class discussion	Chalkboard	Completion item
■ Patients with burn injury	To describe and provide for nursing management of the patient with burn injury as determined by the:			
A. Pathogenesis	A. Pathogenesis of burns			
	1. To describe the current epidemiological findings related to burn injuries	Lecture, discussion	Reading Dimick, AR: Emergency management of the acutely burned patient.	True-false item
	2. To identify the most common causes of burn injury	Class discussion	Slides	Multiple-choice item
	3. To differentiate the various types of burns and the agents usually responsible for each type	Lecture, discussion	Photographs Slides	Multiple-choice item
B. Pathophysiology	B. Pathophysiology of burn injuries			
	1. To identify the factors that determine the degree of burn injury	Lecture, discussion	Reading Jones, CA, and Feller, I: Burns: what to do during the first crucial hours.	True-false item

	Objectives	Method	Media	Evaluation
	2. To differentiate between the factors that determine the degree of burn injury and those that determine the severity of burn injury	Class discussion	Slides	True-false item
	3. To specify at least three general considerations to be made regarding the local effect of a burn injury	Lecture, discussion	Chalkboard	Completion item

	4. To describe the systemic effects of burn injury in the following systems:
	a. Cardiovascular
	  (1) General circulation
	  (2) Cardiac
	b. Pulmonary
	c. Hepatic
	d. Gastrointestinal
	e. Renal
	f. Neuroendocrine
	g. Reproductive
		Lecture, discussion
		Written simulation
			Chalkboard
			Slides
			Readings
			  Dimick.
			  Jones and Feller.
				Essay item

	5. To relate the systemic effects of burn injury to their pathophysiological causes	Written simulation	Chalkboard	Multiple-choice item
	6. To distinguish between partial and full thickness burns in terms of the pathophysiological effects of each	Lecture, discussion	Slides Chalkboard	Multiple-choice item
	7. To describe the pathophysiology of burn shock	Lecture, discussion Written simulation Note: This facility does not care for burn patients requiring hospitalization	Chalkboard Slides	Essay item
C. Clinical assessment	C. To perform clinical and laboratory evaluation of the patient with burn injury			
	1. To identify five parameters used to assess the severity of burn injury and how these may be determined		Slides Handout Burn evaluation.	
	a. Size or extent			

	(1) To describe how the "rule of nines" may be used to estimate the body area involved in a burn and specify its major limitation as an indicator of burn size	Lecture
		Discussion of handout
		Simulated patient
			Readings
			  Dimick.
			  Jones and Feller: pp. 23-24, 29.
				Essay item

	(2) To identify the clinical advantages of the Lund and Browder method of estimating burn area over the "rule of nines"	Lecture Discussion of handout	Handout Burn evaluation.	Multiple-choice item

Continued.

VIII. BURN COMPONENT—cont'd

Topic	Participant objectives	Teaching method	Instructional media	Method of evaluation
Physiological effects of stress— cont'd				
	(3) To describe how the nurse may estimate the area involved in a scattered burn	Lecture, discussion Laboratory practice on simulated patients	Copies of Handout	Clinical demonstration of ability to estimate Checklist
	(4) To demonstrate how to chart accurately a burn evaluation from a case presentation	Classroom practice (case presentation) Written simulation	Copies of Handout	Clinical demonstration of ability to estimate Checklist
b. Depth				
	(1) To distinguish between the clinical characteristics of partial-thickness and full-thickness burn wounds	Lecture, discussion Review of representative slides	Readings Dimick. Jones and Feller. Slides of FTB and PTB	Multiple-choice item
	(2) To differentiate between the clinical characteristics of first and second degree partial-thickness burns and superficial and deep partial-thickness burns	Lecture, discussion Review of slides	Chalkboard Slides of first and second degree burns	Multiple-choice item with slides
	(3) To identify the clinical characteristics of third degree full-thickness burns	Lecture, discussion Review of slides	Chalkboard Slides of third degree burns	True-false item
	(4) To specify the two factors that determine the depth of a burn injury	Lecture	Chalkboard	Completion item
c. Age of patient				
	(1) To specify the age groups associated with comparably higher mortality rates in burn injury and the reasons for their vulnerability	Class discussion	Slides	True-false item
d. Body parts involved				
	(1) To describe how to determine if pulmonary problems are likely to occur as a result of a burn injury	Class discussion Written simulations		Essay item
	(2) To identify the most important body areas that affect the severity of a burn wound	Class discussion	Chalkboard Slides	True-false item

Content	Objectives	Learning activities	Resources	Evaluation
	e. Medical history			
	(1) To specify the chronic medical problems that may be aggravated by burn injury	Class discussion	Chalkboard	Completion item
	(2) To distinguish among the clinical characteristics of minor, moderate, and major burns	Lecture, discussion	Slides Chalkboard	Multiple-choice item
D. Clinical problems	D. To set the priority of clinical problems associated with various burn injuries			
	1. From an enumeration of the systemic effects of burn injury, to identify the clinical problems associated with each pathophysiological effect	Lecture, discussion Written simulations		Multiple-choice item
	2. To specify the most frequent causes of death in burn trauma	Class discussion	Chalkboard	True-false item
	3. To differentiate between the clinical problems of patients with burns who may be treated on an out-patient basis and those who require hospitalization	Class discussion	Chalkboard	Multiple-choice item Written simulation
	4. To differentiate among the clinical problems anticipated during the three major phases of burn management	Class discussion Written simulations	Chalkboard	Multiple-choice item
	5. To identify the priorities of care for effective management of patients with major burn trauma	Class discussion Written simulations	Chalkboard	Multiple-choice item
E. Modes of therapy	E. To describe currently available modes of therapy for the patient with burn trauma			
	1. From the clinical problems identified, to describe acceptable modes of therapy for the patient with minor burns and the rationale for each	Lecture, discussion	Readings Baxter, CR, Marvin, J, and Curreri, PW: Fluid and electrolyte therapy of burn shock. Dimick. Hunt, JL, McGranahan, BG, and Pruitt, BA: Burn-wound management.	Essay item
	2. To describe acceptable ER management of various types of burns	Lecture, discussion		Multiple-choice item

Appendix B

Critical care nursing: level II program

schedule of classes

II. PULMONARY COMPONENT

Day	Date	Time	Room	Topic	Instructor	Readings
Friday	15 June	2:00-4:00	200	Pulmonary: pretest	Ms. Alspach	None
Monday	18 June	8:00-11:30	204	A. Functional anatomy of the pulmonary system. 1. Upper airway 2. Lower airway 3. Alveolus 4. Pulmonary	Ms. Alspach	Wade, JF: Respiratory nursing care, pp. 1-6. Turner, HG: The anatomy and physiology of normal respiration.
		12:30-2:00		5. Lung 6. Pleural space 7. Muscles of ventilation	Ms. Alspach	
		2:00-4:00		B. Pulmonary physiology 1. Ventilation	Ms. Alspach	Wade, pp. 6-9, 26-51. Secor, J: Ventilation: concepts essential to comprehensive nursing care.
Tuesday	19 June	8:00-10:00	204	2. Respiration 3. O_2 and CO_2 transport	Ms. Alspach	Wade, pp. 12-15, 51-53. Wade, pp. 54-63 Waldron, MW: O_2 transport.
		10:00-11:00		4. Pulmonary circulation	Ms. Alspach	Wade, pp. 11-12.
		11:00-12:00		5. Regulation of ventilation	Ms. Alspach	Wade, pp. 9-10.

Day	Date	Time	Location	Session / Topic	Instructor	References
Wednesday	20 June	1:00–4:00	204	*Clinical session* Introduction to Swan-Ganz catheter equipment	Ms. Alspach	
		12:00–4:00	200	6. Acid-base balance	Dr. Allen	Wade, pp. 54–71. Mizgerd, JB: The interpretation of ABG studies. Sharer, JE: Reviewing acid-base balance.
Thursday	21 June	2:00–2:30	ICU	*Clinical session* Skill 3 (V_T, V_C, $\dot{V}_T$)	Ms. Alspach	
		2:30–4:00	ICU-CCU	*Clinical session* Skills 1 Bypassed functions 2 Muscles of respiration 4 Deadspace	Ms. Alspach/preceptors	
Monday	25 June	8:00–10:00	200	7. ABG interpretations and implications for nursing	Ms. Alspach	Robertson, and Guzetta: ABG interpretation in the respiratory ICU.
		10:00–11:00	Lab	*Clinical session ABGs* Skill 11 Drawing ABGs	Preceptors	Wade, pp. 71–76 Lea, A: Obtaining arterial blood samples. Arterial blood gas drawing.
				C. Techniques in clinical assessment of the pulmonary system		Wade, pp. 98–105, 112–123. Barbie, et al: Medical H_x in evaluation of patients with pulmonary disease. Broughton, JO: Chest physical diagnosis for nurses and respiratory therapists. Sweetwood, H: Bedside assessments of respirations. Traver, GA: Assessment of the thorax and lungs.
		12:00–2:00	204	1. Parameters of physical assessment	Ms. Alspach	
		2:00–4:00	ICU-CCU	*Clinical session* Skills 9 Normal ABGs 10 Interpret ABGs	Ms. Alspach	

Continued.

II. PULMONARY COMPONENT—cont'd

Day	Date	Time	Room	Topic	Instructor	Readings
Tuesday	26 June	12:00-12:30	200	Film: Examination of the thorax and lungs	Ms. Alspach	
		12:30-2:30		Tape: Breath sounds	Ms. Alspach	
		2:30-4:00		2. Techniques of physical assessment	Ms. Alspach/preceptors	
				D. Management of care for patients with pulmonary system dysfunction		
				1. Patients with acute respiratory failure		Wade, pp. 140-154, 162-168
Wednesday	27 June	12:00-1:30	204	a. Pathogenesis	Ms. Miller	Rogers, RM, and Tuero, A: Physiologic considerations in the treatment of acute respiratory failure.
				b. Pathophysiology		
				c. Clinical Assessment		
		1:30-3:00		d. Clinical problems	Ms. Alspach	Sheriff, et al: ARF: current concepts of pathophysiology and management.
				e. Modes of therapy		
		3:00-4:00		Clinical conference	Staff	
Thursday	28 June	1:00-4:00	ICU-CCU	Clinical session	Preceptors	None
				Skills		
				5 Assessment		
				6 Reflexes		
				7 Lobes of lungs		
				8 Breath sounds		
Monday	02 July	8:00-10:30	200	2. Patients with acute thoracic trauma	Ms. Alspach	Wade, pp. 188-190. Lance, E: Chest trauma.
				a. Pathophysiology		
				b. Clinical significance		
				c. Initial therapy		
		10:30-11:30		d. Care of patients with chest tubes	Ms. Kelly	Van Meter, M: Chest tubes: basic techniques for better care.

382

Day	Date	Time	Room	Content	Instructor	Reading
		12:30-2:30		3. Patients with adult respiratory distress syndrome a. Pathogenesis b. Pathophysiology c. Clinical assessment	Ms. Jonas	Wade, pp. 186-188. Hopewell, PC: Adult respiratory distress syndrome.
		2:30-3:00		Film: Steroids in ARDS	Ms. Williams	
		3:00-4:00		d. Clinical problems e. Modes of therapy	Ms. Williams	Shinn, AF: Corticosteroids and their use in shock.
Tuesday	03 July	7:30-9:30	204	Artificial airways	Dr. Murphy	Wade, pp. 143-419, 170-177. Stone, EW. and Zuckerman, S: The esophageal obturator airway. Trout, C: Artificial airways: tubes and trachs.
		9:30-12:00	Lab	*Clinical practicum* Skill 34 Techniques of artificial airway insertion	Ms. Alspach	
		1:00-2:30	Lab	Suctioning Principles Techniques Intubated/N-T Manikin practice	Staff preceptors	Wade, pp. 149-151. Demers, RR, and Saklad, M: Minimizing the harmful effects of mechanical aspiration. Sandham, G, and Reid, B: Some Q's and A's about suctioning.
		2:30-4:00	Lab	*Clinical session* Pulmonary hygiene techniques: Breathing exercises Chest pt Postural drainage	Mr. O'Boyle	Wade, pp. 106-112. Tecklin, JS: Positioning, percussing and vibrating patients for bronchial drainage. Ungvarski, P: Mechanical stimulation of coughing.
Thursday	05 July	10:00-12:00	ICU	½ of class for Skills 24-30 to be scheduled with resp. therapy techs		None
		2:00-4:00	ICU-CCU	*Clinical session* (for all) Skills 12-17, 31 Suctioning	Preceptors	
Friday	06 July	10:00-12:00	ICU	Other half of class for Skills 24-30 to be scheduled with resp. therapy techs		None
Monday	09 July	12:00-3:00	204	O₂ and drug therapy	Dr. Hurley	Wade, pp. 125-139. Wade, pp. 154-165.
		3:00-4:00	204	O₂ toxicity	Ms. Alspach	Wade, pp. 132-133. Nett, L, and Petty, TL: O₂ toxicity.

Continued.

II. PULMONARY COMPONENT—cont'd

Day	Date	Time	Room	Topic	Instructor	Readings
Friday	13 July	8:00-12:00	200 Lab	Mechanical ventilation Equipment Principles Types of ventilators IPPB, PEEP, CPAP	Ms. White	Fitzgerald, LM: Mechanical ventilation. Levy, M, and Stubbs, J: Nursing implications in care of patients treated with assisted mechanical ventilation modified with PEEP.
		1:00-3:00	204	Nursing care of patients on mechanical ventilation	Ms. Hennessy	Wade, pp. 200-201, 154. Fitzgerald, LM: Weaning the patient from mechanical ventilation.
		3:00-400	204	Weaning from mechanical ventilation	Ms. Hennessy	Wade, pp. 105-106, 191-200. Moses, R, and Steinberg: Does the MA-1 respirator make you nervous?

Monday	16 July	8:00-10:00	204	4. Patients with status asthmaticus
				   a. Pathogenesis
				   b. Pathophysiology
				   c. Clinical assessment
					Dr. Lane	Wade, pp.86-89.
						Bocles, C: Status asthmaticus.

		10:00-12:00	204	d. Clinical problems e. Modes of therapy	Ms. Harris	Moody, LE: Nursing care of patients with asthma.

		1:00-2:30	204	5. Patients with COPD
				   a. Pathogenesis
				   b. Pathophysiology
				   c. Clinical assessment
				   d. Clinical problems
					Ms. Blake	Wade, pp. 77-86.
						Fuhs, MR: and Stein, AM: Better ways to cope with COPD.

		2:30-4:00	204	e. Modes of therapy	Ms. Parker	Lagerson, J: Nursing care of patients with chronic pulmonary insufficiency. Sedlock, S: Detection of chronic pulmonary disease. Dudley, DL: Psychosocial aspects of care in the COPD patient.

Day	Date	Time	Room	Topic	Instructor	References
Tuesday	17 July	8:00-10:00	200	6. Patients with acute pulmonary embolism a. Pathogenesis b. Pathophysiology c. Clinical assessment d. Clinical problems e. Modes of therapy	Dr. Murrow	Daly, and Kelley: Prevention of pulmonary embolism intracaval devices.
		10:00-12:00	200		Ms. Ulman	Fitzmaurice, J: Current concepts of pulmonary embolism. Wyper, MA: Pulmonary embolism: fighting the silent killer.
		12:30-2:30	ICU-CCU	*Clinical session* Skills 18-20, 41 Trach 21 C & S 22-23 Set-up	Preceptors	
		2:30-4:00	ICU-CCU	Skills 32 Ventilator 33 Weaning	Preceptors	
Wednesday	18 July	1:00-4:00	ICU	*Clinical session* Skills 35-40 O$_2$ devices 42-43 Chest drainage	Preceptors	None
Thursday	19 July	2:00-4:00	204	Review session	Ms. Alspach	None
Monday	23 July	8:00-10:00	200	Pulmonary: posttest	Ms. Alspach	None
		10:00-12:00	200	Posttest review	Ms. Alspach	
		1:00-2:30	200	GI: pretest	Ms. Alspach	
		2:30-4:00	200	Clinical conference	Ms. Alspach	

Continued.

IV. CARDIOVASCULAR COMPONENT

Day	Date	Time	Room	Topic	Instructor	Readings
Monday	06 Aug	2:30-4:00	200	Cardiovascular: pretest	Ms. Alspach	None
Thursday	09 Aug	8:00-10:00	204	A. Functional anatomy of the cardiovascular system 1. Gross anatomy 2. Musculature 3. Chambers 4. Valves	Ms. Alspach	Andreoli, KG, et al: Comprehensive cardiac care, pp. 1-5. CCM: Cardiovascular Physiology, pp. 7-49.
		10:00-12:30	204	5. Vasculature	Ms. Alspach	Handouts (6)
		1:30-3:00	204	6. Conduction system 7. Systemic vasculature	Ms. Alspach	
		3:00-4:00	204	8. ANS Control	Ms. Alspach	Andreoli, pp. 5-7.
Friday	10 Aug	8:00-10:00	204	B. Cardiovascular physiology: Muscle mechanics	Ms. Alspach	Warner, HF, et al: Heart muscle: clinical applications of basic physiology and cellular anatomy, pp. 494-501, 504-506.
		10:00-12:00	204	C. Electrochemical physiology Part I Ionic events Basic electricity	Ms. Alspach	Andreoli, pp. 88-91.
		12:30-2:30	204	Part II Action potentials	Ms. Alspach	Surawicz, B: Input of cellular electrophysiology into the practice of clinical cardiography.
Monday	13 Aug	8:00-9:30	200	Part III, cont'd Electrophysiological properties of the heart	Ms. Alspach	Andreoli, pp. 131-133.
		9:30-12:00	200	E. Clinical assessment of the cardiovascular system	Ms. Alspach	
		1:00-2:00	604	1. History	Dr. Rhiel	Andreoli, p. 14.
		2:00-4:00	604	2. Physical assessment: normal findings a. Inspection b. Palpation c. Percussion d. Auscultation	Dr. Ward	Andreoli, pp. 14-59. Delaney, MT: Examining the chest. Miller, KM: Assessing peripheral purfusion. Winslow, EH: Visual inspection of the patient with cardiopulmonary disease.
Tuesday	14 Aug	8:00-11:30	Lab	3. Techniques of cardiac auscultation (ICU in-service)	Ms. Alspach Preceptors	Andreoli, pp. 34-45. Lehman, J: Auscultation of heart sounds.
		12:30-4:00	Lab	4. Arterial monitoring Peripheral PAP, PAWP CO Techniques and complications	Ms. Henderson	Andreoli, pp. 25-26, 286-287. Smith, RN: Invasive pressure monitoring. Andreoli, pp. 287-290. Lalli, SM: The complete Swan-Ganz.
Wednesday	15 Aug	12:00-2:00	200	5. Physical assessment: some abnormal findings	Ms. Alspach	

Day	Time	Room	Content	Instructor	Readings
	2:00–4:00	Lab	6. CVP monitoring Techniques Complications E. Electrocardiography	Ms. Henderson	Andreoli, pp. 29–32. Haughey, B: CVP lines: monitoring and maintaining.
Monday 20 Aug	8:00–9:30	204	1. ECG paper 2. Standardizations 3. Determining HR and rhythm	Ms. Alspach	Andreoli, pp. 87–90, 128–131, 231, 280–286. Handouts (8) Homework sheets (2)
	9:30–11:15	204	4. Deflections 5. Cardiac cycle	Ms. Alspach	Andreoli, pp. 91–95, 131–132, (tables)
	12:00–4:00	ICU	Clinical practicum Skills Setup Measurements 12 CVP 13 Arterial 14 Swan-Ganz 15 CO	Ms. Alspach/preceptors	
Tuesday 21 Aug	8:00–11:30	200	6. Lead systems	Ms. Alspach	Andreoli, pp. 95–100.
	12:30–1:30	Lab	7. Recording a 12-lead	Ms. Moody	Andreoli, pp. 296–298
	1:30–2:00	200	8. Essentials of echocardiography *Clinical session* Skills Monitoring	Ms. Tierney	Andreoli, pp. 54–56.
	2:00–3:00	CCU	2 Monitor	Preceptors	Andreoli, K: The cardiac monitor.
	3:00–4:00	CCU	1 CCU routine 5 CPR 10 Telemetry	Preceptors	Beaumont, E: ECG telemetry.
Wednesday 22 Aug	12:00–3:00	200	9. Electrical axis	Ms. Alspach	Alspach, J: Electrical axis. Handouts 12-lead ECG Axis homework sheets
	3:00–4:00	CCU	ECG review— rates and rhythms	Ms. Alspach	
Thursday 23 Aug	12:30–4:00	CCU	Clinical practicum Skill 19 Physical assessment of CV system	Ms. Alspach/preceptors	
Monday 27 Aug	8:00–10:00	604	F. Cardiac dysrhythmias 1. Mechanisms 2. Approach to analysis 3. Parameters of NSR 4. Sinus dysrhythmias	Ms. O'Day	Andreoli, pp. 131–133. Fisch, C: Electrophysiologic basis of clinical arrhythmias. Andreoli, pp. 134–139. Andreoli, pp. 140–141. Andreoli, pp. 142–153. Van Meter, and Lavine: Part 1.
	10:00–12:00	604	5. Atrial dysrhythmias	Ms. O'Day	Andreoli, pp. 154–173.
	1:00–4:00	202	ECG review Skill 3 (waves, intervals, axis determinations)	Ms. Alspach	Van Meter, and Lavine: Part 2.

Continued.

Day	Date	Time	Room	Topic	Instructor	Readings
Tuesday	28 Aug	8:00-9:30	200	6. Junctional dysrhythmias	Ms. West	Andreoli, pp. 174-179. Van Meter, and Lavine: Part 3.
		9:30-12:30	200	7. Ventricular dysrhythmias	Ms. West	Andreoli, pp. 180-197. Van Meter, and Lavine: Part 4. Schamroth, L, and Perlman, M: Rule of bigeminy. Conover: 1-1 to 1-14. Conover: 2-1 to 2-30.
		1:30-4:00	200	ECG review Sinus Dysrhythmias Atrial dysrhythmias	Ms. Alspach	

Wednesday	29 Aug	12:00-2:00	204	8. ECG Phenomena of mixed origin
				  a. Re-entry phenomena
				  b. Anomalous A-V conduction
				
				  c. Parasystole
				  d. A-V dissociation
				  e. Fusion beats
				  f. Escape beats
				  g. Aberration vs. ectopy
				  h. Premature beats
				  i. Pauses
					Ms. Finney	Andreoli, pp. 131-133. Segal, I, and Schamroth, L: Basic forms of reciprocal rhythm. Andreoli, pp. 216-221.
						
						Andreoli, pp. 214-215.
						Andreoli, p. 222.
						Andreoli, p. 181.
						Andreoli, pp. 132, 180.
						Andreoli, pp. 223-226.
						Conover: 8-1 to 8-20.
						Sweetwood, H, and Boak, J: Aberrant conduction.
						Conover: 3-1 to 3-25.
						Conover: 4-1 to 4-34.

		2:00-4:00	204	ECG review Junctional dysrhythmias Ventricular dysrhythmias	Ms. Alspach	
Thursday	30 Aug	2:00-4:00	ICU-CCU	Clinical session Skill 3 ECG strips	Ms. Alspach	
Wednesday	31 Aug	7:30-9:00	ICU-CCU-PCU	Skill 4 ECG recording	Nursing staff	
Tuesday	04 Sept	8:00-10:00	604	9. ECG changes in electrolyte imbalances	Ms. Stein	Andreoli, pp. 227-230. Handouts (2)
		10:00-12:00	604	G. Cardiac conduction defects 1. A-V conduction defects	Ms. Murphy	Andreoli, pp. 129 (Fig. 6-1), 198-206, 230. Van Meter, and Lavine: Part 3, pp. 21-25.

Day	Date	Time	Room	Topic	Instructor	Reading
Wednesday	05 Sept	1:00-4:00	204	2. I-V conduction defects	Ms. Murphy	Andreoli, pp. 206-213. Castellanos, A, et al: Hemiblock and BBB.
		12:00-2:00	204	ECG review A-V conduction defects	Ms. Alspach	Conover: 5-1, 5-2, 5-4, 5-6, 5-7, 5-13, 5-15 to 5-22, 5-25, 5-27.
Thursday	06 Sept	2:00-4:00	204	I-V Conduction defects	Ms. Alspach	Conover: 7-1 to 7-18.
Friday	07 Sept	1:00-4:00	200	Review for midterm	Ms. Alspach	Andreoli, pp. 233-257.
		7:30-10:00	200	Cardiovascular component: Midterm exam	Ms. Alspach	
		10:00-11:30	200	Review of midterm exam	Ms. Alspach	
		12:30-2:30	204	H. Management of care for patients with: 1. Acute MI a. Pathogenesis	Dr. Shien	Andreoli, pp. 8-13; 61-68. Epstein, FH: Predicting, explaining and preventing coronary heart disease. Oliver, MF: The metabolic response to a heart attack.
				b. Pathophysiology		Andreoli, pp. 53, 69-73, 115-127. Smith, AM, et al: Serum enzymes in MI.
				c. Clinical assessment		Van Meter, and Lavine: Part 4, pp. 32, 35.
		2:30-4:00	204	d. Cardiovascular drugs	Ms. Parker	Andreoli, pp. 335-373.
Monday	10 Sept	8:00-9:30	604	e. Clinical problems f. Modes of therapy	Ms. Fowler	Andreoli, pp. 290-332.
		9:30-12:00	604	g. Psychosocial aspects of care for MI patient	Psych clinician	Andreoli, pp. 311-317. Cassem, and Hackett: Psychological rehabilitation of MI patients in the acute phase. Scalzi, C: Nursing management of behavioral responses following an acute MI.
		1:00-4:00	CCU	Clinical session Skills 6 Drugs/code blue cart 7 Defibrillator cardioverter	Ms. Alspach	

Continued.

IV. CARDIOVASCULAR COMPONENT—cont'd

Day	Date	Time	Room	Topic	Instructor	Readings
Tuesday	11 Sept	8:00-10:00	202	2. Cardiac conduction system failure	Ms. Morton	Andreoli, pp. 258-261.
				a. Indications for pacing		
				b. Pacemaker components		Andreoli, pp. 261-265. Friedberg, HD: Crucial measurements during pacemaker implantation.
				c. Methods of insertion		
				d. Lead systems		
				e. Features and concepts of pacing		Andreolia, pp. 266-271.
				f. Modalities of pacing		Andreolia, pp. 271-272. Spence, and Lemberg Cardiac pacemakers IV. Complications.
				g. Complications of pacemakers		Andreoli, pp. 272-278. Barold, SS: Modern concepts of cardiac pacing.
	10:00-1:00		202	h. Nursing management	Ms. Alspach	
				i. Interpretation of pacemaker rhythms		
				Clinical session		
	2:00-3:00		ICU-CCU	Skills	Ms. Fowler and Ms. Alspach	
				8 Pacing cart		Conover: 5-3, 5-5, 5-14, 5-23, 5-24, 5-28, 5-29. Hammond, CE: Protecting patients with temporary transvenous pacemakers.
				9 T/V pacers, paced rhythms		
Wednesday	12 Sept	12:00-2:00	200	3. Syndromes of cardiac pump failure	Dr. Jones	Andreoli, pp. 78-86. Evans, RW: Cardiogenic shock: can the prognosis be improved?
				a. Cardiogenic shock		
				(1) Pathogenesis		
				(2) Pathophysiology		Shinn, AF: Concurrent use of dopamine and nitroprusside.
				(3) Clinical assessment		Stude, C: Cardiogenic shock.
	2:00-4:00		200	(4) Clinical problems	Ms. Hennessy	
				(5) Modes of therapy		
Thursday	13 Sept	2:00-3:00	204	ECG review	Ms. Alspach	Conover: 9-1 to 9-13.
				MI patterns		
	3:00-4:00			Clinical conference	Staff	
Monday	17 Sept	8:00-9:30	604	b. Acute CHP	Dr. O'Brien	Andreoli, pp. 73-78, 108-115. Larsen, EL: The patient with acute pulmonary edema.
				(1) Pathogenesis		
				(2) Pathophysiology		

Day	Date	Time	Room	Topic	Leader	Reading
		9:30–11:00	604	(3) Clinical assessment (4) Clinical problems (5) Modes of therapy	Ms. Stein	Andreoli, pp. 45, 375-378.
		12:00–1:00	604	4. Other CV dysfunctions a. Pericarditis/acute pericardial tamponade	Dr. Richard	Hancock, EW: Management of pericardial disease.
		1:00–2:00	604	Related nursing care	Ms. Howard	Moore, SJ: Pericarditis after acute MI.
		2:00–4:00	604	b. Peripheral arterial insufficiency	Ms. Hewitt	Andreoli, p. 378. Breslau, RC: Intensive care following vascular surgery. Long, G: Managing the patient with abdominal aortic aneurysm. Roberts, R: The acutely ischemic limb.
Tuesday	18 Sept	8:00–9:30	204	c. Hypertensive crisis	Mr. Westphal	Finnerty, FA: Aggressive drug therapy in accelerated hypertension.
		9:30–11:00	204	Related nursing care	Mr. Westphal	
		12:00–2:00	204	d. DIC	Ms. Preston	Coleman, et al: DIC: a problem in critical care medicine. Witmer, SE: DIC. Handout (1)
		2:00–4:00	CCU	Clinical session Skills 11 Ivac 15 Doppler 16 Tourniquets 17 Pericardiocentesis 18 Scale	Preceptors	Frantz, A, and Gladys, H: Keeping up with automatic rotating tourniquets.
Wednesday	19 Sept	12:00–2:00	200	Review of CV component	Ms. Alspach	
		2:00–4:00	200	Clinical session	Ms. Alspach	
Monday	24 Sept	12:00–2:00	200	Cardiovascular: posttest	Ms. Alspach	None
		2:00–3:30	200	Review of posttest	Ms. Alspach	
		3:30–4:00	200	Metabolic: pretest	Ms. Alspach	

Continued.

VI. NEUROLOGICAL COMPONENT

Day	Date	Time	Room	Topic	Instructor	Readings
Thursday	11 Oct	2:30-4:00	200	Neurological: pretest	Ms. Alspach	None
Monday	15 Oct	8:00-11:00	204	A. Functional neuroanatomy	Ms. Alspach	Hewitt, W: Functional neuroanatomy for nurses. Handouts (3)
		12:00-2:00	204	B. Nursing responsibilities in radiological exams of neurological system	Dr. Wheatley	Stone, B: Computerized transaxial brain scan.
		2:00-4:00	ICU-CCU	Clinical session Skills 2 Hypothermia 5 Air mattress 6 Range of motion	Ms. Davis	
				C. Clinical assessment of the neurological system		Alexander, and Brown: Neurological examination, parts 17 and 18.
Tuesday	16 Oct	8:00-9:30	200	1. Physical and laboratory exam	Ms. Finney	Mitchell, and Mauss: Increased intracranial pressure an update.
		9:30-11:00	200	2. Clinical assessment	Ms. Alspach	
Tuesday	16 Oct	12:00-2:00	200	C. Neurological physiology 1. Impulse transmission 2. Reflex arc and reflexes 3. Neurotransmitters 4. Spinal cord tracts 5. Functions of nervous system structures 6. Cerebral metabolism 7. CSF physiology	Ms. Michaels	None
		2:00-4:00	ICU	Clinical session Skills 7 Positioning 8 Decubiti	Preceptors	None
Wednesday	17 Oct	12:00-4:00	ICU	Clinical session Skill 1 Assessment	Preceptors	Gifford, and Plant: Abnormal respiratory patterns in the comatose patient caused by intracranial dysfunction. Gifford, and Plant: On describing altered states of consciousness.
Thursday	18 Oct	3:00-4:00	604	Clinical conference	Staff	
Monday	22 Oct	8:00-10:00	204	D. Management of patients with: 1. Acute spinal cord trauma a. Pathogenesis b. Pathophysiology c. Clinical assessment	Ms. Lord	Larrabee, J: SCI: physical care during early recovery.
		10:00-12:00	204	d. Clinical problems e. Modes of therapy	Mr. Palmer	Pepper, G: SCI: psychological care.

Day	Date	Time	Room	Clinical session	Preceptors	
		1:00–2:30	ICU	*Skills* 3 Circoelectric 4 Stryker 9 LP assist 10 Drugs	Preceptors	Gordon, J: Circoelectric beds.
		2:30–4:00	Lab		Preceptors	McGuckin, M: Tips for assisting with cultures of the CSF and other body fluids.
Tuesday	23 Oct	8:00–10:00	200	2. Acute head trauma a. Pathogenesis b. Pathophysiology c. Clinical assessment d. Clinical problems e. Modes of therapy	Ms. Dreyfus	The battered brain.
Tuesday	23 Oct	10:00–12:00	200		Ms. Patrick	Kunkel, and Wiley: Acute head injury.
		1:00–3:00	204	3. Acute CVA a. Pathogenesis b. Pathophysiology c. Clinical assessment d. Clinical problems e. Modes of therapy	Ms. Alspach	Breining: After the blow up . . . how to care for the patient with ruptured cerebral aneurysm. Elwood: Nursing the patient with a CVA. Keller, and Truscorr: TIA.
		3:00–4:00	204	4. Acute meningitis a. Pathogenesis b. Pathophysiology c. Clinical assessment d. Clinical problems e. Modes of therapy	Ms. Simpson	Meade, Ross, and Wehrle: Re-learning to cope with meningitis.
Wednesday	24 Oct	1:00–2:30	604	5. Seizure disorder a. Pathogenesis b. Pathophysiology c. Clinical assessment d. Clinical problems e. Modes of therapy	Dr. Badger	Handout: Describing a seizure.
		2:30–4:00	604		Ms. Gregory	Swift, N: Helping patients live with seizures.
Monday	29 Oct	1:00–2:30	202	6. Guillain–Barré syndrome a. Pathogenesis b. Pathophysiology c. Clinical assessment d. Clinical problems e. Modes of therapy	Ms. Alspach	Sodaro, and Perlick: Guillain-Barre: the syndrome, patient care and some case findings.
Monday	29 Oct	2:30–4:00	202	7. Myasthenia gravis a. Pathogenesis b. Pathophysiology c. Clinical assessment d. Clinical problems e. Modes of therapy	Ms. Dexter	Stackhouse: Myasthenia gravis.
Tuesday	30 Oct	2:30–4:00	200	Review of neurological component	Ms. Alspach	None
Friday	02 Nov	12:00–2:00	200	Neurological: posttest	Ms. Alspach	None
		2:00–3:00	200	Review of posttest	Ms. Alspach	None
		3:00–4:00	200	Renal: pretest	Ms. Alspach	None

Appendix C

Critical care nursing internship program
management and clinical skills inventory

INSTRUCTIONS: As each skill is successively achieved please record date of attainment and signature of staff verifying attainment level. Skills marked with an asterisk must be attained to "Independently performed" level.

MANAGEMENT SKILLS INVENTORY

	Level of attainment					
	Performed only with assistance		Performed with minimal assistance		Independently performed	
Skill	Date	Signature	Date	Signature	Date	Signature
Is able accurately and correctly to:						
1. Admit a patient						
*a. From the ER to CCU						
*b. To ICU						
*c. To PCU						
2. Transfer a patient to						
*a. Another unit within the hospital						
b. Another care facility						

*3. Transport a patient to X-ray, Radioisotope, or the OR					
4. Discharge a patient to					
a. Another care facility					
b. Home					
5. Provide postmortem care related to					
*a. Preparation of patient					
*b. Preparation of requisite forms, charting					
*c. Transfer of patient to morgue					
*d. Notification of Information Desk, Nursing Office					
6. Transcribe medical orders on ICU or CCU (minimum of 3 days)					
*a. Day 1					
*b. Day 2					
*c. Day 3					
7. Function as "monitor watcher" (minimum of 3 days):					
*a. Day 1 PCU					
*b. Day 2 PCU					
*c. Day 1 CCU					

Continued.

CLINICAL SKILLS INVENTORY: Pulmonary component

| Skill | Level of attainment | | | | | |
| | Performed only with assistance | | Performed with minimal assistance | | Independently performed | |
	Date	Signature	Date	Signature	Date	Signature
Is able accurately and correctly to:						
*1. Identify pulmonary system functions that are lost through bypassing with artificial airways						
*2. Locate and name the accessory muscles or respiration						
3. Determine a patient's tidal volume, vital capacity, and minute ventilation						
*4. Clinically differentiate anatomical from mechanical deadspace in an intubated patient						
*5. Perform and record a clinical assessment of the pulmonary system by:						
a. Inspection						
b. Palpation						
c. Percussion						
d. Auscultation						
*6. Determine presence and quality of the four airways reflexes: (a) sneeze, (b) gag, (c) cough, and (d) swallow						
*7. Locate approximate borders of pulmonary lobes						
8. Locate and identify:						
*a. Bronchial (tubular) breath sounds						
*b. Bronchovesicular breath sounds						
*c. Vesicular breath sounds						
*d. Diminished breath sounds						
*e. Fine and coarse rales						
*f. Rhonchi						
*g. Wheezes/asthmatic breath sounds						

*9. State normal arterial blood gas values					
*10. Interpret three arterial blood gas reports in terms of the patient's					
a. Primary acid-base disturbance					
b. Origin of the disturbance (respiratory, metabolic, mixed)					
c. Degree of compensation					
d. Chronic vs acute processes					
e. Alveolar ventilation					
f. Oxygenation					
*11. Draw arterial blood gases					
*12. Demonstrate how to preoxygenate a patient when suctioning is required					
a. Intubated patient					
b. Nonintubated patient					
*13. Demonstrate measures to prevent complications of suctioning procedure					
14. Perform sterile nasotracheal suctioning of secretions from nonintubated patient					
*15. Perform sterile nasotracheal suctioning of secretions from intubated patient					
*16. Perform sterile endotracheal suctioning					
*17. Perform oropharyngeal suctioning					
18. Deflate and reinflate endotracheal tube cuff, using minimal leak technique					
*19. Change tracheostomy dressings (including tie strings)					
*20. Provide tracheostomy care					
*21. Obtain sterile sputum specimen					
*22. Remove, clean, and replace wall suction unit					
*23. Set up and use portable suction machine					
*24. Turn patient side-back-side					

Continued.

CLINICAL SKILLS INVENTORY: Pulmonary component—cont'd

Skill	Level of attainment								
	Performed only with assistance			Performed with minimal assistance			Independently performed		
	Date	Signature		Date	Signature		Date	Signature	
*25. Teach patient to do effective coughing									
*26. Teach patient to do diaphragmatic breathing									
27. Position patient for postural drainage of specific lung areas									
28. Perform chest PT:									
a. Cupping maneuver									
b. Clapping maneuver									
c. Vibrating maneuver									
*29. Demonstrate use of incentive spirometer									
*30. Teach patient to use incentive spirometer									
*31. Mechanically stimulate coughing by endotracheal and external techniques									
32. MA-1 Ventilator									
*a. Empty corregated tubing of excess condensate									
*b. Explain purpose of each dial setting, indicator, light, and alarm									
*c. Demonstrate how to sigh patient using MA-1									
*d. Respond to all ventilator alarms									
*e. Explain purpose of spirometer unit									
*f. Explain rationale for use of PEEP									
*g. Describe complications of artificial ventilation and PEEP									
*h. Identify PEEP pressure used									
33. Weaning									
*a. Wean a patient from mechanical ventilation									
*b. Identify criteria for initiating weaning									

*c. Describe how patient's tolerance for weaning procedure can be evaluated							
*d. Identify indications that patient is *not* tolerating weaning procedure							
34. Insert and remove the following artificial airways in manikin practice: *a. Oropharyngeal							
*b. Nasopharyngeal							
*c. Esophageal obturator							
*d. Endotracheal							
*35. Apply mask O_2							
36. Apply Venti-mask O_2							
*37. Insert nasal cannula O_2							
38. Insert nasal catheter O_2							
*39. Insert and adjust flow rate on wall O_2 unit							
40. Set up portable O_2 tank *a. Turn O_2 tank on and off							
*b. Adjust flow rate of O_2							
*c. Attach appropriate O_2 appliance							
*41. Communicate effectively with intubated patient							
*42. Prepare setup for waterseal chest drainage and verify proper functioning of the system							
*43. Mark and record amount of Pleur-evac chest drainage							
44. Assist physician with: a. Thoracostomy or thoracentesis							
b. Chest tube removal							
c. Chest tube dressing change							
d. Endo- (naso-)tracheal intubation							
e. Tracheostomy insertion							
f. Bronchoscopy							

Continued.

CLINICAL SKILLS INVENTORY: Gastrointestinal component

Skill	Level of attainment					
	Performed only with assistance		Performed with minimal assistance		Independently performed	
	Date	Signature	Date	Signature	Date	Signature
Is able accurately and correctly to:						
1. Demonstrate how the abdomen may be divided into						
*a. 4 quadrants						
*b. 9 areas						
*2. Relate abdominal quadrants and areas to the underlying anatomy						
*3. Determine and describe the following aspects of a patient's abdomen:						
a. Size, shape, symmetry						
b. Presence of peristalsis						
c. Presence of pulsations						
d. Skin condition						
e. Hair distribution						
*4. Perform and describe the findings of auscultation of the abdomen						
*5. Identify normal bowel sounds						
*6. Identify abdominal percussion notes						
*7. Identify the presence or absence of normal abdominal percussion notes						
8. Assess a patient by palpation of the abdomen:						
*a. Superficial palpation						
*b. Deep palpation						

9. Determine the presence or absence of: *a. Asterixis (liver flap)					
*b. Vasomotor instability (via tilt test)					
*10. Demonstrate how to test and interpret NG drainage, emesis, or stool for occult blood (via hemoccult slides)					
11. Demonstrate how to insert a nasogastric tube and secure it in place					
*12. Demonstrate how to connect NG tube to suction apparatus for a. Constant suction					
b. Intermittent suction					
13. Demonstrate how to a. Irrigate an NG tube for iced saline lavage					
b. Accurately record results of lavage					
*14. Demonstrate how to determine if an NG tube is patent and functioning properly					
*15. Demonstrate how to empty and record NG drainage					
16. Care for a patient requiring a Sengstaken-Blakemore tube: a. Check balloons for leaks prior to insertion					
b. Assemble necessary equipment for insertion					
c. Assist and direct patient during insertion					
d. Inflate/deflate gastric and esophageal balloons					
e. Assist in applying traction to tube					

Continued.

CLINICAL SKILLS INVENTORY: Renal component

Skill	Level of attainment					
	Performed only with assistance		Performed with minimal assistance		Independently performed	
	Date	Signature	Date	Signature	Date	Signature
Is able accurately and correctly to:						
1. Determine the degree of normality in a patient's reported						
*a. Urinalysis						
*b. Urine electrolytes						
*c. Serum electrolytes						
*d. Serum BUN, creatinine, uric acid						
e. Serum osmolarity						
f. Urine osmolarity						
2. Identify clinical and laboratory data that signifies renal dysfunction						
3. Measure and record a patient's intake and output						
*4. Determine urine specific gravity with a urometer or refractometer						
*5. Obtain a urine specimen for C+S						
*6. Insert a Foley retention catheter under aseptic technique						
7. Irrigate a Foley catheter						

8. Set up for continuous bladder irrigations using 3 lumen Foley catheter.					
*9. Use a bedscale to obtain a patient's weight					
10. Care for a patient requiring peritoneal dialysis:					
a. Assemble necessary equipment					
b. Weigh patient; take vital signs; prepare patient for procedure					
c. Assist with trocar insertion					
d. Perform peritoneal dialysis					
e. Administer additives to dialysate					
f. Keep cumulative record of fluid balance for every exchange					
11. Care for a patient requiring hemodialysis					
a. Assemble necessary equipment, parenteral therapy, and medications					
b. Weigh patient; take vital signs; obtain necessary laboratory results					
c. Prepare patient for procedure					
d. Assist with shunt insertion					
e. Care for patient during hemodialysis					
f. Keep cumulative record of patient progress					
g. Provide shunt care as ordered					

Continued.

CLINICAL SKILLS INVENTORY: Cardiovascular component

Skill	Level of attainment					
	Performed only with assistance		Performed with minimal assistance		Independently performed	
	Date	Signature	Date	Signature	Date	Signature
Is able accurately and correctly to:						
1. Admission process						
*a. Explain rationale for each element in CCU routine care						
*b. Apply/reapply elastic stockings						
2. Attach cardiac monitor to a patient						
*a. Place and secure electrodes on patient's chest						
*b. Set initial monitor settings for alarm limits						
*c. Obtain clear ECG pattern						
*d. Demonstrate how to change and identify lead being monitored						
*e. Take appropriate actions to remove causes of ECG pattern interference						
*f. Explain reason for each setting and indicator on bedside monitor						
3. Obtain hourly ECG rhythm strips						
*a. Obtain clear ECG pattern on strip						
*b. Determine and record atrial and ventricular rates, P-R interval, QRS duration, Q-T interval from rhythm strip						
*c. Identify ECG rhythm						
*d. State characteristics of normal P wave, P-R interval, and QRS duration						
*e. Demonstrate how to adjust "gain" as necessary for wave differentiation						

404

*f. Demonstrate how to change roll of ECG paper at desk console						
*4. Record a 12-lead ECG and mark (patient's name, date, time, leads) accordingly						
*a. Change roll of paper on ECG machine						
*b. Demonstrate correct technique for standardization						
5. Demonstrate skills of basic cardiac life support						
*a. One-rescuer technique						
*b. Two-rescuer technique						
*c. Monitored arrest procedure						
*d. Obstructed airway technique						
6. Code blue cart and use						
*a. Perform daily check of code cart						
*b. Explain procedure for or obtain replacement of items required on cart						
*c. Demonstrate how to activate code blue clock						
*d. Describe procedure for calling "code blue"						
7. Defibrillator/cardioverter						
*a. Setup for emergency defibrillation						
*b. Test cardioverter output						
*c. Demonstrate appropriate paddle placements used for different types of paddle systems						
d. Explain procedure for or assist with cardioversion						
e. Explain procedure for or assist with defibrillation						

Continued.

CLINICAL SKILLS INVENTORY: Cardiovascular component—cont'd

Skill	Level of attainment					
	Performed only with assistance		Performed with minimal assistance		Independently performed	
	Date	Signature	Date	Signature	Date	Signature
8. Pacemaker cart						
*a. Do daily checking						
*b. Explain procedure for restocking cart						
*c. Explain different types and purposes of cables						
d. Explain how to unipolarize a bipolar pacing system						
*e. Demonstrate how to connect cables to an external pulse generator						
*f. Demonstrate how to change batteries in an external pulse generator						
9. Patients with transvenous pacemakers						
*a. Perform/describe care of dressing site						
*b. Explain precautions taken for electrical safety						
*c. Explain function of each setting on pacemaker unit						
d. Assess from monitor and ECG strip, whether pacemaker is						
*(1) functioning correctly						
(2) Failing to sense						
(3) Failing to capture						

e. Assist with or observe procedure for assisting with insertion of temporary transvenous pacemaker

f. Describe nursing care of a patient with permanent pacemaker

*g. Explain purpose and procedure of magnet use in testing pacemaker

h. Demonstrate or explain how to use gas sterilizer

10. Telemetry
*a. Explain rationale for

*b. Attach patient electrodes for monitoring

*c. Demonstrate how to change batteries

11. Demonstrate how to set up and use IVAC equipment

12. CVP lines
*a. Assist or describe procedure for assisting with CVP line insertion

*b. Demonstrate how to set up CVP manometer

*c. Demonstrate dressing change technique

*d. Demonstrate how to level CVP for readings

*e. Demonstrate how to obtain and record CVP reading

13. Peripheral arterial lines
*a. Demonstrate how to set up, balance, and calibrate transducer

*b. Demonstrate nursing care of insertion site: taping and dressing

Continued

CLINICAL SKILLS INVENTORY: Cardiovascular component—cont'd

Skill	Level of attainment								
	Performed only with assistance			Performed with minimal assistance			Independently performed		
	Date	Signature		Date	Signature		Date	Signature	
13. Peripheral arterial lines—cont'd									
*c. Demonstrate how to immobilize extremity									
*d. Demonstrate how to take BP readings: (systolic, diastolic, and mean arterial pressures)									
e. Assist with insertion of arterial catheter									
14. Care for a patient with pulmonary artery (Swan-Ganz) catheter monitoring									
a. Provide or explain how to assist with insertion of a PA catheter									
b. Demonstrate how to interconnect and prime all equipment and lines									
c. Demonstrate how to set up, balance, and calibrate transducer									
d. Obtain and record the following:									
(1) PA systolic and diastolic pressures									
(2) Mean PAP									
(3) PAWP									
e. Identify the features of a normal arterial wave									
f. Demonstrate or explain how to look for:									

408

(1) Dampened wave				
(2) Loss of tracing				
(3) Inability to obtain wedge tracing				
(4) Inappropriate wedge tracing				
(5) RV tracing				
g. Provide dressing change at catheter insertion site				
15. Set up equipment for cardiac output determinations by thermodilution technique				
a. Describe or demonstrate procedure for determining CO measurements				
b. Record results of CO determinations				
*16. Demonstrate use of Doppler unit for BPs				
17. Set up and demonstrate use of rotating tourniquets				
a. Manual rotation				
*b. Automatic rotation				
18. Assist with pericardiocentesis				
19. Demonstrate how to use bedscale				
20. Perform and accurately record an assessment of CV system by				
*a. Inspection				
*b. Palpation				
*c. Percussion				
*d. Auscultation				

Continued.

CLINICAL SKILLS INVENTORY: Neurological component

Skill	Level of attainment					
	Performed only with assistance		Performed with minimal assistance		Independently performed	
	Date	Signature	Date	Signature	Date	Signature
Is able accurately and correctly to:						
1. Assess a patient's neurological status:						
*a. Orientation to time, place, person, and self						
*b. Memory for recent events						
*c. Memory for long-term events						
*d. Nature and quality of speech						
*e. Respiratory pattern						
*f. Pupil size (mm)						
*g. Pupil reaction (1) Direct light						
(2) Consensual light						
(3) Ciliospinal reflex						
*h. Level of consciousness						
*i. Spontaneous motor responses						
*j. Strength of motor responses (ex. grip)						
*k. Evidence of decorticate posturing						
*l. Evidence of decerebrate posturing						
*m. Sensory response						
*n. In trauma patients: (1) Otorrhea						
(2) Rhinorrhea						
(3) Raccoon eyes						
(4) Battle's sign						

*o. Nuchal rigidity								
p. Intact reflexes								
(1) Deep tendon reflexes								
(2) Superficial								
*q. Pathological reflexes								
*r. Seizure activity								
(1) Focal								
(2) Generalized								
(3) Petit mal vs grand mal								
2. Set up hypothermia machine for patient use								
*a. Explain purpose and use of components								
*b. Adjust temperature								
*3. Demonstrate proper use of Circoelectric bed								
*4. Demonstrate use of Stryker frame								
*5. Set up air mattress for patient use								
*6. Demonstrate how to perform passive range of motion to all extremities								
*7. Demonstrate proper body positioning of comatose/paralyzed patient								
*8. Describe alternative nursing interventions used to prevent or treat decubiti								
9. Set up and assist with lumbar puncture								
10. Provide for care of patient in cervical traction								
11. Assess neurovascular integrity in casted extremities								
*a. Upper extremity								
*b. Lower extremity								

Continued.

411

CLINICAL SKILLS INVENTORY: Metabolic component

Skill	Level of attainment					
	Performed only with assistance		Performed with minimal assistance		Independently performed	
	Date	Signature	Date	Signature	Date	Signature
Is able accurately and correctly to:						
1. Assess a patient for the presence of						
*a. Chvostek's sign						
*b. Trousseau's phenomenon						
*c. Serum Ca^{++} and P abnormalities						
2. Assess a patient for the relative presence of						
*a. Glycosuria						
*b. Ketonuria						
c. Hyperglycemia						
d. Hypoglycemia						
e. Diabetes insipidus						
f. Inappropriate ADH (SIADH)						
3. Demonstrate procedure for urine testing using						
*a. Two-drop method						
*b. Five-drop method						
*c. Testape method						

Index

413